Catecholamine Function in Posttraumatic Stress Disorder: Emerging Concepts

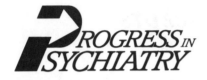

PROGRESS *IN*
PSYCHIATRY

Number 42

David Spiegel, M.D.
Series Editor

Catecholamine Function in Posttraumatic Stress Disorder: Emerging Concepts

Edited by
M. Michele Murburg, M.D.

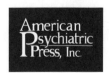

American
Psychiatric
Press, Inc.

Washington, DC
London, England

Note: The authors have worked to ensure that all information in this book concerning drug dosages, schedules, and routes of administration is accurate as of the time of publication and consistent with standards set by the U.S. Food and Drug Administration and the general medical community. As medical research and practice advance, however, therapeutic standards may change. For this reason and because human and mechanical errors sometimes occur, we recommend that readers follow the advice of a physician who is directly involved in their care or in the care of a member of their family.

Books published by the American Psychiatric Press, Inc., represent the views and opinions of the individual authors and do not necessarily represent the policies and opinions of the Press or the American Psychiatric Association.

American Psychiatric Press, Inc.
1400 K Street, N.W., Washington, DC 20005

Library of Congress Cataloging-in-Publication Data
Catecholamine function in posttraumatic stress disorder : emerging
  concepts / edited by M. Michele Murburg.—1st ed.
      p. cm. — (Progress in psychiatry series : #42)
    Includes bibliographical references and index.
    ISBN 0-88048-473-X (alk. paper)
    1. Post-traumatic stress disorder—Endocrine aspects.
  2. Catecholamines. 3. Post-traumatic stress disorder
  —Pathophysiology. I. Murburg, M. Michele, 1952– . II. Series.
    [DNLM: 1. Stress Disorders, Post-Traumatic—physiopathology.
  2. Catecholamines—physiology. 3. Adaptation, Psychological.
  4. Adaptation, Physiological. 5. Neurophysiology. W1 PR6781L no.
  42 1994 / WM 170 C357 1994]
  RC552.P67C376 1994
  616.8521—dc20
  DNLM/DLC   93-5677
  for Library of Congress   CIP

British Library Cataloguing in Publication Data
A CIP record is available from the British Library.

Contents

Section I:
The Role of Catecholaminergic Systems in Stress Response Syndromes

Section II:
Peripheral Autonomic and
Catecholamine Function in PTSD

Section III:
Central Catecholamine Function in PTSD

Section IV: Methodological Issues

Contributors

Seymour M. Antelman, Ph.D.
Professor, Department of Psychiatry, Western Psychiatric Institute and Clinic and Pittsburgh School of Medicine, Pittsburgh, Pennsylvania

E. Alexandra Ashleigh, M.D.
Assistant Professor, Department of Psychiatry and Behavioral Sciences, University of Washington; Chief, Partial Care Program, VA Medical Center, Seattle, Washington

Gary Aston-Jones, Ph.D.
Director, Division of Behavioral Neurobiology; Professor, Department of Mental Health Sciences, Hahnemann University, Philadelphia, Pennsylvania

Avraham Bleich, M.D.
Commanding Officer, Department of Mental Health, Israel Defense Force; Senior Lecturer, Department of Psychiatry, Faculty of Medicine, Sackler Medical School, Tel Aviv University, Tel Aviv, Israel

David Boisoneau, M.D.
Medical Student, University of Connecticut School of Medicine, Farmington, Connecticut

David L. Braff, M.D.
Professor, Department of Psychiatry, University of California at San Diego, San Diego, California

Curtis Breslin, M.S.
Department of Medical Psychology, Uniformed Services University of the Health Sciences, Bethesda, Maryland

Dennis S. Charney, M.D.
Professor, Department of Psychiatry, Yale University
School of Medicine, New Haven, Connecticut; Chief of
Psychiatry, West Haven VA Medical Center; Director,
Clinical Neuroscience Division, National Center for
Post-Traumatic Stress Disorder, West Haven, Connecticut

Michael Davis, Ph.D.
Professor, Department of Psychiatry, Yale University
School of Medicine, New Haven, Connecticut

Ariel Y. Deutch, Ph.D.
Associate Professor, Department of Psychiatry, Yale
University School of Medicine, New Haven, Connecticut

Bruce I. Diamond, Ph.D.
Professor, Department of Psychiatry and Pharmacology,
Medical College of Georgia, Augusta, Georgia

Matthew J. Friedman, M.D., Ph.D.
Professor of Psychiatry and Pharmacology, Dartmouth
University; Executive Director, National Center for
Post-Traumatic Stress Disorder, White River Junction,
Vermont

Mark A. Geyer, Ph.D.
Professor, Department of Psychiatry, University of
California at San Diego, San Diego, California

Earl L. Giller, Jr., M.D., Ph.D.
Professor, Department of Psychiatry, University of
Connecticut Health Center, University of Connecticut
School of Medicine, Farmington, Connecticut

Eitan Gur, M.D.
Resident, Department of Psychiatry, Hadassah-Hebrew
University Medical Center, Jerusalem, Israel

Mark B. Hamner, M.D.
Assistant Professor, Department of Psychiatry, VA Medical
Center and Medical University of South Carolina,
Charleston, South Carolina

Ana Hitri, Ph.D.
Research Pharmacologist, Psychiatry Service,
VA Medical Center, Washington, D.C.

Daniel W. Hommer, M.D.
Chief, Section of Clinical Electrophysiology and
Brain Imaging, Laboratory of Clinical Studies, National
Institute of Alcoholism and Alcohol Abuse, Bethesda,
Maryland

Melissa A. Jenkins, B.A.
Department of Psychiatry, University of California at San
Diego, San Diego, California

Boaz Kahana, Ph.D.
Director, Center for Aging; Professor, Department
of Psychology, Cleveland State University, Cleveland,
Ohio

Grant N. Ko, M.D.
Research Associate Professor, Department of Psychiatry,
New York University, New York, New York; Associate
Director, Experimental Medicine, Pfizer Central Research,
Groton, Connecticut

John H. Krystal, M.D.
Assistant Professor, Department of Psychiatry, Yale
University School of Medicine, New Haven, Connecticut;
Director, Clinical Research, VA Medical Center, West
Haven, Connecticut

Bernard Lerer, M.D.
Professor of Psychiatry, Director, Biological Psychiatry
Laboratory, Hadassah-Hebrew University Medical Center,
Jerusalem, Israel

Xiaowan Ma, B.S.
Sandoz Pharmaceuticals,
East Hanover, New Jersey

John W. Mason, M.D.
Director, Psychoneuroendocrinology Laboratory, Clinical Neurosciences Division, National Center for Post-traumatic Stress Disorder, West Haven VA Medical Center, West Haven, Connecticut; Professor, Department of Psychiatry, Yale University School of Medicine, New Haven, Connecticut

Miles E. McFall, Ph.D.
Associate Professor, Department of Psychiatry and Behavioral Sciences, University of Washington School of Medicine; Director, Post-traumatic Stress Disorder Program, VA Medical Center, Seattle, Washington

Arthur T. Meyerson, M.D.
Professor and Chairman, Department of Mental Health Sciences, Hahnemann University, Philadelphia, Pennsylvania

M. Michele Murburg, M.D.
Associate Professor, Department of Psychiatry and Behavioral Sciences, University of Washington, Seattle, Washington; Visiting Associate Professor, Department of Psychiatry and Behavioral Sciences, Stanford University; Associate Director for Neurobiological Research, National Center for Post-Traumatic Stress Disorder, Education and Clinical Research Division, VA Medical Center, Palo Alto, California

Michael Newman, Ph.D.
Senior Neurochemist, Biological Psychiatry Laboratory, Department of Psychiatry, Hadassah-Hebrew University Medical Center, Jerusalem, Israel

Bruce D. Perry, M.D., Ph.D.
Associate Professor of Psychiatry and Behavioral Sciences, Departments of Psychiatry, Pharamacology, and Pediatrics; Chief of Psychiatry, Texas Children's Hospital; Director, PTSD Clinical Research Programs, Vice Chairman for Research, Baylor College of Medicine and Houston VA Medical Center, Houston, Texas

Jeffrey L. Rausch, M.D.
Professor and Vice Chairman, Department of Psychiatry
and Health Behavior, Medical College of Georgia, Augusta,
Georgia

Peter E. Simson, Ph.D.
Assistant Professor, Department of Psychology, Miami (of
Ohio) University, Oxford, Ohio

Steven M. Southwick, M.D.
Associate Clinical Professor, Department of Psychiatry,
Yale University School of Medicine; Director,
Post-traumatic Stress Disorder Program, National Center
for Post-traumatic Stress Disorder, West Haven VA Medical
Center, West Haven, Connecticut

Elisabeth J. Van Bockstaele, Ph.D.
Department of Neurobiology, Cornell University Medical
College, New York, New York

Richard C. Veith, M.D.
Professor, Department of Psychiatry and Behavioral
Sciences, University of Washington; Director, Geriatrics
Research Educational and Clinical Center, VA Medical
Center, Seattle, Washington

Rita J. Valentino, Ph.D.
Associate Professor, Department of Mental Health Sciences,
Division of Behavioral Neurobiology, Hahnemann
University, Philadelphia, Pennsylvania

Jay M. Weiss, Ph.D.
Professor, Department of Psychiatry, Duke University
Medical Center, Durham, North Carolina

Rachel Yehuda, Ph.D.
Director, Traumatic Stress Studies Program; Assistant
Professor, Department of Psychiatry, Mount Sinai School of
Medicine, Bronx VA Medical Center, Bronx, New York

Robert M. Zacharko, Ph.D.
Associate Professor, Department of Psychology,
Neuroscience Research Unit, Carleton University, Ottawa,
Ontario, Canada

Introduction to the Progress in Psychiatry Series

The Progress in Psychiatry Series is designed to capture in print the excitement that comes from assembling a diverse group of experts from various locations to examine in detail the newest information about a developing aspect of psychiatry. This series emerged as a collaboration between the American Psychiatric Association's (APA) Scientific Program Committee and the American Psychiatric Press, Inc. Great interest is generated by a number of the symposia presented each year at the APA annual meeting, and we realized that much of the information presented there, carefully assembled by people who are deeply immersed in a given area, would unfortunately not appear together in print. The symposia sessions at the annual meetings provide an unusual opportunity for experts who otherwise might not meet on the same platform to share their diverse viewpoints for a period of 3 hours. Some new themes are repeatedly reinforced and gain credence, whereas in other instances disagreements emerge, enabling the audience and now the reader to reach informed decisions about new directions in the field. The Progress in Psychiatry Series allows us to publish and capture some of the best of the symposia and thus provide an in-depth treatment of specific areas that might not otherwise be presented in broader review formats.

Psychiatry is, by nature, an interface discipline, combining the study of mind and brain, of individual and social environments, of the humane and the scientific. Therefore, progress in the field is rarely linear—it often comes from unexpected sources. Furthermore, new developments emerge from an array of viewpoints that do not necessarily provide immediate agreement but rather expert examination of the issues. We intend to present innovative ideas and data that will enable you, the reader, to participate in this process.

We believe the Progress in Psychiatry Series will provide you with an opportunity to review timely, new information in specific fields of interest as they are developing. We hope you find that the excitement of the presentations is captured in the written word and that this book proves to be informative and enjoyable reading.

David Spiegel, M.D.
Series Editor
Progress in Psychiatry Series

Progress in Psychiatry
Series Titles

Clinical Advances in Monoamine Oxidase Inhibitor Therapies (#43)
Edited by Sidney H. Kennedy, M.D., F.R.C.P.C.

Catecholamine Function in Posttraumatic Stress Disorder: Emerging Concepts (#42)
Edited by M. Michele Murburg, M.D.

Management and Treatment of Insanity Acquittees: A Model for the 1990s (#41)
Edited by Joseph D. Bloom, M.D., and Mary H. Williams, M.S., J.D.

Chronic Fatigue and Related Immune Deficiency Syndromes (#40)
Edited by Paul J. Goodnick, M.D., and Nancy G. Klimas, M.D.

Psychopharmacology and Psychobiology of Ethnicity (#39)
Edited by Keh-Ming Lin, M.D., M.P.H., Russell E. Poland, Ph.D., and Gayle Nakasaki, M.S.W.

Electroconvulsive Therapy: From Research to Clinical Practice (#38)
Edited by C. Edward Coffey, M.D.

Multiple Sclerosis: A Neuropsychiatric Disorder (#37)
Edited by Uriel Halbreich, M.D.

Biology of Anxiety Disorders (#36)
Edited by Rudolf Hoehn-Saric, M.D., and Daniel R. McLeod, Ph.D.

Psychoimmunology Update (#35)
Edited by Jack M. Gorman, M.D., and Robert M. Kertzner, M.D.

Family Environment and Borderline Personality Disorder (#23)
Edited by Paul Skevington Links, M.D.

Amino Acids in Psychiatric Disease (#22)
Edited by Mary Ann Richardson, Ph.D.

Serotonin in Major Psychiatric Disorders (#21)
Edited by Emil F. Coccaro, M.D., and Dennis L. Murphy, M.D.

Personality Disorders: New Perspectives on Diagnostic Validity (#20)
Edited by John M. Oldham, M.D.

Biological Assessment and Treatment of Posttraumatic Stress Disorder (#19)
Edited by Earl L. Giller, Jr., M.D., Ph.D.

Depression in Schizophrenia (#18)
Edited by Lynn E. DeLisi, M.D.

Depression and Families: Impact and Treatment (#17)
Edited by Gabor I. Keitner, M.D.

Depressive Disorders and Immunity (#16)
Edited by Andrew H. Miller, M.D.

Treatment of Tricyclic-Resistant Depression (#15)
Edited by Irl L. Extein, M.D.

Current Approaches to the Prediction of Violence (#14)
Edited by David A. Brizer, M.D., and Martha L. Crowner, M.D.

Tardive Dyskinesia: Biological Mechanisms and Clinical Aspects (#13)
Edited by Marion E. Wolf, M.D., and Aron D. Mosnaim, Ph.D.

Eating Behavior in Eating Disorders (#12)
Edited by B. Timothy Walsh, M.D.

Cerebral Hemisphere Function in Depression (#11)
Edited by Marcel Kinsbourne, M.D.

Psychobiology of Bulimia (#10)
Edited by James I. Hudson, M.D., and
Harrison G. Pope, Jr., M.D.

Psychiatric Pharmacosciences of Children and Adolescents (#9)
Edited by Charles Popper, M.D.

Biopsychosocial Aspects of Bereavement (#8)
Edited by Sidney Zisook, M.D.

Medical Mimics of Psychiatric Disorders (#7)
Edited by Irl Extein, M.D., and Mark S. Gold, M.D.

Can Schizophrenia Be Localized in the Brain? (#6)
Edited by Nancy C. Andreasen, M.D., Ph.D.

The Psychiatric Implications of Menstruation (#5)
Edited by Judith H. Gold, M.D., F.R.C.P.C.

Post-Traumatic Stress Disorder in Children (#4)
Edited by Spencer Eth, M.D., and
Robert S. Pynoos, M.D., M.P.H.

Treatment of Affective Disorders in the Elderly (#3)
Edited by Charles A. Shamoian, M.D.

Premenstrual Syndrome: Current Findings and Future Directions (#2)
Edited by Howard J. Osofsky, M.D., Ph.D., and
Susan J. Blumenthal, M.D.

The Borderline: Current Empirical Research (#1)
Edited by Thomas H. McGlashan, M.D.

Foreword

The organism's response to environmental threats was conceptualized by Cannon (1914) as the "fight or flight" reaction and by Selye (1936) as the "general adaptation syndrome." These responses constitute a state of coordinated cognitive, affective, and physiological arousal that optimizes the organism's ability to respond to life-threatening situations and then to return to the arousal levels appropriate for daily activities. In addition, remembering danger signals and effective responses provides the nervous system with the ability to respond more specifically and rapidly to similar threatening conditions, just as the cellular memory of exposure to antigens permits the immune system to respond more effectively upon reexposure to similar agents. The fact that markedly stressful situations, or traumatic stress, can also cause long-term physiological (DaCosta 1871) and psychological (van der Kolk and van der Hart 1989) problems has been recognized for centuries, and the clinical syndrome engendered by extreme stressors is currently called posttraumatic stress disorder (PTSD).

Although it has been studied most extensively in combat veterans, PTSD is more than a "veteran's problem." Recent studies have shown that the incidence of exposure to traumatic stress in the general population is high, that the lifetime prevalence of PTSD in those exposed to traumatic events is 24% to 69%, and that civilian samples are similar to Vietnam combat veterans in that approximately half the persons with acute PTSD develop chronic PTSD (Breslau and Davis 1992). Trauma occurring in childhood can result in a variety of dissociative disorders with symptoms that are not as circumscribed as those seen in PTSD resulting from later-life trauma. There may, however, be some overlap in the biological changes seen after early versus later life trauma, such as the catecholaminergic findings described in the chapter by Dr. Perry (Chapter 12).

The understanding of PTSD requires a synthesis of information from several different areas of study. First, one must have an understanding of the psychobiology of the acute normal stress response, because some elements of PTSD appear to reflect a prolongation of this response. Second, one must consider the extent to which PTSD may be composed of additional elements not found in the acute stress response, or result from the failure of homeostatic mechanisms to return the organism to baseline. This overlapping relationship between normal and pathological mechanisms is not unique to PTSD, and is also a problem in applying concepts of day-to-day emotions such as anxiety and depression to clinical anxiety and affective disorders. Third, further progress in our understanding of the pathophysiology of neuropsychiatric disorders requires stimulation across animal and human studies, with an integration of both sets of results into an evolving conceptual framework. Because both human and animal studies have limitations, both are needed in order to synthesize conceptual paradigms that can describe psychopathological states more accurately. Animal studies can provide concurrent behavioral and neurochemical measures of systems that are thought to be involved, and can allow for their manipulation, but are weak in evaluating psychological constructs. In turn, clinical studies provide psychological measures and peripheral biological correlates but allow only limited access to brain chemical measures, although new metabolic imaging techniques are promising. Finally, drug studies in both animals and humans may contribute to the validation of specific psychobiological formulations of disorders.

Dr. Murburg has assembled state-of-the-art reviews of the functional significance of catecholamines in animal central nervous system (CNS) function and models of PTSD; the use of these concepts to guide clinical studies of catecholamine function in PTSD; the clinical biological findings (primarily peripheral to date); and a review of antidepressant treatment. Each chapter is excellent alone, and the range allows for some integration across paradigms. Although the understanding of neuropsychiatric disorders such as PTSD in terms of brain pathophysiology is limited by the lack of satisfactory models of cognitive and affective processing as normal brain functions, we do know that the catecholaminergic systems constitute a critical element of the stress response. Dr. Murburg, in her introduction, provides an overview of the rationale for examining catecholamine function in the interaction of the organism with the environment.

The function of the locus coeruleus (LC) (and other noradrenergic nuclei) in responding to meaningful environmental stimuli, the association between LC activity and the organism's state of arousal, and the changes in central catecholaminergic systems after high-magnitude stress not only indicate that central catecholaminergic systems are involved in PTSD, but suggest what the neuronal mechanisms may be for some of the symptoms, and why some medications may be effective. Multiple systems, however, are likely to be involved in the clinical syndrome of PTSD, as emphasized by studies such as those investigating the effects of stress on peptides and other neurotransmitters influencing catecholaminergic systems.

The strengths and weaknesses of methodologies in which peripheral measures are used to investigate neuropsychiatric disorders are discussed in subsequent chapters. While understanding the CNS abnormalities underlying disorders such as PTSD is critical, considering peripheral measures solely as an approximation of brain activity misses the fact that the purpose of much brain activity is to direct at least three effector systems: musculoskeletal, endocrine, and autonomic. Thus, peripheral measures are not simply murky ways of trying to understand what is going on in the brain, but more importantly the end-point measurements of what the brain works to accomplish (Mason et al. 1990). Psychophysiological studies of PTSD, showing increased autonomic responsiveness to trauma-specific stimuli, have been well formulated in classical and operant conditioning terms even though the brain mechanisms involved in conditioning are not completely known. Subsequent chapters suggest that baseline sympathoadrenal activity may not be consistently elevated, but that the sympathetic nervous system (SNS) may instead show increased reactivity in response to specific episodic stimuli in PTSD. Repeated, frequent phasic SNS hyperactivity when summed over time, however, can look like increased tonic activity, and patients with PTSD often clinically appear to be more sensitive to nonspecific low-magnitude stressors in addition to trauma-related stimuli. Full investigation of the nature of SNS activation in PTSD will require multiple time-point measurements of sympathoadrenal activity. Finally, monitoring of catecholamine receptor changes, especially in the CNS, is essential in evaluating catecholamine activity. Whether such receptor alterations represent primary or secondary changes, they are important determinants of catecholaminergic system function.

These studies of the pathophysiology of PTSD have resulted in exciting developments and a renaissance of interest in the interaction of the organism with the environment. Abnormalities in the stress response, however, likely constitute a complex spectrum of disorders. To minimize confusion, the subject populations in clinical studies need to be described completely with respect to the presence or absence of symptom(s) and the severity of those symptoms in terms of frequency, intensity, and duration. It is also essential to specify other stress parameters in basic animal studies and human studies. It is necessary to know the lifetime history of stress exposure, especially high-magnitude trauma (not simply the current stressor), and the time(s) of life at which the stressor(s) occurred. Animal studies have shown that single traumatic events can cause changes that intensify over time, as shown by Antelman and Yehuda's review of time-dependent sensitization. On the other hand, repeated stress exposure may be necessary for the development of such sequelae as learned helplessness. Thus, the pattern of stress in terms of timing, repetition, and chronicity should be specified. The type of stressor—including, in humans, whether it resulted from human activity, and whether it was controllable or uncontrollable—is an important parameter. Mediating variables are important in determining the relationship of stressors to symptoms. Such variables can either increase or decrease the risk of developing PTSD given a particular stressor. Thus, not only previous trauma history but genetics and character traits may mediate trauma response, although character traits are difficult to study posttrauma in humans because character changes may result from trauma and/or the presence of chronic PTSD. Such variables and others not yet specified may help to explain why particular individuals do *not* develop PTSD when exposed to a severe trauma.

The course of the stress-response disorders needs to be more clearly delineated. In humans, acute, chronic, and recurrent patterns are seen, and PTSD for many is a life-long diagnosis. Given the evidence presented in this book for the complex biological changes engendered by stress in human beings and animals, and given the evidence that such changes may evolve over time, reduction of symptoms may not be simple desensitization with repetition, but an active process reducing the strength of intrusive, and possibly avoidant, symptoms. This process may be the basis for the repetition of trauma-related situations variously described as addiction to the trauma and working through.

Posttraumatic stress disorder has reemerged as a neuropsychiatric disorder for which biological formulations are strongly grounded in previous and current understanding of CNS function and neurochemistry. Subsequent studies in this area will, it is hoped, capitalize on advances made in the past while avoiding past mistakes made in studying other disorders. Oversimplifying theories of brain function in terms of neurochemistry alone, and ignoring the reality that all results are obtained in the context of specific experimental paradigms, can result in trivial results or confusing conclusions. Further careful research into the psychobiology of PTSD can also contribute to our understanding of normal brain function and may add to a more sophisticated formulation of how catecholamines and stress affect the pathophysiology and expression of schizophrenia (van Kammen et al. 1990) and depression (Gold et al. 1988).

Dr. Murburg has provided a comprehensive summary of data and theories about catecholamine function in PTSD from multiple animal and human studies, which makes this an essential volume for researchers and clinicians interested in stress and PTSD. Moreover, the book engages the reader in an active process of deciding where different workers and models fit together or clash so that one can see demonstrated the process by which our current concepts of catecholamine function in PTSD are emerging.

Earl L. Giller, Jr., M.D., Ph.D.

REFERENCES

Breslau N, Davis GC: PTSD in an urban population of young adults: risk factors for chronicity. Am J Psychiatry 149:671–675, 1992

Cannon WB: The emergency function of the adrenal medulla in pain and the major emotions. Am J Physiol 3:356–372, 1914

DaCosta JM: On irritable heart: a clinical study of a form of functional cardiac disorder and its consequences. Am J Med Sci 61:17–52, 1871

Gold PW, Goodwin F, Chrousos GP: Clinical and biochemical manifestations of depression: relationship to the neurobiology of stress. N Engl J Med 319:348–353, 413–420, 1988

Mason JW, Giller EL Jr, Kosten TR, et al: Psychoendocrine approaches to the diagnosis and pathogenesis of PTSD, in The Biological Assessment and Treatment of Posttraumatic Stress Disorder. Edited by Giller EL Jr. Washington, DC, American Psychiatric Press, 1990, pp 65–86

Selye H: A syndrome produced by diverse noxious agents. Nature 138:32, 1936

van der Kolk BA, van der Hart O: Pierre Janet and the breakdown of adaptation in psychological trauma. Am J Psychiatry 146:1530–1540, 1989

van Kammen DP, Peters J, Yao J, et al: Norepinephrine in acute exacerbations of chronic schizophrenia: negative symptoms revisited. Arch Gen Psychiatry 47:161–168, 1990

Introduction

In both human and nonhuman species, central and peripheral catecholaminergic systems are important components of the body's stress response apparatus. An increase in vigilance and attention mediated in part through central nervous system (CNS) noradrenergic pathways, diversion of bloodflow to key tissues and organs and increased heart rate in response to localized activation of peripheral sympathetic noradrenergic neurons, and increased mobilization of energy stores in response to epinephrine released from the adrenal medulla all contribute to the ability to respond successfully to stressful situations (see Charney et al., Chapter 6; Perry, Chapter 12). The effects of stress on central and peripheral catecholaminergic systems in nonhuman species have been studied in some detail and are profound. Normally, upon termination of an acute stressor, these systems return to a homeostatic level of function. However, under conditions of chronic stress, a number of changes may occur. Catecholamine synthesis increases to compensate for increased utilization by repeatedly activated systems. Additionally, complex processes such as behavioral conditioning and sensitization appear to maximize the animal's ability to perceive and respond to identical or similar situations. Although animal studies using stressors such as electric shock or forced swims in cold water cannot predict with certainty how parallel human systems will respond under conditions of exposure to very different stressors, such as combat, they provide critically important paradigms for scientists investigating the biological effects of stress in humans.

The short- and long-term effects of stress on human catecholaminergic systems have been less extensively investigated. Symptoms of posttraumatic stress disorder (PTSD) develop in many persons exposed to massive stress or trauma, although they may occur quite some time after exposure. Some symptoms of PTSD, particularly intrusive recollections, flashbacks, and nightmares of the trauma, may themselves serve as chronic stressors. A number of PTSD symptoms, such as exaggerated startle response, hypervigilance, sleep disturbance, difficulty with attention and concentration, irritability, loss of interest in activities, and physiological reactivity upon exposure to stimuli similar to the trauma, suggest that central and peripheral catecholamine function may be altered in this disorder. In the past several years, a number of studies have examined catecholaminergic systems function in PTSD. The results of some of those studies were presented in May 1990, in a symposium given at the annual meeting of the American Psychiatric Association in New York. This book expands on the content of that symposium.

In this volume, we include chapters from researchers investigating many different aspects of catecholaminergic systems in PTSD. In addition, we have included chapters from several basic scientists whose contributions to our knowledge of the neuroanatomy of catecholaminergic systems, the neurophysiology of stress, animal models of stress response, and the anatomy and physiology of behaviors potentially relevant to PTSD, add importantly to our ability to conceptualize the biological alterations that may underlie human PTSD.

Because human studies are necessarily limited in their scope and invasiveness, the paradigms that we construct to explain our clinical findings are largely dependent upon our knowledge of how related systems and processes operate in nonhuman species that have been more exhaustively studied. Conversely, the appropriateness of animal models to the study of PTSD must be judged largely in terms of the "fit" between animal-derived paradigms and the clinical syndromes and human biological alterations that such paradigms are meant to help clarify. As Kuhn has described (Kuhn TS: *The Structure of Scientific Revolutions*. Chicago, IL, University of Chicago Press, 1970), scientific paradigms evolve as new data fail to be accommodated by existing models. A dynamic interchange between basic and clinical researchers is, then, key to the progressive refinement of our understanding of human disorders, including PTSD. We hope to communicate a sense of that interchange in this book.

In the first chapter, we have attempted to provide some background information for readers coming to this topic from different disciplines. Some clinicians may not have a working knowledge of the biology of catecholaminergic systems, and scientists researching the biology of stress in animals may not be familiar with the clinical syndrome of PTSD. Next, we present five chapters by scientists investigating the anatomy and physiology of stress response in animals. In Chapter 2, Dr. Aston-Jones and his colleagues present a review of the biology of the brain's major noradrenergic nucleus, the locus coeruleus (LC), and the systems that regulate it. Included in this chapter are some extremely important data that this group and others have generated regarding regulation of the LC by the nucleus paragigantocellularis (PGi). Next, Drs. Simson and Weiss, in Chapter 3, detail some of the physiological alterations induced by stress in the LC. Their findings, which suggest that tonic and stress-induced LC activity may be regulated differently, may shed light on some of the clinical findings described later in the book. Next, Drs. Antelman and Yehuda describe the intriguing phenomenon of time-dependent change, including sensitization and desensitization by a stimulus of the subsequent response to similar and unrelated stimuli. They discuss the relevance of such time-dependent change to PTSD. In Chapter 5, Dr. Zacharko provides an extensive analysis of the effects of stress on central dopaminergic systems and on some of the behaviors subserved in part by these systems. Importantly, some of the "negative" behaviors produced by chronic stress exposure in animals, such as impairment in motivation, may have relevance to some of the "negative symptoms" of PTSD, including loss of interest in people and activities. In Chapter 6, Dr. Charney and colleagues review the key models of PTSD that emerge from consideration of clinical observations together with animal studies.

The focus of the book then turns to clinical findings that suggest altered catecholamine function in PTSD. Dr. McFall, in Chapter 7, reviews the psychophysiological studies that first suggested altered autonomic function in PTSD. Our group then provides chapters describing basal sympathetic nervous system (SNS) function in PTSD and depression (Chapter 8), and SNS responses to trauma-related versus trauma-unrelated stimuli (Chapter 9). In Chapter 10, Dr. Yehuda and colleagues provide data suggesting a relationship between the severity of PTSD symptoms and the magnitude of some peripheral catecholaminergic alterations not only in combat veterans but in survivors of the Holocaust. Their data suggest that catecholaminergic alterations are seen following a variety of traumas and persist for as long as half a century after stress exposure. In Chapter 11, Dr. Hamner and associates describe plasma catecholamine responses to exercise in PTSD patients, providing an important example of catecholamine response to physiological challenge. Then, in Chapter 12, Dr. Perry presents some of his pioneering work investigating the effects of childhood trauma on autonomic activity and platelet noradrenergic receptors. He also describes the effects of clonidine on autonomic and psychological symptoms in childhood PTSD. Dr. Lerer and colleagues, in Chapter 13, provide an extensive description of adrenergic receptors and the results of two studies investigating alterations in these receptors and postreceptor mechanisms in patients with PTSD.

The book then moves to descriptions of data directly supporting the concept that CNS catecholamine function is altered in PTSD. Dr. Rausch and colleagues, in Chapter 14, discuss the biology of the startle response and their own data documenting altered startle response in patients with PTSD. Then, in Chapter 15, Dr. Southwick and colleagues review and analyze studies of antidepressant effects on PTSD symptoms and draw conclusions of both clinical and theoretical importance. Dr. Veith (Chapter 16) highlights some important methodological issues that need to be kept in mind when interpreting peripheral catecholamine measurements in humans, particularly with respect to the "stress response." Finally, in a closing comment, Drs. Yehuda and Antelman discuss the applicability of animal models to clinical PTSD. Taken together, these chapters contain clear evidence of alterations in a number of aspects of central and peripheral catecholamine function in PTSD.

Although not totally unexpected, these findings are exciting for a number of reasons. First, although they cannot directly replicate the results of studies of stress effects in nonhuman species, many of the research findings in patient populations are compatible with conceptual paradigms of stress response that have emerged from the animal literature. It would therefore appear that some animal models of stress, although limited in what they can predict about human responses, may indeed be applicable to the study of PTSD. Second, these studies provide a body of evidence for central and peripheral neurotransmitter alterations in a disorder that is experientially, rather than genetically, based. The studies therefore have important implications for research approaches to other psychiatric illnesses that, although they may have genetic components, may be modified in their expression by experiential factors. Third, these studies form an initial basis for the conceptualization of specific alterations in catecholamine function in PTSD and point to the need for further research into factors that may contribute to these alterations. Last, and perhaps most important for our patients, they provide new insights into biological features of PTSD that may in the future be addressed by more specific pharmacological interventions than are currently available.

Although catecholaminergic systems play an important role in the stress response and may undergo alteration in PTSD, they do not operate in a vacuum. Many other neurotransmitter and neuroendocrine systems, including those constituting the hippocampo-hypothalamo-pituitary-adrenal axis, respond profoundly to stress and may also exhibit altered function in PTSD. Moreover, although for convenience we study, discuss, and tend to treat these systems as discrete entities, they are not functionally isolated but rather interact at multiple levels. To date, few studies have been performed to investigate how these systems and their interactions may be altered in PTSD. Such questions clearly point to important directions for future research.

As editor, I would like to express my appreciation to the authors who so carefully prepared their contributions to this volume, and to the veterans and other volunteers who participated in our studies so that we could all learn. The helpful comments of Dr. Richard Veith concerning earlier versions of this manuscript, as well as his mentorship and collegial support, deserve special thanks. Dr. Rachel Yehuda's input as this volume was being prepared is also very much appreciated. Additionally, I would like to acknowledge Regina R. Warmoth for her skillful secretarial assistance. Finally, I would like to thank my family for their patience and support while this book was being prepared.

M. Michele Murburg, M.D.

Section I

The Role of Catecholaminergic Systems in Stress Response Syndromes

Chapter 1

Biology of Catecholaminergic Systems and Their Relevance to PTSD

M. Michele Murburg, M.D.
E. Alexandra Ashleigh, M.D.
Daniel W. Hommer, M.D.
Richard C. Veith, M.D.

In an effort to make this book "user-friendly" to readers from a variety of disciplines, we provide in this chapter some background information not given elsewhere in this volume on both the biology of catecholaminergic systems and the phenomenology of posttraumatic stress disorder (PTSD). The information presented below is not meant to be an exhaustive treatment of any of the topics discussed, and readers who would like further details may want to consult some of the sources referenced herein. A description of peripheral catecholamines and the sympathetic nervous system (SNS) is provided in Chapter 16 by Drs. Veith and Murburg.

SYNTHESIS, STORAGE, RELEASE, METABOLISM, AND REUPTAKE OF CATECHOLAMINES

The catecholamines that act as neurotransmitters in mammalian central and peripheral nervous systems are the related compounds dopamine, norepinephrine, and epinephrine. As shown in Figure 1–1, dopamine is formed from the amino acid precursor tyrosine and in turn serves as a precursor for norepinephrine, which may be transformed into epinephrine (Nagatsu et al.

1964). The reactions by which each of these compounds is formed occur in the brain, sympathetic nerves and ganglia, the heart and arterial and venous tissue, and the adrenal medulla (Cooper et al. 1991). Because each step in the synthesis of these compounds is catalyzed by a specific enzyme, the profile of catecholamine end products synthesized in a particular tissue reflects, in part, the relative expression of genes for those enzymes in that tissue under a given set of conditions. Catecholamine synthesis may thus be regulated by a variety of factors influencing enzyme synthesis and activity. For example, catecholamines exert feedback inhibition over tyrosine hydroxylase activity (Nagatsu et al. 1964), while steroid hormones increase phenylethanolamine-N-methyltransferase activity (Cooper et al. 1986). Other factors, including the availability of tyrosine substrate, may be important under certain conditions such as increased neuronal impulse flow (Milner and Wurtman 1986).

Once synthesized, catecholamines are stored in specialized storage vesicles, or granules, in sympathetic nerve endings, chromaffin cells, and central nervous system (CNS) catecholaminer-

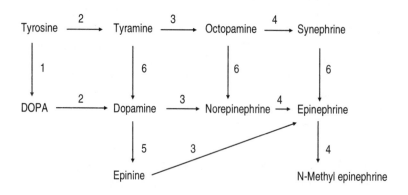

Figure 1–1. Synthesis of catecholamines. 1, tyrosine hydroxylase; 2, aromatic amino acid decarboxylase; 3, dopamine ß-hydroxylase; 4, phenylethanolamine-N-methyltransferase; 5, nonspecific N-methyltransferase in lung/folate-dependent N-methyltransferase in brain; 6, catechol-forming enzyme. DOPA = dihydroxyphenylalanine. For a full discussion, see Cooper et al. 1991.

gic neurons (Hillarp et al. 1953). These storage vesicles protect the catecholamines from degradation by intraneuronal enzymes such as monoamine oxidase (MAO) (see Carlsson 1987 for review), and then permit them to be released upon depolarization of the nerve cell. Release of catecholamines from nerve terminals is subject to local feedback inhibition by catecholamines acting at presynaptic autoreceptors, and also by the actions of certain other neurotransmitters, neuropeptides, and prostaglandins (see Cooper et al. 1991 for review).

The catecholamines undergo metabolic degradation by the enzymes MAO and catechol-O-methyltransferase (COMT) (for review, see Axelrod 1973; Carlsson 1987). The products of catecholamine metabolism are shown in Figures 1–2 and 1–3. In

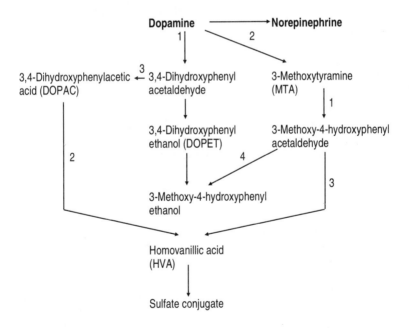

Figure 1–2. Metabolism of dopamine. 1, monoamine oxidase (MAO); 2, catechol-O-methyltransferase (COMT); 3, aldehyde dehydrogenase; 4, aldehyde reductase. For a full discussion, see Cooper et al. 1991.

addition to inactivation by metabolic degradation, catecholamine activity at the synapse is terminated by an active, energy-dependent process called *reuptake,* whereby neurotransmitters are taken back into the presynaptic nerve terminals and then into the storage granules (Axelrod 1973; Carlsson 1987; Cooper et al. 1986). Reuptake and enzymatic degradation are important mechanisms in both the CNS and the peripheral SNS for removal of active catecholamine neurotransmitter from the synaptic terminal areas. In addition, catecholamines released from SNS neurons into the bloodstream are removed from circulation by the kidneys.

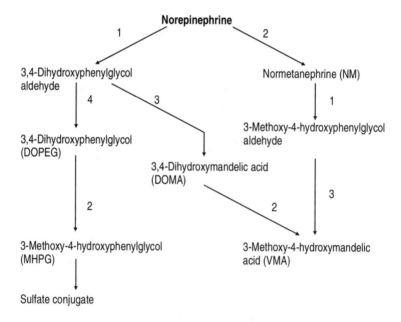

Figure 1–3. Metabolism of norepinephrine. 1, monoamine oxidase (MAO); 2, catechol-O-methyltransferase (COMT); 3, aldehyde dehydrogenase; 4, aldehyde reductase. For a full discussion, see Cooper et al. 1991.

CATECHOLAMINE-RECEPTOR INTERACTIONS

Like other neurotransmitters, catecholamines exert their effects on target cells by binding to receptors, or specialized macromolecules on the surface of the postsynaptic cell membrane, that recognize specific transmitters. This binding then triggers a number of effects on the target cell through a series of *postreceptor* mechanisms. Norepinephrine and epinephrine bind to several subtypes of adrenergic receptors, referred to as α_{1A}, α_{1B}, α_{2A}, α_{2B}, α_{2C}, and β_1, β_2, and β_3 (Harrison et al. 1991; see Lerer et al., Chapter 13, this volume, for a full discussion). Dopamine binds to a family of receptors (D_{1A}, D_{1B}, D_{2A}, D_{2B}, D_3, D_4, D_5) (see Strange 1991 for review; Sunahara et al. 1991). These receptors are coupled via guanine nucleotide-binding proteins to second messenger systems such as adenylate cyclase/cyclic AMP or phosphatidylinositol. Binding of the catecholamine to the receptor results in either activation or inhibition of such second messenger systems (see Lerer et al., Chapter 13, this volume), which in turn regulate intracellular calcium mobilization and protein kinase C activation (Berridge 1984a, 1984b; Nishizuka 1984). These "third messengers" in turn affect neuronal activity, gene expression, and protein activation. In general, β and D_1 receptors stimulate adenylate cyclase, α_2 and D_2 receptors inhibit adenylate cyclase, and α_1 receptors stimulate hydrolysis of phosphatidylinositol (see Cooper et al. 1986 for review).

FUNCTIONAL ANATOMY OF CENTRAL CATECHOLAMINERGIC SYSTEMS

Norepinephrine

The brain's major noradrenergic nucleus is the locus coeruleus (LC), a cell group in the central gray of the caudal pons. From the LC, fibers course through five major tracts to innervate structures throughout the neuraxis such as the brain stem, neocortex, hypothalamus, cerebellum, spinal cord (including parasympathetic nuclei), amygdala, and hippocampus, among many others (for reviews, see Aston-Jones et al., Chapter 2, this volume; Murburg et al. 1990). The structures to which the LC projects include areas known to participate in responses to fear and pain, as well as areas involved in vigilance, cardiovascular regulation, and the mediation of motor activity.

Direct input to the LC, once thought to be extensive, has more recently been shown to be limited (see Aston Jones et al., Chapter 2, this volume, for review). The LC appears to receive direct input mainly from the nucleus paragigantocellularis (PGi) and the nucleus prepositus hypoglossi (Aston-Jones et al. 1986; Pieribone et al. 1987, 1988). These nuclei in turn receive sensory and autonomic input from a number of sources and may serve as relays to the LC (Andrezik et al. 1981; Van Bockstaele et al. 1988). In addition, there is evidence for parallel activation of the LC and the SNS by the PGi (Svensson 1988), suggesting that the LC and the SNS may serve, respectively, as the central and peripheral limbs of a catecholaminergic stress effector system (see Aston-Jones et al., Chapter 2, this volume, for review).

The other CNS noradrenergic system is the lateral tegmental system (LTS), consisting of two major groups of noradrenergic neurons, one medullary and one pontine (Moore and Bloom 1979). These areas innervate the basal forebrain, septal areas, the central amygdaloid nucleus (Fallon et al. 1978; Moore and Bloom 1979), and the paraventricular nucleus of the thalamus (Lindvall and Bjorklund 1974). These areas also receive input from the LC (Moore and Bloom 1979). The LTS provides noradrenergic input to the hypothalamus, and also innervates brain-stem areas other than associational and primary sensory nuclei (Moore and Bloom 1979), as well as sympathetic and somatic motor areas of the spinal cord (Westlund and Coulter 1980). The LTS appears to play a role in sympathoregulation (Granata et al. 1986), but its physiology is not completely understood.

Epinephrine

Adrenergic cells in the CNS are found in three brain-stem groups, designated C_1, C_2, and C_3 (Hokfelt et al. 1984). From these two nuclei, which are intermingled with noradrenergic cells, adrenergic neurons send projections to the hypothalamus, the nuclei of visceral efferent and afferent systems, the intermediolateral columns of the spinal cord, the periventricular region, and the LC (Cooper et al. 1986). These cell groups are thought to participate in autonomic and neuroendocrine regulation (Cooper et al. 1991).

Dopamine

The long-length dopaminergic systems include the mesocortical and mesolimbic projections, and the nigrostriatal pathway. The mesocortical system arises in the ventral tegmentum and substantia nigra, and projects to the prefrontal (including the supplementary motor area), cingulate, and entorhinal cortices. The mesolimbic system sends projections from these same origins to the septum, olfactory tubercle, nucleus accumbens, amygdala, and piriform cortex. The nigrostriatal pathway, which arises in these same areas and terminates in the caudate and putamen (see Cooper et al. 1986 for review), is involved in sensorimotor integration and control of motor output. Although their functions are not as well understood as those of the nigrostriatal dopaminergic projections, the mesolimbic and mesocortical dopaminergic systems also appear to be involved in sensorimotor integration. In these latter systems the information being integrated involves higher-order sensory representations and motivational or emotional states rather than information about muscle tone, limb position, and target location (Goldman-Rakic and Selemon 1990).

The intermediate-length systems include the tuberohypophyseal system, which originates in the arcuate and periventricular nuclei and projects to the intermediate pituitary lobe and to the tuberoinfundibular vascular system, which supplies the anterior pituitary lobe. These systems are involved in pituitary regulation. The incertohypothalamic system and the medullary periventricular group (including dopaminergic cells in the dorsal motor nucleus of the vagus, the nucleus tractus solitarius, and the tegmental radiation of the periaqueductal gray) are intermediate-length systems (Cooper et al. 1986) involved in neuroendocrine and possibly autonomic functions. Ultrashort dopaminergic systems in the brain include the periglomerular cells of the olfactory bulb and the interplexiform amacrine-like neurons that connect the inner and outer plexiform layers of the retina (Cooper et al. 1986) and are involved in primary sensory processing.

Table 1–1.   DSM-III-R diagnostic criteria for posttraumatic stress
             disorder

A. The person has experienced an event that is outside the range of
   usual human experience and that would be markedly distressing to
   almost anyone, e.g., serious threat to one's life or physical integrity;
   serious threat or harm to one's children, spouse, or other close
   relatives and friends; sudden destruction of one's home or
   community; or seeing another person who Has recently been, or is
   being, seriously injured or killed as the result of an accident or
   physical violence.

B. The traumatic event is persistently reexperienced in at least one of
   the following ways:
   1. Recurrent and intrusive distressing recollections of the event (in
      young children, repetitive play in which themes or aspects of the
      trauma are expressed)
   2. Recurrent distressing dreams of the event
   3. Sudden acting or feeling as if the traumatic event were recurring
      (includes a sense of reliving the experience, illusions,
      hallucinations, and dissociative [flashback] episodes, even those
      that occur upon awakening or when intoxicated)
   4. Intense psychological distress at exposure to events that
      symbolize or resemble an aspect of the traumatic event, including
      anniversaries of the trauma

C. Persistent avoidance of stimuli associated with the trauma or
   numbing of general responsiveness (not present before the
   trauma), as indicated by at least three of the following:
   1. Efforts to avoid thoughts or feelings associated with the trauma
   2. Efforts to avoid activities or situations that arouse recollections
      of the trauma
   3. Inability to recall an important aspect of the trauma (psychogenic
      amnesia)
   4. Markedly diminished interest in significant activities (in young
      children, loss of recently acquired developmental skills such as
      toilet training or language skills)
   5. Feelings of detachment or estrangement from others
   6. Restricted range of affect, e.g., unable to have loving feelings
   7. Sense of a foreshortened future, e.g., does not expect to have a
      career, marriage, or children, or a long life

D. Persistent symptoms of increased arousal (not present before the
   trauma), as indicated by at least two of the following:

(continued)

Table 1–1. DSM-III-R diagnostic criteria for posttraumatic stress disorder *(continued)*

1. Difficulty falling or staying asleep
2. Irritability or outbursts of anger
3. Difficulty concentrating
4. Hypervigilance
5. Exaggerated startle response
6. Physiologic reactivity upon exposure to events that symbolize or resemble an aspect of the traumatic event (e.g., a woman who was raped in an elevator breaks out in a sweat when entering any elevator)

E. Duration of the disturbance (symptoms in B, C, and D) of at least 1 month.

Specify delayed onset if the onset of symptoms was at least 6 months after the trauma.

Source. Reprinted from American Psychiatric Association: *Diagnostic and Statistical Manual of Mental Disorders,* 3rd Edition, Revised. Washington, DC, American Psychiatric Association, 1987, pp. 250–251. Copyright 1987, American Psychiatric Association. Used with permission.

EFFECTS OF STRESS ON CATECHOLAMINERGIC SYSTEMS

Stressors of various types cause changes in central and peripheral catecholaminergic systems. The effects of stress exposure can vary depending on the brain area studied, the nature and chronicity of the stressor, and the species and strain of animal utilized. In many animal studies, acute stressors, particularly those that are uncontrollable, cause an increase in CNS norepinephrine and epinephrine release, with a consequent transient decrease in norepinephrine and epinephrine content in a number of brain areas (see Murburg et al. 1990 for review). With chronic stress, in most cases, compensatory increases in synthesis occur, so this decrease in content is not seen. Similarly, the number of CNS ß-adrenergic receptors decreases and the number of α_2-adrenergic receptors increases in a number of brain areas following chronic stress, probably in response to increased catecholamine levels (see Murburg et al. 1990 for review).

Stress effects on central dopaminergic systems are more complex and less uniform, as described in detail by Dr. Zacharko in Chapter 5 of this volume. The nigrostriatal, mesolimbic, and mesoprefrontal systems—but not the mesopiriform, tuberoinfundibular, or tuberohypophyseal systems—manifest an increase in dopamine synthesis and catabolism in response to mild acute stress (Cooper et al. 1986). With chronic stress, the increase in dopamine turnover seen with acute stress is attenuated (see Chapter 5). Thus, in general, the transient depletion in catecholamine stores seen with acute stress exposure is not seen with chronic stress exposure because of compensatory mechanisms such as increased catecholamine synthesis and/or decreased catecholamine turnover that occur under conditions of chronic stress.

CATECHOLAMINES AND PTSD

The findings mentioned above indicating prominent changes in central catecholaminergic systems under conditions of acute and chronic stress in animals have suggested to many investigators that similar alterations may occur in patients with PTSD. This hypothesis is buttressed by recent clarifications in the anatomy and physiology of specific behaviors that are related to PTSD symptoms and are mediated in part by catecholamines. Examples of such symptoms are exaggerated startle response (see Rausch et al., Chapter 14, this volume); physiological reactivity—including increased activity of the SNS—to stimuli that resemble the etiological trauma (see McFall and Murburg, Chapter 7, and Murburg et al., Chapters 8 and 9); diminished interest in significant activities (see Zacharko, Chapter 5); difficulty with sleep and concentration, and hypervigilance (see Aston-Jones et al., Chapter 2); and possibly even flashbacks (see Charney et al., Chapter 6). This book constitutes a current compendium of much of the currently available data regarding involvement of catecholamine function in the pathophysiology of PTSD.

DIAGNOSTIC CRITERIA FOR PTSD

For those unfamiliar with the diagnostic criteria, or the cardinal symptoms, currently used in making the diagnosis of PTSD, these criteria (American Psychiatric Association 1987) are detailed in Table 1–1. These symptoms may occur immediately or long after the precipitating event, and may persist for decades. Although we are far from being able to provide definitive treatment for PTSD, a number of approaches have been utilized with varying degrees of success. Both psychotherapeutic and biological interventions are humane and reasonable, although there is a great need for well-controlled studies of short- and long-term outcome, and both types of interventions may impact dually upon the psychology and biology of the disorder.

REFERENCES

American Psychiatric Association: Diagnostic and Statistical Manual of Mental Disorders, 3rd Edition, Revised. Washington, DC, American Psychiatric Association, 1987

Andrezik JA, Chan-Palay V, Palay SL: The nucleus paragigantocellularis lateralis in the rat: demonstration of afferents by the retrograde transport of horseradish peroxidase. Anat Embryol (Berl) 161:373–390, 1981

Aston-Jones G, Ennis M, Pieribone VA, et al: The brain nucleus locus coeruleus: restricted afferent control of a broad afferent network. Science 234:734–737, 1986

Axelrod J: The fate of noradrenaline in the sympathetic neurone. Harvey Lect 67:175, 1973

Berridge MJ: Cellular control through interactions between cyclic nucleotides and calcium. Advances in Cyclic Nucleotide Protein Phosphorylation Research 17:329–335, 1984a

Berridge MJ: Inositol triphosphate and diacylglycerol as second messengers. Biochem J 220:345–60, 1984b

Carlsson A: Monoamines of the central nervous system: a historical perspective, in Psychopharmacology: The Third Generation of Progress. Edited by Meltzer HY. New York, Raven, 1987, pp 39–48

Cooper JR, Bloom FE, Roth RE: The Biochemical Basis of Neuropharmacology, 5th Edition. New York, Oxford University Press, 1986

Cooper JR, Bloom FE, Roth RE: The Biochemical Basis of Neuropharmacology, 6th Edition. New York, Oxford University Press, 1991

Fallon JH, Koziell DA, Moore RY: Catecholamine innervation of the basal forebrain, II: amygdala, suprarhinal cortex and enterorhinal cortex. J Comp Neurol 180:508–532, 1978

Goldman-Rakic PS, Selemon LD: New frontiers in basal ganglia research. Trends Neurosci 13:241–244, 1990

Granata AR, Numao Y, Kumada M, et al: A1 noradrenergic neurons tonically inhibit sympathoexcitatory neurons of the C1 area in rat brainstem. Brain Res 377:127–146, 1986

Harrison JK, Pearson WR, Lynch KR: Molecular characterization of alpha-1 and alpha-2 adrenoceptors. Trends Pharmacol Sci 12:62–67, 1991

Hillarp NA, Lagerstedt S, Nilson B: Isolation of granular fraction from suprarenal medulla, containing sympathomimetic catecholamines. Acta Physiol Scand 29:251–263, 1953

Hokfelt T, Johansson O, Goldstein M: Chemical anatomy of the brain. Science 225:1326–1334, 1984

Lindvall O, Bjorklund A: The organization of the ascending catecholamine neuron systems in the rat brain as revealed by the glyoxylic acid fluorescence method. J Comp Neurol 154:317–348, 1974

Milner JD, Wurtman RJ: Catecholamine synthesis: physiological coupling to precursor supply. Biochem Pharmacol 35:875–881, 1986

Moore RY, Bloom FE: Central catecholamine neural systems: anatomy and physiology of the norepinephrine and epinephrine systems. Annu Rev Neurosci 2:113–168, 1979

Murburg MM, McFall ME, Veith RC: Catecholamines, stress, and posttraumatic stress disorder, in Biological Assessment and Treatment of Posttraumatic Stress Disorder. Edited by Giller EL, Jr. Washington, DC, American Psychiatric Press, 1990, pp 29–64

Nagatsu T, Levitt M, Udenfriend S: Tyrosine hydroxylase: the initial step in norepinephrine biosynthesis. J Biol Chem 239:2910–2917, 1964

Nishizuka Y: Turnover of inositol phospholipids and signal transduction. Science 225:1365–1370, 1984

Pieribone VA, Aston-Jones G, Bohn MC, et al: Double labeling using fluorogold reveals neurotransmitter identity of afferents to locus coeruleus: a fluorescent double labeling study. Society for Neuroscience Abstracts 13:1458, 1987

Pieribone VA, Aston-Jones G, Bohn MC: Adrenergic and noradrenergic neurons in the C1 and C3 areas project to locus coeruleus: a fluorescent double labeling study. Neurosci Lett 85:297–303, 1988

Strange PG: Interesting times for dopamine receptors. TINS 14:43–45, 1991

Sunahara RK, Guan HC, O'Dowd BF, et al: Cloning of the gene for a human dopamine D_5 receptor with higher affinity for dopamine than D_1. Nature 350:614–619, 1991

Svensson TH: Peripheral regulation of locus coeruleus neurons: implications for drug effects. Paper presented at the 18th annual meeting of the Society for Neuroscience, Toronto, Ontario, November 1988

Van Bockstaele EJ, Pieribone VA, Aston-Jones G, et al: Anatomic evidence that autonomic and visceral areas converge on paragigantocellularis, a major afferent to locus coeruleus. Abstracts of the 18th annual meeting of the Society for Neuroscience, Toronto, Ontario, 1988, p 1318

Westlund KN, Coulter JD: Descending projections of the locus coeruleus and subcoeruleus/medial parabrachial nuclei in monkeys: axonal transport studies and dopamine-beta-hydroxylase immunocytochemistry. Brain Res Rev 2:235–264, 1980

Chapter 2

Locus Coeruleus, Stress, and PTSD: Neurobiological and Clinical Parallels

Gary Aston-Jones, Ph.D.
Rita J. Valentino, Ph.D.
Elisabeth J. Van Bockstaele, Ph.D.
Arthur T. Meyerson, M.D.

Some of the cardinal symptoms of posttraumatic stress disorder (PTSD)—including hypervigilance, enhanced startle reactions, increased physiological response to stress-related stimuli, irritability, and sleep abnormalities, as well as the increased incidence of substance abuse seen in PTSD patients—may be viewed as manifestations of overactivity or overreactivity of a central alerting or vigilance system. Several levels of evidence suggest that the brain's major noradrenergic nucleus, the locus coeruleus (LC), which is known to mediate many brain and behavioral responses to stress as well as vigilance and sleep, may be such a system (Aston-Jones 1985; Aston-Jones et al. 1990). Symptoms of anxiety, panic, and depression, which commonly accompany PTSD, are also associated with alterations in LC function (Aston-Jones et al. 1984). Hyperreactivity of the sympathetic nervous system (SNS) has also been described in PTSD (see McFall and Murburg, Chapter 7; Murburg et al., Chapters 8 and 9, this volume). Recent data, to be described in this chapter, demonstrate close links between the LC and the SNS. Importantly, the major input to the LC derives from the nucleus paragigantocellularis (PGi), a key brain area for control of sympathetic activity. These considerations suggest that altered function of the PGi may serve as a neurobiological basis for salient central (via the LC) and peripheral (via the SNS) manifestations of PTSD.

Our purpose in this chapter is to review the neurobiology of the LC system and to explore the possibility that this system provides the neural substrate for some of the clinical manifestations of PTSD. We will conclude that when recent developments in our understanding of LC neurobiology are considered, the connections between the LC system and PTSD prove even closer than had been previously suspected, and that the LC system may well be involved in the mediation of at least some key elements of PTSD.

First, in reviewing the anatomic, physiological, neurochemical, and connectional properties of LC neurons and their targets and afferents, we assess the evidence that the LC serves as a vigilance system in the brain. We focus on recent findings that the major afferent to the LC, the PGi, is a key sympathoexcitatory region in the rostral medulla, considering this evidence of a neurobiological basis for parallel activation of the sympathetic and LC systems by imperative stimuli. We then outline a possible role for such a vigilance system in the increased emotional and physiological reactivity and exaggerated startle response characteristic of PTSD. We next describe the close association between the LC system and responses to stress, including afferent regulation of the LC by corticotropin-releasing factor inputs in response to stressful stimuli. Finally, we consider aspects of PTSD symptomatology that may be especially linked to LC dysfunction and approachable by pharmacological manipulation of the noradrenergic LC system.

CELLULAR PROPERTIES OF THE NORADRENERGIC LOCUS COERULEUS: NEUROBIOLOGY OF A VIGILANCE SYSTEM

Global Efferent Projections

Intense interest in the LC was first stimulated by Swedish researchers (Dahlström and Fuxe 1964; Ungestedt 1971) who discovered that the cells in this nucleus give rise to an extensive set of efferent projections. These and subsequent studies have established that the LC projects throughout the cerebral cortex, hippocampus, thalamus, midbrain, brain stem, cerebellum, and spinal cord (Foote et al. 1983). In fact, this small nucleus innervates a greater variety of brain areas than does any other single nucleus yet described. This extensive efferent projection network and the fact that LC neurons appeared to use the then recently discovered neurotransmitter norepinephrine to communicate with their target cells generated great enthusiasm for understanding LC function(s).

Although some investigators have argued that norepinephrine may be released from LC fibers in a nonsynaptic manner, providing a hormone-like, paracrine influence on many neurons within a diffusion-limited area (Beaudet and Descarries 1978), more recent studies have shown that LC terminals in several brain structures make conventional synapse-like appositions with postsynaptic specializations on target neurons (Koda et al. 1978; Olschowka et al. 1981; Papadopoulos and Parnavelas 1990; Papadopoulos et al. 1989). There is, in fact, a great deal of both regional and laminar specificity in the innervation of target structures by LC axons (e.g., Morrison et al. 1982). Finally, while some investigators have reported norepinephrine fibers in apposition with blood vessels (Edvinsson et al. 1973; Hartman 1973; Swanson et al. 1977), more recent studies in LC terminal areas do not find a preference for apposition of dopamine beta-hydroxylase (DBH)–containing fibers on capillaries (Olschowka et al. 1981; Papadopoulos and Parnavelas 1990; Papadopoulos et al. 1989). Although such findings do not rule out the possibility that LC projections participate in the regulation of blood flow and metabolism in target areas, they indicate that this system is structured to provide conventional synaptic input to brain neurons.

Increase in Signal-to-Noise Ratio of Postsynaptic Neurons

Using microiontophoresis, early studies (Hoffer et al. 1973; Segal and Bloom 1974) found that norepinephrine inhibited basal discharge of cerebellar or hippocampal neurons in anesthetized rats. However, subsequent experiments by Foote, Segal, and colleagues (Foote et al. 1975; Segal and Bloom 1976) found that, in addition to decreasing basal discharge, norepinephrine may also enhance the selectivity of target cell discharge so that in the presence of this neurotransmitter, neurons respond with increased preference to their most strongly determined inputs. In these studies and in studies by others (see Foote et al. 1983 for review), norepinephrine, presumably acting at beta receptors, decreased spontaneous impulse activity to a greater extent than activity evoked by strong afferent input or sensory stimulation. It is noteworthy that in many cases norepinephrine has been found to augment evoked activity (either excitatory or inhibitory) while decreasing spontaneous discharge of the same neuron (Waterhouse and Woodward 1980; Waterhouse et al. 1980, 1984). Such selective enhancement of responses to strong inputs relative to low-level or basal activity has been likened to an increase in the "signal-to-noise" ratio of target neurons by norepinephrine. Although other effects of norepinephrine have been described for various target areas, such biasing of target cells to respond preferentially to their strongest inputs is most significant for the present analysis.

Variance in Tonic Locus Coeruleus Discharge With Behavioral State

One hypothesized function of LC neurons is the control of various stages of the sleep-waking cycle (Hobson et al. 1975; Jouvet 1969; McCarley and Hobson 1975). We have found that spontaneous LC discharge covaries consistently with stages of the sleep-waking cycle, firing fastest during waking, more slowly during slow-wave sleep, and becoming virtually silent during paradoxical sleep (Aston-Jones and Bloom 1981a). These observations, the first of their kind for known norepinephrine-containing neurons, support proposals that a similar subpopulation of unidentified cat LC neurons may be noradrenergic (Hobson et al. 1975; Rasmussen et al. 1986).

Further analysis revealed that LC impulse activity also changes *within* stages of the sleep-waking cycle in anticipation of the subsequent stage (Figure 2–1). That is, during waking, LC neurons progressively decrease in activity as slow-wave sleep approaches, and likewise during slow-wave sleep, LC neurons decrease in activity before the onset of paradoxical sleep (Aston-Jones and Bloom 1981a; Hobson et al. 1975). If waking rather than paradoxical sleep follows slow-wave sleep, LC neurons abruptly emit phasically robust activity 100 to 500 msec prior to waking. The one exception to such stage-anticipation in LC discharge occurs in the transition from paradoxical sleep to waking. Rat LC neurons return to waking activity either coincident with or slightly after the cessation of paradoxical sleep as measured by electroencephalography. Thus, although anticipatory LC activity during most stage transitions is consistent with a role in generating the subsequent stage, this nucleus cannot be responsible for

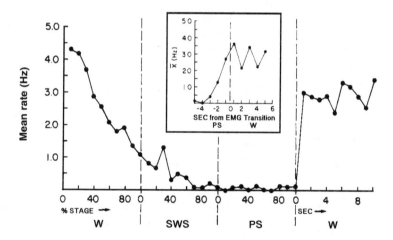

Figure 2–1. Locus coeruleus discharge rate during sleep-waking cycle progression. Mean discharge rates for multiple cell recordings during epochs normalized for the percentage of sleep-waking cycle stage completion are plotted consecutively for complete sleep-waking cycles. Note that when paradoxical sleep-to-waking transitions are judged by the EEG (main plot), cellular activity does not anticipate the transition; however, enhanced discharge does anticipate these same transitions scored by EMG criteria (inset). Reprinted from Aston-Jones G, Bloom FE: "Activity of Norepinephrine-Containing Locus Coeruleus Neurons in Behaving Rats Anticipates Fluctuations in the Sleep-Waking Cycle." *Journal of Neuroscience* 1:876–886, 1981a. Used with permission.

the termination of paradoxical sleep (Aston-Jones and Bloom 1981a; Aston-Jones et al. 1984; however, see also Hobson et al. 1975). These sleep-related changes in LC activity have been observed across a number of species. We have observed similar discharge properties of LC neurons during waking and drowsiness in unanesthetized, chair-restrained primates (Alexinsky and Aston-Jones 1990; Aston-Jones et al. 1988; Foote et al. 1980; Grant et al. 1988), and others have reported similar results for cats (Hobson et al. 1975; Rasmussen et al. 1986).

We have noted that LC discharge is altered during certain spontaneous waking behaviors. During both consumption of a glucose solution and grooming, rat LC discharge decreased compared with during other epochs of similar arousal on the electroencephalogram (EEG) (Aston-Jones and Bloom 1981a). Similar results were obtained for LC activity in behaving primates (Alexinsky and Aston-Jones 1990; Aston-Jones et al. 1988; Grant et al. 1988). These results indicate that LC discharge is reduced not only for periods of low arousal (drowsiness or sleep) but also during certain behaviors (grooming and consumption) when animals are in an active waking, but inattentive (nonvigilant), state.

Locus coeruleus discharge also varies strongly with orienting behavior. In both rat (Aston-Jones and Bloom 1981a, 1981b) and monkey (Alexinsky and Aston-Jones 1990; Aston-Jones et al. 1988; Foote et al. 1980; Grant et al. 1988), the highest discharge rates we observed for LC neurons were consistently associated with spontaneous or evoked behavioral orienting responses. LC discharge associated with orienting behavior is phasically most intense when automatic, tonic behaviors (i.e., sleep, grooming, or consumption) are suddenly disrupted and the animal orients toward the external environment (Aston-Jones and Bloom 1981a, 1981b). Thus, as is found following sleep, grooming, or consumption, there is close correspondence between spontaneous bursts of discharge and interruption of automatic, preprogrammed behaviors, with an increase in attentiveness and vigilance.

Polymodal Sensory Responsiveness in Locus Coeruleus Neurons

In addition to the above fluctuations in LC spontaneous discharge, we found that LC neurons in unanesthetized rats and monkeys were responsive to non-noxious environmental stimuli (Figure 2–2) (Aston-Jones and Bloom 1981b; Foote et al. 1980). In waking rats, LC activity is markedly phasic, yielding short-latency (15 to 50 msec) responses to simple stimuli in each modality tested (i.e., auditory, visual, somatosensory, and olfactory). Responses were most consistently evoked by intense, conspicuous stimuli, although sporadic responses were observed for non-conspicuous stimuli as well. These responses, which were similar for the different sensory modalities, consisted of a brief excitation followed by diminished activity lasting a few hundred milliseconds. Similar results have been found in cat LC (Rasmussen et al. 1986; Reiner 1986).

In general, stimuli effective in eliciting LC responses in rats and monkeys were also those that disrupted ongoing behavior and elicited a behavioral orienting response. We have quantified this linkage between behavioral disruption/orientation and LC sensory responses for rat LC neurons (Aston-Jones and Bloom 1981b). The largest responses were elicited by stimuli that caused an abrupt transition from sleep to waking, with associated behavioral orientation. Responses evoked during uninterrupted slow-wave sleep were much smaller in magnitude, while no LC response occurred to stimuli that did not interrupt paradoxical sleep. In addition, we found that response magnitudes during uninterrupted grooming or consumption of sweet water were reduced, whereas stimuli that disrupted such activity and generated orienting behavior elicited strong responses. Thus, there was a strong correspondence in rat, as in monkey, between sensory-evoked responsiveness in behavior and LC discharge, and a common factor for stimulus-responsivity in the two species is *behavioral disruption and reorientation*. In sum, in both rat and monkey, stimuli that disrupt behavior and evoke an orienting response evoke LC activity.

Response of Locus Coeruleus Neurons in Monkeys to Meaningful Stimuli During an "Oddball" Discrimination/Vigilance Task

The above results suggested that the essential property of stimuli to elicit LC responses was *meaningfulness*. Intense stimuli elicited responses because their intensity made them meaningful, but

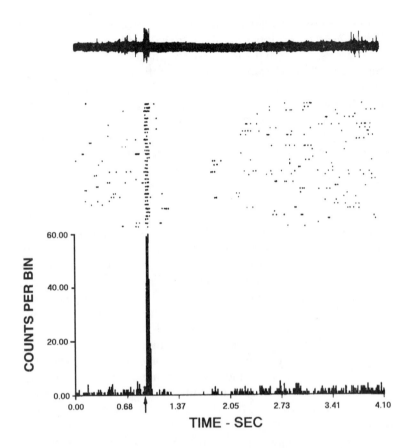

Figure 2–2. Tone pip-evoked discharge in a locus coeruleus (LC) multiple cell recording. *Upper panel:* Single oscilloscope sweep of analog discharge trace for one trial. Dots were generated for spikes meeting waveform discriminator criteria. *Middle panel:* Raster display of impulse activity for 40 consecutive trials, in sequence from *top* to *bottom.* *Lower panel:* Poststimulus time histogram accumulated for 50 consecutive trials (bin width = 8 msec). Time axis and tone pip onsets (*arrow*) apply to all panels. Light flash and tactile stimuli evoked similar responses, except that flash responses were weaker. Reprinted from Aston-Jones G, Bloom FE: "Norepinephrine-Containing Locus Coeruleus Neurons in Behaving Rats Exhibit Pronounced Responses to Non-Noxious Environmental Stimuli." *Journal of Neuroscience* 1:887–900, 1981b. Used with permission.

nonintense, meaningful stimuli may also reliably elicit responses of LC cells. To explicitly test this possibility, we recorded LC activity in unanesthetized primates trained in an "oddball" visual discrimination task (Alexinsky and Aston-Jones 1990; Alexinsky et al. 1990; Aston-Jones et al. 1988, 1991a). The task involved discriminating differently colored light cues for juice reward. A target stimulus (S+) was presented on 10% of trials, intermixed in a semirandom random fashion with nontarget lights of a different color (S–). Neurons in the LC area were recorded along with cortical surface slow waves (averaged event-related potentials, or AERPs) and behavioral responses (i.e., hits, misses, false alarms, and correct omissions). Although some cells in the LC area showed responses that were purely sensory or motor in nature, most neurons exhibited activity specifically linked to the target stimulus. That is, responses for most cells were evoked selectively by S+ stimuli but not by S– stimuli, or by bar release or reward that followed S+ stimuli on successful trials (Figure 2–3).

Recordings during reversal training revealed that these responses were specifically related to the *meaningfulness* of the stimuli, not to their physical attributes. After reversal training, neurons in the LC region reversed their stimulus preference, so that responses were selectively elicited for the new S+ (previous S–), while responses for the old S+ (new S–) faded. A second period of reversal training rapidly reestablished the original stimulus selectivity of primate LC neurons. Interestingly, these changes varied closely with behavioral performance: responses to the new S+ increased (and responses to the new S– decreased) as the percentage of correct behavioral responses to the new S+ increased (and behavioral responses to the new S– decreased). In addition, cortical event-related potentials (similar to the "P300 attention waves" reported for humans) exhibited a similar set of properties (see Aston-Jones et al. 1991a for more details).

Therefore, there is a close relationship between 1) neurons in the LC area, 2) cortical activity, and 3) behavioral responding to meaningful sensory cues. These results indicate that LC responses can be conditioned to salient stimuli and events in the environment, a potentially important attribute for understanding the role of this system in PTSD.

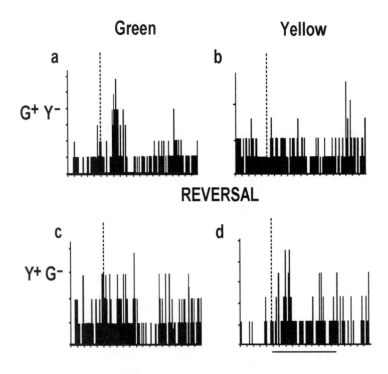

Figure 2–3. A reversal procedure in a visual discrimination task reveals responses for locus coeruleus (LC) neurons of a behaving monkey specific to meaningful stimuli. Target stimuli occur on 10% of trials, and nontarget stimuli on 90% of trials. The animal receives a drop of juice when it responds after a target stimulus. *Upper panels:* Poststimulus time histograms (PSTHs) for response of an LC neuron to green (target), but not yellow (nontarget), stimuli. *Lower panels:* Similar PSTHs for the same LC neuron but after reversal training, so that target stimuli are now yellow and nontarget stimuli are green. Note that green stimuli (*lower left panel*) no longer elicit responses, whereas yellow stimuli (*lower right panel*) now elicit a small response. Thus, the response is selectively elicited by meaningful stimuli. Calibration bar = 1 second. Reprinted from Aston-Jones G, Chiang C, Alexinsky T: "Discharge of Noradrenergic Locus Coeruleus Neurons in Behaving Rats and Monkeys Suggests a Role in Vigilance." *Progress in Brain Research* 85:501–520, 1991a. Copyright 1991, Elsevier Science Publishers. Used with permission.

A VIEW OF LOCUS COERULEUS FUNCTION BASED ON CELLULAR ATTRIBUTES: THE VIGILANCE/RESPONSE INITIATION HYPOTHESIS

We have thus far reviewed some key cellular anatomic and physiological attributes of the LC system, including 1) the efferent projections of LC neurons, 2) the effects of norepinephrine released from LC terminals on target neuron activity, and 3) the conditions under which LC neurons are active and their transmitter is being released. When viewed together, these cellular properties have broad functional implications.

First, the broad efferent trajectory of the LC system implies that it has a global function, with physically distant and functionally disparate brain areas receiving similar input from the LC. This notion is underscored by our physiological studies revealing that LC neurons are markedly homogeneous in their discharge characteristics; for example, LC neurons throughout the nucleus exhibit very similar rates and patterns of spontaneous or sensory-evoked impulse activity (Aston-Jones and Bloom 1981a, 1981b). Thus, our data, in combination with the efferent anatomic results reviewed above, indicate that robust LC discharge results in globally synchronized release of norepinephrine onto target neurons located throughout the neuraxis.

Postsynaptically, norepinephrine influences target cells so as to relatively promote responses to other strong afferent input while reducing spontaneous or low-level activity. Such an enhancement of postsynaptic "signal-to noise" ratios can lead to increased selectivity of target cell discharge to favor specific aspects of target neuron response profiles.

In the context of these previous findings, the specific conditions of LC activation in unanesthetized behaving animals led us to hypothesize a role for the LC system in the control of vigilance and initiation of adaptive behavioral responses (Aston-Jones and Bloom 1981a, 1981b; Aston-Jones et al. 1984). We have proposed that the LC is strongly influenced by two general classes of extrinsic afferents: 1) excitatory inputs mediating sensory-evoked activity in LC neurons, and 2) a more tonically active set of inhibitory afferents serving to modulate overall LC excitability in accordance with the vigilance state. Recent findings concerning major inputs to LC from two rostral medullary nuclei (reviewed below) suggest candidate structures for these theoretical inputs.

The level of LC activity at any time may be a consequence of the relative influence of each of these two classes of inputs. Strong tonic inhibition (such as that found during paradoxical sleep) could serve to prevent LC neurons from responding to environmental stimuli during this state, so that LC inactivity permits paradoxical sleep to occur. Conversely, we propose that intense LC activity interrupts automatic, internally oriented or vegetative behaviors (such as sleep, grooming, or consumption) that are incompatible with phasic, adaptive behavioral responding, and instead engages a mode of activity characterized by a high degree of alertness, vigilance, and interaction with diverse environmental stimuli. This theoretical framework is consistent with our observation that LC activity is most intense just before interruption of low-vigilance behaviors such as sleep, grooming, or consumption, giving rise to alert orienting behaviors.

Intense LC activation may occur when either tonic inhibition of LC neurons (engaged for automatic or vegetative behaviors) has suddenly decreased, or the excitatory input impinging on these cells (in response to an unexpected, imperative sensory event) is sufficiently intense to overcome concurrent tonic inhibitory inputs. Conversely, low-vigilance programs may predominate in behavior when either LC discharge is effectively inhibited from responding to unexpected external stimuli, or the stimulus environment is highly predictable. In this way, the LC may serve as a gate to determine the relative influences of two mutually exclusive sets of behavioral programs. In general terms, the LC may function to influence the overall orientation of behavior or mode of sensorimotor activities, to favor either automatic, vegetative behavioral programs, or phasic adaptive responding to salient environmental stimuli (Aston-Jones 1985; Aston-Jones et al. 1984; Aston-Jones et al. 1991b). Our recent results with monkeys indicate that LC neurons easily become conditioned to respond to even low-intensity stimuli linked to a behavioral imperative to respond. Such activity may underlie some aspects of the stimulus conditioning and sensitization seen in PTSD.

These neurobiological attributes of the LC system suggest cellular substrates for certain symptoms associated with PTSD, including hypervigilance, sensitization to stimuli, increased startle, nervousness, and sleep disturbances. As we will discuss below, this possible role of the noradrenergic LC system in PTSD is consistent with the finding that noradrenergic drugs such as clonidine, propranolol, and desmethylimipramine may be effective in treating this disorder (see Southwick et al., Chapter 15, this volume). However, what is the cause of LC dysfunction? What promotes sympathetic hyperreactivity in PTSD? Insights into these questions may yield new perspectives on this problem and suggest new approaches to therapy. Recent results indicate that a highly integrative nucleus in the ventral rostrolateral medulla may play a pivotal role in controlling both LC and sympathetic activities.

THE NUCLEUS PARAGIGANTOCELLULARIS, A KEY REGULATOR OF LOCUS COERULEUS AND SYMPATHETIC ACTIVITIES

Receptor binding, immunocytochemical, and pharmacological studies indicated that a multitude of transmitter systems impinge on the LC, implying that this nucleus receives inputs from a wide variety of central sites (Foote et al. 1983). This belief was strongly reinforced by the fact that LC projects throughout the neuraxis, and therefore it was felt that this nucleus was likely to be under similarly widespread afferent regulation. This viewpoint was further supported by tract-tracing studies published over a decade ago (Cedarbaum and Aghajanian 1978; Clavier 1979; Morgane and Jacobs 1979) which showed that the LC receives inputs from a wide array of brain areas, including several telencephalic and other forebrain regions.

However, our recent reexamination of LC afferents found that this view of multiple-source projections to LC was unwarranted (Aston-Jones et al. 1986, 1990, 1991b; Chiang et al. 1987; Pieribone and Aston-Jones 1991; Pieribone et al. 1988, 1990). Using discrete injections of sensitive retrograde tract-tracers into the LC proper, we found that only two areas contained numerous heavily labeled neurons: the nucleus paragigantocellularis (PGi) in the ventrolateral rostral medulla, and the medial nucleus prepositus hypoglossi (PrH) and adjacent perifascicular reticular formation in the dorsomedial rostral medulla (Figure 2–4).

Anterograde tracing from these areas confirmed that they provide major inputs to the LC and that other previously reported afferents terminate nearby but outside of the LC nucleus. Details of our anatomic and physiological studies confirming the very restricted afferentation of LC are found elsewhere (Aston-Jones et al. 1986, 1990, 1991b; Pieribone and Aston-Jones 1991) and will not be reviewed here. Also, for the purposes of this chapter, we will focus on the PGi input to LC; details on the PrH input can be found in the publications referenced above.

Excitatory Amino Acid Pathway From the Nucleus Paragigantocellularis to the Locus Coeruleus

Single-pulse stimulation of the PGi activated 78% of LC neurons (Ennis and Aston-Jones 1986, 1988). Cholinergic antagonists had no effect on activation of the LC by the PGi or sciatic nerve stimulation. This finding is consistent with recent observations that the LC proper appears to be nearly devoid of cholinergic fibers (Ruggerio et al. 1990). However, as shown in Figure 2–5, the excitatory amino acid antagonists kynurenic acid or D-glutamyl glycine (DGG) consistently blocked both PGi- and sciatic-induced activation of the LC (Aston-Jones and Ennis 1988; Ennis and Aston-Jones 1988).

Similar results have recently been obtained with local application of kynurenic acid or the non-NMDA antagonist CNQX (Ennis et al. 1992; Shiekhattar and Aston-Jones 1992). These results have now been replicated by several groups (Chen and Engberg 1989; Rasmussen and Aghajanian 1989a; Svensson et al. 1989; Tung et al. 1989). The NMDA antagonists AP5 and AP7 were only modestly effective on either response, indicating that PGi-induced excitatory amino acid activation of LC neurons takes place primarily at a non-NMDA receptor in the LC.

Nucleus Paragigantocellularis Mediation of the Locus Coeruleus Response to Sensory Stimulation

As the major excitatory input to the LC, the PGi is a natural candidate for relaying the multimodal sensory-evoked activation

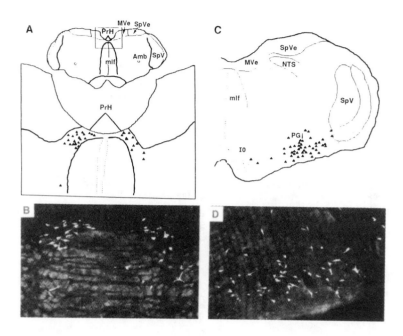

Figure 2–4. Major retrogradely labeled locus coeruleus (LC) afferents, in nucleus prepositus hypoglossi (PrH) (A and B) and the nucleus paragigantocellularis (PGi) (C and D). (A) Video computer–aided plot of retrogradely labeled neurons in a coronal section through the rostral medulla after an injection of the retrograde tracer WGA-HRP into LC. Low- (*upper*) and high-power (*lower*) views of the same section are given for orientation. Amb, nucleus ambiguous; mlf, medial longitudinal fasciculus; MVe, medial vestibular nucleus; SpV, spinal trigeminal nucleus; SpVe, superior vestibular nucleus. (B) High-power, dark-field, polarized-light photomicrograph of retrogradely labeled neurons in PrH. Same orientation as in A. (C) Computer-aided plot of retrogradely labeled neurons in a coronal section through the PGi (slightly caudal to section in A) after an injection of WGA-HRP into LC ipsilaterally. Midline is at left. IO, inferior olive; NTS, nucleus tractus solitarius. Other abbreviations are as in A. (D) High-power, dark-field, polarized-light photomicrograph of retrogradely labeled neurons in the PGi. Same orientation as in C. Reprinted from Aston-Jones G, Ennis M, Pieribone VA, et al: "The Brain Nucleus Locus Coeruleus: Restricted Afferent Control of a Broad Efferent Network." *Science* 234:734–737, 1986. Copyright 1986, American Association for the Advancement of Science. Used with permission.

of LC neurons described above. To test the hypothesis that sciatic-evoked activation of LC is mediated through the PGi, we (Chiang and Aston-Jones 1993) recorded LC neuron activity while stimulating the contralateral footpad subcutaneously (FS) to activate the sciatic nerve, and slowly infused the local anesthetic lidocaine (100–400 nl) into the PGi region. Such lidocaine

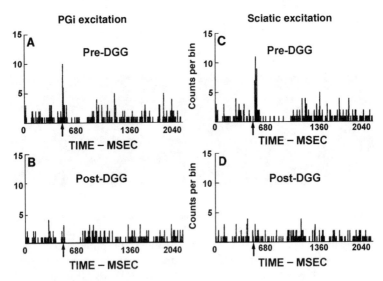

Figure 2–5. Blockade of nucleus paragigantocellularis (PGi)– and sciatic nerve–evoked excitation of LC neurons by the excitatory amino acid antagonist D-glutamyl glycine (DGG). (A) Poststimulus time histogram (PSTH) showing PGi-evoked excitation of an LC neuron. (B) PSTH for the same cell, revealing that excitation shown in A is completely blocked 1.5 min after 0.32 μmol DGG (administered icv). Note purely inhibitory response of this neuron to PGi stimulation is revealed after blockade of excitation by DGG. Stimulation intensity in A and B, 600 μA. Similarly, after this same dose of DGG, footshock (FS)–evoked excitation of this same cell (C, predrug) was simultaneously and completely abolished, (D, 3 min postdrug). Stimulation amplitude in C and D, 40 V. Stimuli (50 in each PSTH) at arrows. Reprinted from Ennis M, Aston-Jones G: "Activation of Locus Coeruleus From Nucleus Paragigantocellularis: A New Excitatory Amino Acid Pathway in Brain." *Journal of Neuroscience* 8:3644–3657, 1988. Used with permission.

infusions consistently blocked responses of LC neurons to sciatic nerve activation. Similar infusions of gamma-aminobutyric acid (GABA) or of a synaptic decoupling solution, 10 mM Cd^{++} plus 20 mM Mn^{++} (to antagonize Ca^{++} effects and prevent transmitter release), produced similar attenuation of footpad responses in LC neurons. These results indicate that the PGi forms a critical synaptic link in this sensory response. It is noteworthy that lesions of the PGi area by others have failed to block sciatic-evoked activation of LC (Rasmussen and Aghajanian 1989a). This result may reflect topographic specificity within the PGi for LC-projecting neurons that mediate responses to sciatic stimulation. Indeed, infusions of lidocaine, GABA, or the Cd^{++}/Mn^{++} solution were all most effective when injected into the ventromedial retrofacial PGi area (Chiang and Aston-Jones 1993). Further experiments are under way to test the hypothesis that other modalities for sensory responses in the LC are also mediated by excitatory amino acid inputs from the PGi.

Interestingly, other experiments indicate that the excitatory amino acid pathway from the PGi to the LC may also mediate LC response to certain systemically administered drugs. Engberg and colleagues found that systemic nicotine potently activates LC neurons via an unknown, indirect influence (Engberg and Svensson 1980; Svensson and Engberg 1980). Recent evidence indicates that nicotine stimulates peripheral sensory (presumably visceral) afferents that in turn activate the excitatory amino acid pathway from the PGi to the LC (Chen and Engberg 1989; Engberg 1989; Hajos and Engberg 1988). One other example of a potent drug effect on LC neurons that has been found to be mediated through the PGi is hyperactivity of LC neurons during withdrawal from morphine. We (Akaoka et al. 1990) and others (Rasmussen and Aghajanian 1989b) have found that the characteristic opiate-withdrawal activation of LC neurons can be blocked by excitatory amino acid antagonists or lesion of the PGi; because similar projections exist from the PGi to the sympathetic region of the spinal cord, a similar pathway may underlie sympathetic hyperactivity associated with opiate withdrawal as well. These results, and the close connection of the PGi to visceral stimuli (via, e.g., vagal inputs to nucleus tractus solitarius [NTS] to PGi), suggest a new pathway for some psychopharmacological effects. Such knowledge of the mechanisms of drug influences on LC neurons is a significant advance, because it opens the way for modulation of these effects, which are thought to be important for the psychological and behavioral impact of many systemically administered drugs. Together, these findings indicate that the PGi may be an integrative "final common pathway" for activating the LC by any of a variety of means.

The Nucleus Paragigantocellularis as Key Brain Region for Control of the Sympathetic Nervous System

The medulla and pons have been recognized as being essential for the regulation of sympathetic activity and the normal maintenance of blood pressure since the work of Dittmar in the 1870s (Dittmar 1873). Following these initial experiments, many studies attempted to localize discrete sites in the reticular formation involved in regulating autonomic processes. During the past decade, a specific group of brain nuclei have come to be seen as important in the central regulation of vascular tone (for review, see Ruggiero et al. 1989).

The PGi in the rostral ventral medulla, first described anatomically for the human brain (Olzewski and Baxter 1954) and later for the rat (Andrezik et al. 1981), is a cardinal component in the mediation of autonomic processes (Barman 1987; Ciriello et al. 1986; Loewy and McKellar 1980; McAllen and Blessing 1987). Specifically, neurons in the PGi project to the intermediolateral cell column of the spinal cord to influence sympathetic preganglionic neurons (Dampney and Moon 1980; Feldman 1986; Guertzenstein and Silver 1974; Ross et al. 1981). Neurons in the lateral aspect of the PGi are involved in 1) the control of resting arterial pressure (Ross et al. 1984), 2) cardiopulmonary reflexes, 3) respiration (Feldman 1986), and 4) parasympathetic function (Bieger and Hopkins 1987; Nosaka et al. 1979). Neurons in the medial aspect of the PGi have also been implicated in blood pressure regulation (Howe et al. 1983; Minson et al. 1987) as well as in antinociception and analgesia (Azami et al. 1982; Punnen et al. 1984; Satoh et al. 1979; Sun and Guyenet 1986).

These considerations indicate that the PGi is an important brain region for preparing the body to respond to urgent stimuli in the environment (defense response, "fight or flight" response), as sympathetic responses to such stimuli are mediated, at least in part, through this area. Because such unexpected or urgent stimuli are also the most reliable stimuli for activating LC neurons in rats or monkeys (described above), this function for the PGi suggests that it may be involved in simultaneously activating LC neurons as well as peripheral sympathetic neurons in response to such stimuli. In fact, there is a remarkable temporal correlation between evoked LC discharge and sympathetic nerve activity (Elam et al. 1981, 1984, 1985, 1986; Reiner 1986). This led us to test whether sensory responses of LC neurons are mediated through the PGi. Indeed, as described above, we found that blockade of the excitatory amino acid pathway from the PGi eliminated responses to sciatic nerve activation (Aston-Jones and Ennis 1988; Ennis and Aston-Jones 1988), as did disruption of synaptic transmission within the PGi (Aston-Jones and Ennis 1988; Aston-Jones et al. 1990; Chiang and Aston-Jones 1993). Thus, it appears that the peripheral sympathetic system is activated in parallel with the central LC system by projections to both areas from the PGi area. As illustrated in Figure 2–6, the PGi appears to be a key area for integration and coordination of activities in the LC and the sympathetic systems.

This analysis of the PGi has led us to extend our hypothesis of LC function, from serving to control vigilance to acting as the cognitive limb of a *global* sympathetic system. Thus, the LC may optimize behavioral state (via heightened attention to environmental stimuli) for making adaptive *decisions* concerning phasic behavioral responses at the same time that the peripheral sympathetic system prepares the animal physically to *execute* phasic responses to urgent stimuli. Because PTSD patients often display symptoms related both to *central* noradrenergic hyperactivity/hyperreactivity (e.g., hypervigilance, sleep disturbances, etc.) as well as peripheral sympathetic hyperactivity (e.g., sweating, tachycardia, hypertension), it seems possible that the overall syndrome may be related to control of the *global* state of "readiness to respond," perhaps by alteration of control mechanisms emanating from the PGi (Figure 2–6). These mechanisms could involve excitatory amino acid pathways, well known to strongly activate both LC and the preganglionic sympathetic neurons in the spinal

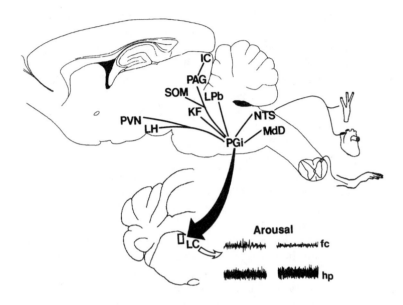

Figure 2–6. Schematic illustration of a sagittal section through rat brain depicting afferents to the retrofacial nucleus paragigantocellularis (PGi). Cardiovascular information is conveyed to neurons in the nucleus tractus solitarius (NTS) via the IXth and Xth cranial nerves. NTS neurons then project to the PGi and form part of the baroreflex circuit. Noxious stimuli, such as sciatic nerve stimulation, are carried through the spinal cord and reach the PGi either monosynaptically or polysynaptically. PGi neurons, in turn, can influence sympathetic preganglionic neurons (cardiovascular) or dorsal horn neurons (analgesia) in the spinal cord via their descending efferents, or influence rostral brain structures via their ascending efferents. In particular, the projection from the PGi to the locus coeruleus (LC) may be responsible for the increased arousal and vigilance that accompanies peripheral sympathetic activity. Activation of LC neurons causes desynchronization in electroencephalographic recordings as seen at the open arrow. Abbreviations: IC, inferior colliculus; PAG, periaqueductal gray; SOM, supraoculomotor nucleus of the central gray; LPb, lateral parabrachial nucleus; KF, Kölliker-Fuse nucleus; MdD, medullary reticular formation; PVN, paraventricular nucleus of the hypothalamus; LH, lateral hypothalamus; fc, frontal cortex; hp, hippocampus.

cord. However, this dysregulation could also involve other neurotransmitters innervating the LC and the preganglionic cells from the PGi, such as epinephrine (see Pieribone and Aston-Jones 1991; Aston-Jones et al. 1990, for details of adrenergic innervation of the LC from the PGi).

Afferents to the Nucleus Paragigantocellularis

If there is dysregulation of the LC and sympathetic systems in PTSD from their common major afferent, the PGi, as the foregoing analysis suggests, it becomes important to understand the circuits and mechanisms involved in regulation of the PGi. As summarized in Figure 2–6, anatomic studies have revealed widespread afferents to the PGi from many diverse brain areas as well as topographic specificity of afferent terminations within the PGi (Van Bockstaele et al. 1989). Retrograde transport studies have revealed that many afferent nuclei with autonomic and integrative properties project to the PGi. In the spinal cord, cervical and lumbosacral segments exhibit the greatest density of retrogradely labeled neurons. Areas containing the greatest number of retrogradely labeled neurons, centrally, include the caudal medullary reticular formation (MdD) just dorsal to the lateral reticular nucleus, the NTS, the lateral parabrachialis, the Kölliker-Fuse nucleus, the periaqueductal gray, and the supraoculomotor nucleus of the central gray. These regions have all been associated with sympathetic and autonomic regulation. Areas with more moderate retrograde labeling include the contralateral PGi, the area postrema, the caudal raphe nuclei, the nucleus gigantocellularis, the medial vestibular nucleus, the accessory nucleus of the VIth and VIIth cranial nerves, the LC, the inferior colliculus, and the region of A5 noradrenergic neurons. Certain areas of the di- and telencephalon contain retrograde labeling following large injections of tracer into the PGi. Such areas include the paraventricular nucleus of the hypothalamus, the lateral hypothalamus, and the infralimbic cortex, structures that have been implicated in limbic-autonomic regulation (Ruggiero et al. 1989). A small number of retrogradely labeled neurons were observed in the insular cortex. Finally, as noted above, neurons in the PGi provide the major input to the nucleus LC (Aston-Jones et al. 1986, 1990,

1991b; Guyenet et al. 1987; Pieribone and Aston-Jones 1991). These LC-projecting neurons are broadly distributed throughout the PGi but with some topographical organization. LC afferent neurons are preferentially medially located in rostral PGi, but also become laterally distributed in caudal PGi.

Certain afferents to the PGi stand out as potentially important in the context of PTSD. In particular, recent studies by LeDoux and colleagues have elucidated much of the brain circuitry important for conditioned emotional responses (CERs), which seem to be similar to the conditioned, aversive emotional states encountered in PTSD. These studies have found that the central nucleus of the amygdala is a critical area for conditioning neutral stimuli to become emotionally significant. Furthermore, projections from the amygdala to the PAG and the lateral hypothalamus are key elements in the expression of CER behavior (LeDoux et al. 1988). These results are intriguing, as both the PAG and the lateral hypothalamus are major inputs to the PGi (as discussed above). Therefore, it seems possible that these pathways not only are involved in generating CER behavior but also may transfer such emotionally important information to the LC through the PGi, perhaps providing a pathway for the conditioned stimulus responding found in primate LC neurons (see subsection on response of LC neurons in monkeys earlier in this chapter). Although the role of the LC in CER behavior is not yet known, these results suggest avenues for future work that could yield insights into the neurobiology of PTSD and other emotional disorders.

CORTICOTROPIN-RELEASING FACTOR AS A MEDIATOR OF PTSD

One neurotransmitter recently identified in the projections from the PGi to the LC is the peptide corticotropin-releasing factor (CRF) (Valentino et al. 1990), an important peripheral and central mediator of stress responses that may be significant in the etiology of PTSD and depression. Recent evidence strongly implicates CRF as a neurotransmitter in the LC during stress (Valentino 1989). Additional evidence suggests that CRF neurotransmission in the LC may be important in depression, which is often associated with PTSD, and in the mechanism of action of antidepressants, which are used in the treatment of PTSD (Curtis and Valentino 1991; Valentino et al. 1990). Moreover, many of the effects of centrally administered CRF mimic many of the symptoms of PTSD, and some of these actions may be mediated by the direct effects of CRF on LC neurons (see below). It is important to determine whether CRF neurotransmission in the LC plays a role in symptoms of PTSD, because this would allow us to predict that CRF antagonists would be useful in treatment. A review of the evidence supporting this link is given in the following subsections.

Corticotropin-Releasing Factor as a Brain Neurotransmitter

Corticotropin-releasing factor was identified and characterized by Vale and colleagues (1981) and is now considered to serve as the primary neurohormone responsible for ACTH release during stress. However, much evidence has accumulated suggesting that CRF has a more global role in the stress response. This expanded role is evidenced by the extrahypothalamic distribution of CRF cells and fibers (Merchenthaler et al. 1982; Olschowka et al. 1982; Sakanaka et al. 1987; Swanson et al. 1983; Valentino et al. 1992) and CRF binding sites (DeSouza 1987; DeSouza et al. 1985), and the finding that central administration of CRF mimics many of the autonomic (Brown et al. 1982; Fisher et al. 1982; Tache et al. 1983) and behavioral (Britton et al. 1982, 1985; Eaves et al. 1985; Kalin 1985; Sutton et al. 1982) aspects of stress even when administered to hypophysectomized rats. These data suggest that CRF functions outside of the hypothalamic-pituitary axis as a neurotransmitter. Consistent with this concept, many autonomic (Brown et al. 1985; Lenz et al. 1988) and behavioral (Kalin et al. 1988; Tazi et al. 1987) aspects of stress are attenuated by pretreatment with a CRF antagonist, alpha-helical CRF_{9-41}. Taken together, these data are consistent with a role for CRF as a neurohormone in hypophyseal circuits to mediate the endocrine branch of the stress response, and as a neurotransmitter in extrahypophyseal circuits to mediate autonomic and behavioral components of stress. Assuming that hypophyseal and extrahypophyseal CRF circuits are equisensitive to stressors, a single stressor would be predicted to initiate coordinated simultaneous release of CRF throughout the brain, resulting in the coordinated multicomponent stress response.

Effects of Corticotropin-Releasing Factor That Mimic PTSD

Many of the effects elicited by central administration of CRF mimic symptoms of PTSD. For example, CRF produces sympathetic activation characterized by increased blood pressure, heart rate, glucose utilization, and oxygen consumption, and these effects are thought to be mediated by extrahypophyseal systems (Brown et al. 1982; Fisher et al. 1982). Likewise, the effects of CRF on the gastrointestinal tract are similar to those observed during stress (i.e., decreased gastric acid secretion and diminished motility) (Lenz et al. 1988; Tache et al. 1983). Consumptive behaviors are inhibited by CRF, and this may be related to the decreased appetite observed in PTSD patients (Morley and Levine 1990). Reproductive behaviors are also decreased by CRF, and such decrease is thought to be due to inhibition of secretion of gonadotropic hormones (Rivier and Vale 1984).

Corticotropin-releasing factor has very potent effects on the EEG, with low doses producing arousal and higher doses resulting in seizure-like activity. Interestingly, these effects on the EEG are very long-lasting and have been related to kindling (Ehlers et al. 1983). Although some of these effects are thought to be mediated within the amygdala, the LC may also be a site of action for CRF-induced effects on arousal. This hypothesis is based on the association of LC discharge with EEG correlates of arousal (as discussed earlier in this chapter) and the finding that CRF increases LC discharge (see below). The effects of CRF in many behavioral paradigms suggest that CRF is anxiogenic. For example, CRF potentiates the CER (Cole and Koob 1988) and the acoustic startle response (Swerdlow et al. 1986). Similarly, CRF acts as if it were an anxiogenic agent in the Gellert-Seifert conflict procedure, enhancing the effects of punishment (Britton et al. 1985). The LC-norepinephrine system may be involved in some of the anxiogenic effects of CRF, because propranolol antagonizes CRF effects on the CER (Cole and Koob 1988). Consistent with this finding, CRF is much more potent in producing certain anxiogenic effects when injected directly into the LC than when injected intracerebroventricularly (Butler et al. 1990).

These findings demonstrate a potential relationship between the effects of CRF and symptoms of PTSD. The administration of the CRF antagonist alpha-helical CRF_{9-41} attenuates some of the sympathetic activation associated with stress (Brown et al. 1985) as well as some of the gastrointestinal effects. Decreases in consumptive behaviors induced by restraint stress can also be ameliorated by administration of a CRF antagonist (Tazi et al. 1987). Finally, certain stress-induced behaviors such as stress-induced aggression are attenuated by prior administration of a CRF antagonist. These results support a role for endogenous CRF in the stress-induced responses that are seen in PTSD. Moreover, they suggest that agents that interfere with CRF may be useful in treating PTSD. Although the site of action for the elicitation of the autonomic and behavioral effects by CRF has not been established, the elucidation of these sites could be critical to the understanding of PTSD.

Corticotropin-Releasing Factor Localization in the Locus Coeruleus

The LC is one region for which substantial evidence implicates CRF as a neurotransmitter, and this site may be a target for CRF in producing PTSD-like symptoms. Several anatomic studies of CRF distribution have demonstrated the existence of CRF-immunoreactive (CRF-ir) fibers in rat LC (Cummings et al. 1983; Sakanaka et al. 1987). Our own studies support those of others and have detailed CRF-ir innervation of the LC region (Valentino et al. 1992). A high density of CRF-ir fibers is visualized just lateral to the anterior pole of the LC and medial to the mesencephalic nucleus of the fifth nerve (Valentino et al. 1992). This area is of interest because the dendrites of LC neurons overlap this region (Fu et al. 1989). Without analysis with electron microscopy it is impossible to determine whether CRF neurons synapse with LC cells or dendrites in this region. Although the electrophysiological studies described below suggest that CRF serves as a neurotransmitter in the LC, it is possible that CRF from pericoerulear regions may act on LC neurons in a neurohormone capacity. Alternatively, CRF may act as a neurotransmitter on other pericoerulear neurons that project to the LC. In addition to rat LC, CRF-ir fibers have been described in monkey (Foote and Cha 1988) and human (Pammer et al. 1990) LC.

The source of CRF innervation of the LC region was recently investigated in double-labeling studies utilizing CRF immuno-histochemistry and retrograde tract-tracing (Valentino et al. 1992). Many CRF-immunoreactive neurons found in the PGi were also labeled with retrograde tract-traces after LC injection (Figure 2–7). In contrast, no double-labeled neurons were localized in the PrH. The results of this study suggest that sources of CRF innervation of the LC region include the nucleus PGi and perhaps pericoerulear CRF neurons.

Effects of Corticotropin-Releasing Factor on Locus Coeruleus Discharge

Prior to the isolation and characterization of CRF, the LC had been implicated in stress response by studies which showed that stressors increase norepinephrine turnover in brain regions having the LC as their sole source of norepinephrine (Cassens et al. 1980; Korf et al. 1973). Taken together with recent studies demonstrating that the LC spontaneous discharge rate is increased by certain stressors (Abercrombie and Jacobs 1987a, 1987b; Elam et al. 1981, 1984; Morilak et al. 1987a, 1987b, 1987c; Svensson 1987; Svensson and Thorén 1979), these findings indicate that stressors activate the LC-norepinephrine system. However, the circuitry and/or neurotransmitters involved in LC activation remain to be elucidated. Because of its role in stress and its localization in fibers in LC, CRF is a potential mediator of LC activation.

The effects of CRF on LC activity have now been characterized in anesthetized and unanesthetized rats. Central CRF administration (icv) increases LC spontaneous discharge rate in a dose-dependent manner (Valentino and Foote 1987, 1988; Valentino et al. 1983) and is more potent and efficacious in unanesthetized vs. halothane-anesthetized rats (Valentino and Foote 1988). Interestingly, in unanesthetized, but not anesthetized, rats, the dose-response curve for CRF activation of the LC determined 40 minutes after injection is shifted to the left of that determined 10 minutes after injection (Valentino and Foote 1988). As mentioned above, this increased effect with time has also been reported for electro-encephalographic effects of CRF, although the mechanisms for these effects are not clear. Direct application of CRF to LC neurons by pressure application also increases the LC spontaneous discharge rate, at least in anesthetized rats, supporting a neurotransmitter role for CRF in the LC (Valentino et al. 1983).

Responsiveness to phasic sensory stimuli is an important characteristic of LC discharge that has been part of the evidence implicating the LC in arousal. Central CRF administration alters LC responses to phasic sensory stimuli in both anesthetized and

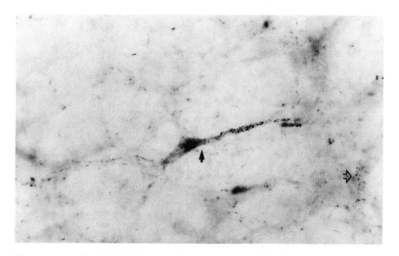

Figure 2–7. Bright-field photomicrograph of a neuron (at closed arrow) in the nucleus paragigantocellularis (PGi) retrogradely labeled from the locus coeruleus (LC) that is immunoreactive for corticotropin-releasing factor. Overall, about 10% of LC-projecting cells in the PGi also contained CRF. The retrograde label, colloidal gold, appears as black granules, and the immunoreactivity is the diffuse staining of the neuron. A non-CRF neuron that is retrogradely labeled from LC is shown at the open arrow. Calibration bar = 25 μm. Reprinted from *Neuroscience,* Vol. 48, Valentino RJ, Page M, Van Bockstaele EJ, et al: "Corticotropin-Releasing Factor–Immunoreactive Cells and Fibers in the Locus Coeruleus Region: Distribution and Sources of Input," pp. 689–705, Copyright 1992, with permission from Pergamon Press Ltd., Headington Hill Hall, Oxford 0X3 0BW, UK.

unanesthetized rats. In anesthetized rats in which repeated sciatic nerve stimulation is used to elicit LC discharge, CRF increases nonstimulated discharge and decreases stimulus-evoked discharge (Valentino and Foote 1987). The net effect is that LC neurons discharge at a greater frequency throughout a trial of stimulus presentations, and discharge is not temporally correlated to a phasic stimulus. When CRF is administered to unanesthetized rats that are presented with repeated auditory stimuli (20-millisecond tones), nonstimulated LC discharge increases to a much greater degree than does evoked discharge (Valentino and Foote 1988). The net effect is similar to that observed in anesthetized rats—that is, LC discharge is greater throughout a trial of sensory stimulation and shows less temporal correlation to the sensory stimulus.

The effect of CRF on LC sensory responses is difficult to interpret because the pattern of LC discharge to phasic sensory stimuli has yet to be translated to norepinephrine release in targets, to effects on target cell discharge, or to any function. Presumably, the burst of LC discharge that is elicited by a sensory stimulus would cause a pulse of norepinephrine release in targets, the end result of which may be to enhance information processing about the sensory stimulus. The production by CRF of a more general increase in the LC discharge rate that is not specifically correlated to a phasic sensory stimulus would be predicted to result in a more persistent release of norepinephrine and a general tuning of all targets toward receipt of information that is not limited to a specific sensory stimulus. These effects may be adaptive in stress because it may be more important to respond to the stressor (which is usually a more tonic stimulus) and to be less responsive to more phasic stimuli that may be less important. However, persistent release of norepinephrine may also sensitize targets to many irrelevant sensory stimuli, and such sensitization may be involved in the enhanced startle or enhanced responses to stimuli seen in PTSD.

Stress Effects on Locus Coeruleus Activity

The effects of various physiological and environmental stressors on LC discharge have been well studied in unanesthetized cats

(Abercrombie and Jacobs 1987a, 1987b; Morilak et al. 1987a, 1987b, 1987c). Most of the challenges presented increased the LC spontaneous discharge rate as well as autonomic activity, indicating that stress-induced LC activation is accompanied by autonomic activation. This process has not been as thoroughly studied in the rat. However, hypercarbia, hypovolemia, hypotension, and bladder distension all increase LC discharge rates of halothane-anesthetized rats (Elam et al. 1981, 1984; Svensson 1987; Svensson and Thorén 1979), which is consistent with the findings of increased norepinephrine turnover in LC target areas during stress.

Because of its localization and its effects on LC discharge, CRF is one likely mediator of stress-induced LC activation. In support of this, CRF levels have been demonstrated to increase in the LC region in acutely and chronically stressed rats, although it is not known whether the CRF levels measured reflect increases in processing or changes in CRF release (Butler et al. 1990). Moreover, certain stressors induce tyrosine hydroxylase expression in the LC, and these effects are prevented by the CRF antagonist alpha-helical CRF_{9-41}, suggesting that stressors activate LC by a CRF-dependent mechanism (Melia et al. 1990).

Electrophysiological evidence strongly supports the hypothesis that CRF is a mediator of LC activation by at least one stressor, hemodynamic stress. Hypotension induced by nitroprusside infusion, which has been used as an autonomic stress because it elicits hypophyseal CRF release (Plotsky and Vale 1984; Plotsky et al. 1986), mimics many of the neuronal effects of CRF on LC discharge. For example, nitroprusside increases LC spontaneous discharge by approximately 30%, and the time course of this effect is correlated to the time course of hypotension (Valentino 1989; Valentino and Wehby 1988). The LC sensory response to sciatic nerve stimulation during nitroprusside infusion is disrupted in a manner similar to that observed after CRF injection (i.e., unstimulated discharge is enhanced and evoked discharge is decreased) (Valentino 1989). These changes in LC discharge elicited by nitroprusside are now thought to be mediated by CRF release within the LC, because LC activation is completely prevented by prior icv administration of alpha-helical CRF_{9-41} (Valentino 1989) or by direct application of alpha-helical CRF_{9-41}

(100–150 ng) into the LC (Valentino et al. 1990) (Figure 2–8).

The antagonism by alpha-helical CRF$_{9-41}$ is specific in that the CRF antagonist has no effect on LC responses to sciatic nerve stimulation or LC spontaneous discharge rates (Valentino et al. 1990). In contrast to alpha-helical CRF, prior administration of dexamethasone, which prevents hypophyseal CRF release by hemodynamic stress, does not prevent LC activation by nitroprusside (Valentino 1989). Likewise, intracerebroventricular administration of kynurenic acid in a dose sufficient to block LC activation by sciatic nerve stimulation or PGi stimulation has no effect on LC activation by nitroprusside (Valentino et al. 1990). These results strongly suggest that LC activation by hemodynamic stress and perhaps other stressors is mediated by CRF release within the LC.

The function of LC activation during hemodynamic stress is not clear, particularly because this activation is not dramatic (i.e., approximately 30% increase above baseline discharge rates). It is not known if an increase of this magnitude for even a sustained length of time would result in increased norepinephrine release in LC targets. Microdialysis studies that parallel electrophysiological studies would be needed to determine if such increases in LC discharge rate are translated to norepinephrine release in targets. However, it is likely that such increases are translated, because increases in LC discharge rates of halothane-anesthetized rats that are administered nitroprusside are temporally correlated to changes on the EEG recorded from cortical and hippocampal leads (Valentino et al. 1990). Thus, cortical EEG becomes desynchronized and is characterized by low-amplitude, high-frequency activity characteristic of arousal. Consistent with this, a strong theta rhythm becomes apparent in EEG activity recorded from the hippocampus. The onset of the EEG changes is temporally correlated to the onset of LC activation. These findings suggest that LC activation associated with stress may be important in increasing or maintaining arousal and that CRF is involved in this effect. These findings support the concept that the increased arousal in PTSD may be related to CRF effects on LC discharge.

The finding of CRF-ir fibers in LC, the effects of CRF on LC neurons, and evidence linking stress-induced LC activation with

CRF release in the LC implicate CRF as a neurotransmitter that mediates LC activation by stressors. The anatomic and physiological features of the LC give it the potential to serve as an amplifier for CRF, or provide a way for CRF to simultaneously alter activity of targets whose function varies from autonomic, motor, or behavioral. This may be adaptive when the response to a stimulus requires the coordinated activity of endocrine, autonomic, motor, and behavioral systems. Based upon the effects of LC activation on target cells, LC activation by CRF would be predicted to bias the central nervous system toward focusing on the stressor. In PTSD, LC neurons may be hypersensitive to CRF, or CRF may be hypersecreted as is thought to occur in depression. This would be predicted to result in a pathological persistent activation of the LC-norepinephrine system and exaggerated symptoms of arousal and inappropriate responses to stimuli.

The Link Between Corticotropin-Releasing Factor and the Locus Coeruleus in Depression

The syndrome of major depression accompanies PTSD in a high percentage of patients, and the symptoms of both disorders may respond, at least in part, to antidepressant agents (see Southwick et al., Chapter 15, this volume). Because several lines of data suggest that CRF is hypersecreted in major depression, this peptide may also be hypersecreted in patients with PTSD and depression. Such CRF hypersecretion may be the major cause of the hypothalamic-pituitary abnormalities, such as hypercortisolemia, that characterize depression (see Stokes and Sikes 1987 for review). The findings that pituitary corticotrophs are responsive to inhibition by glucocorticoid administration (Gold et al. 1984), that CRF levels in the CSF of depressed patients are increased (Nemeroff et al. 1984), and that chronic infusion of CRF can mimic the same neuroendocrine profile as that observed in depression (Schulte et al. 1985)—all support the hypothesis that CRF hypersecretion plays an important role in depression. It is not clear whether CRF hypersecretion in depression is limited to the hypophyseal portal system or is a general feature of all CRF neurons. CRF hypersecretion in the LC would be predicted to result in profound changes in LC physiology and consequent

Figure 2–8. *(at right)* Nitroprusside-elicited locus coeruleus (LC) activation is blocked by local LC injection of alpha-helical CRF_{9-41}. The abscissa indicates the time (minutes) before and after intravenous infusion of nitroprusside, which occurred from 0 to 15 minutes, as shown by the line. The ordinate indicates LC discharge rate as a percentage of the mean discharge rate determined over 9 minutes prior to nitroprusside infusion. Each point is the mean of seven cells in which 150 nl of saline was injected into the LC (*solid circles*) and 6 to 11 cells in which 150 ng alpha-helical CRF_{9-41} (*open squares*) was injected into the LC (6 minutes, $n = 9$; 9–15 minutes, $n = 6$). The 18-minute time point is the mean of two cells for saline and six cells for alpha-helical CRF_{9-41}. Vertical lines indicate ± 1 SEM. Variability appears high for the saline group because the increase in LC discharge rate occurred at different times for different cells (usually between 3 and 9 minutes). Because of this variability, the effect of nitroprusside in saline-pretreated rats was not statistically significant as determined by a one-way analysis of variance with repeated measures ($F_{(5,30)} = 1.73$, $P = 0.16$). However, significant increases in LC discharge occurred at the 3-minute ($P < 0.005$) and 6-minute ($P < 0.05$) time points determined by the Student's t test for matched pairs (two-tailed). The decrease in LC discharge rate in rats administered nitroprusside after alpha-helical CRF_{9-41} was statistically significant ($F_{(7,35)} = 10.6$, $P = 0.0001$). There was a statistically significant difference between saline– and alpha-helical CRF_{9-41}–pretreated groups ($F_{(1,11)} = 6.5$, $P < 0.05$). The inset shows the mean maximum increase in LC discharge rate occurring at any time during nitroprusside infusion. Vertical lines indicate ± 1 SEM. Nitroprusside effects were not different between saline-pretreated ($n = 7$) and untreated control rats ($n = 8$). In contrast, the effects of nitro- prusside in rats pretreated with alpha-helical CRF_{9-41} were different compared with untreated rats ($n = 11$, $P < 0.001$) and saline-pretreated rats ($P < 0.05$) (Student's t test for independent samples). The mean LC spontaneous discharge rates prior to nitroprusside infusion for the saline and alpha-helical CRF_{9-41} groups were $2.35 ± 0.5$ and $2.77 ± 0.2$, respectively. $*P < 0.05$; $**P < 0.01$. Modified from Valentino RJ, Page ME, Curtis AL: "Activation of Noradrenergic Locus Coeruleus Neurons by Hemodynamic Stress Is Due to Local Release of Corticotropin Releasing Factor. *Brain Research* 555:25–34, 1991. Copyright 1991, Elsevier Science Publishers. Used with permission.

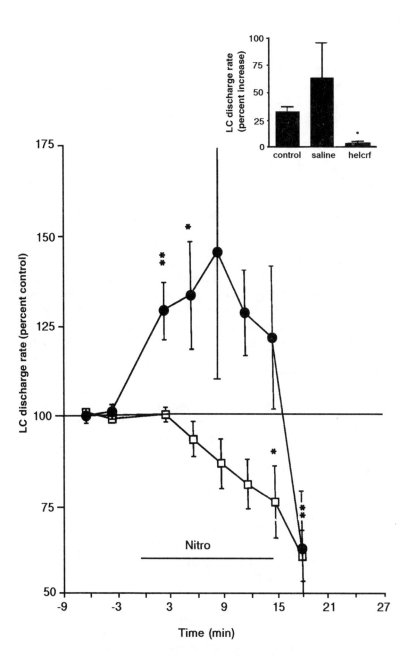

changes in LC targets throughout the brain. For example, persistent exposure of LC cells to CRF should result in higher baseline spontaneous discharge rates and decreased responses to phasic sensory stimuli, assuming that LC cells do not adapt to chronic CRF exposure. This in turn could result in increased arousal and altered responses to discrete stimuli. Interestingly, these are characteristic features of both depression and PTSD.

The hypothesis that CRF hypersecretion in the LC leads to behavioral or physiological changes that characterize depression has not been directly tested. However, a corollary of this hypothesis—that antidepressants act by interfering with CRF in the LC—is being tested. In characterizing and quantifying the acute and chronic effects of antidepressants on LC discharge it was found that some antidepressants attenuate LC activation by stress that is dependent on CRF release in the LC, whereas others alter LC discharge in a manner opposite to CRF and may be able to functionally antagonize hypersecreted CRF (Curtis and Valentino 1991; Valentino et al. 1990). It is not known whether interference with CRF neurotransmission in the LC is a common feature of all antidepressants. Further tests of the hypothesis will reveal whether this is an important mechanism of antidepressant action and whether CRF hypersecretion in the LC contributes to symptoms of depression or PTSD. Thus, the link between CRF and LC may be important in the normal behavioral and physiological response to stressors and also in the pathology underlying depression and PTSD. The response of PTSD patients to antidepressant agents may be related to the ability of these drugs to interfere with CRF neurotransmission in the LC.

CONCLUSIONS

Several features of the noradrenergic LC system suggest that hyperactivity or hyperreactivity of this nucleus may be an important contributor to PTSD:

1. Considerable cellular, physiological, and anatomic data indicate that the LC system may function to regulate vigilance or sensitivity to the general sensory environment.

2. The major afferent to the LC, the PGi in the rostral ventral medulla, is a major sympathoexcitatory brain region. There is potent parallel activation of the LC and the peripheral SNS by this integrative medullary area.
3. Additional evidence indicates that CRF may link the LC to stress and that this system may be an important component in the brain's adaptive responding to stressful stimuli.
4. Evidence suggests that disorders such as depression and drug abuse, which are highly linked to the LC system, commonly coexist with PTSD, and that pharmacotherapy of these symptoms may be acting at the norepinephrine-LC system.

In sum, these findings strengthen the hypothesis that the noradrenergic LC system may be a key area in which dysregulation leads to at least some aspects of PTSD. Further research is called for to explore this possibility more fully. Such additional research, along with the recently acquired knowledge of major afferents controlling the LC (e.g., amino acids and CRF), may give new insights into treatments to help alleviate this disorder.

REFERENCES

Abercrombie ED, Jacobs BL: Single unit response of noradrenergic neurons in locus coeruleus of freely moving cats, I: acutely presented stressful and nonstressful stimuli. J Neurosci 7:2837–2843, 1987a

Abercrombie ED, Jacobs BL: Single unit response of noradrenergic neurons in locus coeruleus of freely moving cats, II: adaptation to chronically presented stressful stimuli. J Neurosci 7:2844–2848, 1987b

Akaoka H, Drolet G, Chiang C, et al: Local, naloxone-precipitated withdrawal in the ventrolateral medulla activates locus coeruleus neurons via an excitatory amino acid pathway. Society for Neuroscience Abstracts 16:1027, 1990

Alexinsky T, Aston-Jones G: Physiological correlates of adaptive behavior in the reversal of a light discrimination task in monkeys. Eur J Pharmacol 3(suppl):149, 1990

Alexinsky T, Aston-Jones G, Rajkowski J, et al: Physiological correlates of adaptive behavior in a visual discrimination task in monkeys. Society for Neuroscience Abstracts 16:164, 1990

Andrezik JA, Chan-Palay V, Palay SL: The nucleus paragigantocellularis lateralis in the rat: comformation and cytology. Anat Embryol (Berl) 161:355–371, 1981

Aston-Jones G: Behavioral functions of locus coeruleus derived from cellular attributes. Physiological Psychology 13:118–126, 1985

Aston-Jones G, Bloom FE: Activity of norepinephrine-containing locus coeruleus neurons in behaving rats anticipates fluctuations in the sleep-waking cycle. J Neurosci 1:876–886, 1981a

Aston-Jones G, Bloom FE: Norepinephrine-containing locus coeruleus neurons in behaving rats exhibit pronounced responses to non-noxious environmental stimuli. J Neurosci 1:887–900, 1981b

Aston-Jones G, Ennis M: Sensory-evoked activation of locus coeruleus may be mediated by a glutamate pathway from the rostral ventrolateral medulla, in Frontiers in Excitatory Amino Acid Research. Edited by Cavalheiro A, Lehmann J, Turski L. New York, AR Liss, 1988, pp 471–478

Aston-Jones G, Foote SL, Bloom FE: Anatomy and physiology of locus coeruleus neurons: functional implications, in Norepinephrine (Frontiers of Clinical Neuroscience). Edited by Ziegler M, Lake CR. Baltimore, MD, Williams & Wilkins, 1984, pp 92–116

Aston-Jones G, Ennis M, Pieribone VA, et al: The brain nucleus locus coeruleus: restricted afferent control of a broad efferent network. Science 234:734–737, 1986

Aston-Jones G, Alexinsky T, Grant S: Activity of locus coeruleus neurons in behaving primates: relationship with vigilance. Society for Neuroscience Abstracts 14:407, 1988

Aston-Jones G, Shipley MT, Ennis M, et al: Restricted afferent control of locus coeruleus neurons revealed by anatomic, physiologic and pharmacologic studies, in The Pharmacology of Noradrenaline in the Central Nervous System. Edited by Marsden CA, Heal DJ. Oxford, UK, Oxford University Press, 1990, pp 187–247

Aston-Jones G, Chiang C, Alexinsky T: Discharge of noradrenergic locus coeruleus neurons in behaving rats and monkeys suggests a role in vigilance. Prog Brain Res 85:501–520, 1991a

Aston-Jones G, Shipley MT, Chouvet G, et al: Afferent regulation of locus coeruleus neurons: anatomy, physiology and pharmacology. Prog Brain Res 85:47–75, 1991b

Azami J, Llewelyn MB, Roberts MHT: The contribution of nucleus reticularis paragigantocellularis and nucleus raphe magnus to the analgesia produced by systemically administered morphine, investigated with the microinjection technique. Pain 12:229–246, 1982

Barman SM: Electrophysiological analysis of the ventrolateral medullospinal sympathoexcitatory pathway, in Organization of the Autonomic Nervous System: Central and Peripheral Mechanisms. Edited by Ciriello J, Calaresu FR, Renaud LP, et al. New York, AR Liss, 1987, pp 239–249

Beaudet A, Descarries L: The monoamine innervation of rat cerebral cortex: synaptic and nonsynaptic axons terminals. Neuroscience 3:851–860, 1978

Bieger D, Hopkins DA: Viscerotopic representation of the upper alimentary tract in the medulla oblongata in the rat: the nucleus ambiguus. J Comp Neurol 262:546–562, 1987

Britton D, Koob G, Rivier J, et al: Intraventricular corticotropin-releasing factor enhances behavioral effects of novelty. Life Sci 31:363–367, 1982

Britton K, Morgan J, Rivier J, et al: Chlordiazepoxide attenuates CRF-induced response suppression in the conflict test. Psychopharmacology (Berlin) 86:170–174, 1985

Brown M, Fisher L, Speiss J, et al: Corticotropin-releasing factor (CRF): actions on the sympathetic nervous system and metabolism. Endocrinology 111:928–931, 1982

Brown MR, Fisher LA, Webb V, et al: Corticotropin-releasing factor: a physiologic regulator of adrenal epinephrine secretion. Brain Res 328:355–357, 1985

Butler P, Weiss J, Stout J, et al: Corticotropin-releasing factor produces fear-enhancing and behavioral activating effects following infusion into the LC. J Neurosci 10:176–183, 1990

Cassens G, Roffman G, Kuruc A, et al: Alterations in brain norepinephrine metabolism induced by environmental stimuli previously paired with inescapable shock. Science 209:1138–1139, 1980

Cedarbaum JM, Aghajanian GK: Afferent projections to the rat locus coeruleus as determined by a retrograde tracing technique. J Comp Neurol 178:1–16, 1978

Chen Z, Engberg G: The rat nucleus paragigantocellularis as a relay station to mediate peripherally induced central effects of nicotine. Neurosci Lett 101:67–71, 1989

Chiang C, Aston-Jones G: Response of locus coeruleus neurons to footshock stimulation is mediated by neurons in the rostral ventral medulla. Neuroscience 53:705–715, 1993

Chiang C, Ennis M, Pieribone VA, et al: Effects of prefrontal cortex stimulation on locus coeruleus discharge. Society for Neuroscience Abstracts 13:912, 1987

Ciriello J, Caverson MM, Polosa C: Function of the ventrolateral medulla in the control of the circulation. Brain Res 11:359–391, 1986

Clavier RM: Afferent projections to the self-stimulation regions of the dorsal pons, including the locus coeruleus, in the rat as demonstrated by the horseradish peroxidase technique. Brain Res Bull 4:497–504, 1979

Cole B, Koob G: Propranolol antagonizes the enhanced conditioned fear produced by corticotropin-releasing factor. J Pharmacol Exp Ther 247:902–910, 1988

Cummings E, Elde R, Ells J, et al: Corticotropin-releasing factor immunoreactivity is widely distributed within the central nervous system of the rat: an immunohistochemical study. J Neurosci 3:1355–1368, 1983

Curtis A, Valentino R: Acute and chronic effects of the atypical antidepressant, mianserin on brain noradrenegic neurons. Psychopharmacology (Berlin) 103:330–338, 1991

Dahlström A, Fuxe K: Evidence for the existence of monoamine-containing neurons in the central nervous system, I: demonstration of monoamines in the cell bodies of brain stem neurons. Acta Physiol Scand Suppl 62:5–55, 1964

Dampney RA, Moon EA: Role of ventrolateral medulla in vasomotor response to cerebral ischemia. Am J Physiol 239:H349–H358, 1980

DeSouza E: Corticotropin-releasing factor receptors in the rat central nervous system: characterization and regional distribution. J Neurosci 7:88–100, 1987

DeSouza E, Insel T, Perrin M, et al: Corticotropin-releasing factor receptors are widely distributed within the rat central nervous system: an autoradiographic study. J Neurosci 5:3189–3203, 1985

Dittmar C: Ein neuer Beweis für die Reizbarkeit der centripetalen Endfarsen des Ruckenmarks. Akad Wissenschaft 22:18–45, 1873

Eaves M, Thatcher-Britton K, Rivier J, et al: Effects of corticotropin-releasing factor on locomotor activity in hypophysectomized rats. Peptides 6:923–926, 1985

Edvinsson L, Lindvall M, Nielsen KC, et al: Are brain vessels innervated also by central (non-sympathetic) adrenergic neurons? Brain Res 63:496–499, 1973

Ehlers C, Henricksen S, Wong M, et al: Corticotropin-releasing factor produces increases in brain excitability and convulsive seizures in the rat. Brain Res 278:332–336, 1983

Elam M, Yao T, Thorén P, et al: Hypercapnia and hypoxia: chemoreceptor-mediated control of locus coeruleus neurons and splanchnic, sympathetic nerves. Brain Res 222:373–381, 1981

Elam M, Yao T, Svensson TH, et al: Regulation of locus coeruleus neurons and splanchnic, sympathetic nerves by cardiovascular afferents. Brain Res 290:281–287, 1984

Elam M, Svensson TH, Thorén P: Differentiated cardiovascular afferent regulation of locus coeruleus neurons and sympathetic nerves. Brain Res 358:77–84, 1985

Elam M, Svensson TH, Thorén P: Locus coeruleus neurons and sympathetic nerves: activation by cutaneous sensory afferents. Brain Res 366:254–261, 1986

Engberg G: Nicotine-induced excitation of locus coeruleus neurons is mediated via release of excitatory amino acids. Life Sci 44:1535–1540, 1989

Engberg G, Svensson TH: Pharmacological analysis of a cholinergic receptor mediated regulation of brain norepinephrine neurons. J Neural Transm 49(3):137–150, 1980

Ennis M, Aston-Jones G: A potent excitatory input to the nucleus locus coeruleus from the ventrolateral medulla. Neurosci Lett 71:299–305, 1986

Ennis M, Aston-Jones G: Activation of locus coeruleus from nucleus paragigantocellularis: a new excitatory amino acid pathway in brain. J Neurosci 8:3644–3657, 1988

Ennis M, Aston-Jones G, Shiekhattar R: Activation of locus coeruleus by nucleus paragigantocellularis or noxious sensory stimulation is mediated by intracoerulear excitatory amino acid neurotransmission. Brain Res 598:185–195, 1992

Feldman JL: Neurophysiology of breathing in mammals, in Handbook of Physiology, Section 1: The Nervous System, Volume IV, Intrinsic Regulatory Systems of the Brain. Edited by Bloom FE. Washington, DC, American Physiological Society, 1986, pp 463–524

Fisher L, Rivier J, Rivier C, et al: Corticotropin-releasing factor (CRF): central effects on mean arterial pressure and heart rate in rats. Endocrinology 110:2222–2224, 1982

Foote S, Cha C: Distribution of corticotropin-releasing factor-like immunoreactivity in brainstem of two monkey species (Saimiri sciureus and Macaca facsicularis): an immunohistochemical study. J Comp Neurol 276:239–264, 1988

Foote SL, Freedman R, Oliver AP: Effects of putative neurotransmitters on neuronal activity in monkey auditory cortex. Brain Res 86:229–242, 1975

Foote SL, Aston JG, Bloom FE: Impulse activity of locus coeruleus neurons in awake rats and monkeys is a function of sensory stimulation and arousal. Proc Natl Acad Sci U S A 77:3033–3037, 1980

Foote SL, Bloom FE, Aston-Jones G: Nucleus locus ceruleus: new evidence of anatomical and physiological specificity. Physiol Rev 63:844–914, 1983

Fu L, Shipley MT, Aston-Jones G: Dendrites of rat locus coeruleus are asymmetrically distributed: immunocytochemical LM and EM studies. Society for Neuroscience Abstracts 15:1013, 1989

Gold P, Chrousos G, Kellner C: Overview: psychiatric implications of basic and clinical studies with corticotropin-relealing factor. Am J Psychiatry 141:619–627, 1984

Grant SJ, Aston-Jones G, Redmond DJ: Responses of primate locus coeruleus neurons to simple and complex sensory stimuli. Brain Res Bull 21:401–410, 1988

Guertzenstein PG, Silver A: Fall in blood pressure produced from discrete regions of the ventral surface of the medulla by glycine and lesions. J Physiol (Lond) 242:489–503, 1974

Guyenet PG, Filtz TM, Donaldson SR: Role of excitatory amino acids in rat vagal and sympathetic baroreflexes. Brain Res 407:272–284, 1987

Hajos M, Engberg G: Role of primary sensory neurons in the central effects of nicotine. Psychopharmacology (Berlin) 94:468–470, 1988

Hartman BK: The innervation of cerebral blood vessels by central noradrenergic neurons, in Frontiers in Catecholamine Research. Edited by Usdin E, Snyder SH. New York, Pergamon, 1973, pp 91–96

Hobson J, McCarley R, Wyzinski P: Sleep cycle oscillation: reciprocal discharge by two brainstem groups. Science 189:55–58, 1975

Hoffer BJ, Siggins GR, Oliver AP, et al: Activation of the pathway from locus coeruleus to rat cerebellar Purkinje neurons: pharmacological evidence of noradrenergic central inhibition. J Pharmacol Exp Ther 184:553–569, 1973

Howe PRC, Kuhn DM, Minson JB, et al: Evidence for a bulbospinal serotonergic pressor pathway in the rat brain. Brain Res 270:29–36, 1983

Jouvet M: Biogenic amines and the states of sleep. Science 163:32–41, 1969

Kalin N: Behavioral effects of ovine corticotropin-releasing factor administered to rhesus monkeys. Federation Proceedings 44:249–254, 1985

Kalin N, Sherman J, Takahashi L: Antagonism of endogenous corticotropin-releasing hormone systems attenuates stress-induced freezing behaviors in rats. Brain Res 457:130–135, 1988

Koda LY, Schulman JA, Bloom FE: Ultrastructural identification of noradrenergic terminals in the rat hippocampus: unilateral destruction of the locus coeruleus with 6-hydroxydopamine. Brain Res 145:190–195, 1978

Korf J, Aghajanian G, Roth R: Increased turnover of norepinephrine in the rat cerebral cortex during stress: role of the locus coeruleus. Neuropharmacology 12:933–938, 1973

LeDoux JE, Iwata J, Cichetti P, et al: Different projections of the central amygdaloid nucleus mediate autonomic and behavioral correlates of conditioned fear. J Neurosci 8:2517–2529, 1988

Lenz H, Raedler A, Geten H, et al: Stress-induced gastrointestinal secretory and motor responses in rats are mediated by endogenous corticotropin-releasing factor. Gastroenterology 95:1510–1517, 1988

Loewy AD, McKellar S: The neuroanatomical basis of central cardiovascular control. Federation Proceedings 39:2495–2503, 1980

McAllen RM, Blessing WW: Neurons (presumably A1-cells) projecting from the caudal ventrolateral medulla to the region of the supraoptic nucleus respond to baroreceptor inputs in the rabbit. Neurosci Lett 73:247–252, 1987

McCarley RW, Hobson JA: Neuronal excitability modulation over the sleep cycle: a structural and mathematical model. Science 189:58–60, 1975

Melia K, Nestler E, Haycock J, et al: Regulation of tyrosine hydroxylase (TH) in the locus coreuleus (LC) by corticotropin-releasing factor (CRF): relation to stress and depression. Society for Neuroscience Abstracts 16:444, 1990

Merchenthaler I, Vigh S, Petrusz P, et al: Immunocytochemical localization of corticotropin-releasing factor (CRF) in the rat brain. Am J Anat 165:386–396, 1982

Minson JB, Chalmers JP, Caon AC, et al: Separate areas of rat medulla oblongata with populations of serotonin- and adrenaline-containing neurons alter blood pressure after L-glutamate stimulation. J Auton Nerv Syst 19:39–50, 1987

Morgane PJ, Jacobs MS: Raphe projections to the locus coeruleus in the rat. Brain Res Bull 4:519–534, 1979

Morilak DA, Fornal CA, Jacobs BL: Effects of physiological manipulations on locus coeruleus neuronal activity in freely moving cats, I: thermoregulatory challenge. Brain Res 422:17–23, 1987a

Morilak DA, Fornal CA, Jacobs BL: Effects of physiological manipulations on locus coeruleus neuronal activity in freely moving cats, II: cardiovascular challenge. Brain Res 422:24–31, 1987b

Morilak DA, Fornal CA, Jacobs BL: Effects of physiological manipulations on locus coeruleus neuronal activity in freely moving cats, III: glucoregulatory challenge. Brain Res 422:32–39, 1987c

Morley J, Levine A: Corticotropin-releasing factor and ingestive behaviors, in Basic and Clinical Studies of a Neuropeptide. Edited by DeSouza EB, Nemeroff CB. Boca Raton, FL, CRC Press, 1990, pp 267–274

Morrison JH, Foote SL, O'Connor D, et al: Laminar, tangential and regional organization of the noradrenergic innervation of monkey cortex: dopamine-beta-hydroxylase immunohistochemistry. Brain Res Bull 9:309–319, 1982

Nemeroff C, Widerlov E, Bissette G, et al: Elevated concentrations of CSF corticotropin-releasing factor-like immunoreactivity in depressed patients. Science 226:1342–1344, 1984

Nosaka S, Yamamoto T, Yasunuga K: Localization of vagal cardioinhibitory preganglionic neurons within rat brain stem. J Comp Neurol 186:79–92, 1979

Olschowka JA, Grzanna R, Rice F, et al: Ultrastructural demonstration of noradrenergic synapses in the rat central nervous system by dopamine-beta-hydroxylase immunocytochemistry. J Histochem Cytochem 29:271–280, 1981

Olschowka JA, O'Donohue TL, Mueller GP, et al: The distribution of corticotropin-releasing factor–like immunoreactive neurons in rat brain. Peptides 3:995–1015, 1982

Olzewski J, Baxter D: Cytoarchitecture of the Human Brain Stem. Basel, S Karger, 1954

Pammer C, Gorcs T, Palkovits M: Peptidergic innervation of the locus coeruleus cells in the human brain. Brain Res 515:247–255, 1990

Papadopoulos GC, Parnavelas JG: Distribution and synaptic organization of serotoninergic and noradrenergic axons in the lateral geniculate nucleus of the rat. J Comp Neurol 294:345–355, 1990

Papadopoulos GC, Parnavelas JG, Buijs RM: Light and electron microscopic immunocytochemical analysis of the noradrenaline innervation of the rat visual cortex. J Neurocytol 18:1–10, 1989

Pieribone VA, Aston-Jones G: Adrenergic innervation of the rat nucleus locus coeruleus arises from the C1 and C3 cell groups in the rostral medulla: an anatomic study combining retrograde transport and immunofluorescence. Neuroscience 41:525–542, 1991

Pieribone VA, Aston-Jones G, Bohn MC: Adrenergic and non-adrenergic neurons of the C1 and C3 areas project to locus coeruleus: a fluorescent double labeling study. Neurosci Lett 85:297–303, 1988

Pieribone VA, Shipley MT, Ennis M, et al: Anatomic evidence for GABAergic afferents to the rat locus coeruleus in the dorsal medial medulla: an immunocytochemical and retrograde transport study. Society for Neuroscience Abstracts 16:300, 1990

Plotsky P, Vale W: Hemorrhage-induced secretion of corticotropin-releasing factor–like immunoreactivity into the rat hypophyseal portal circulation and its inhibition by glucocorticoids. Endocrinology 114:164–169, 1984

Plotsky P, Otto S, Sapolsky R: Inhibition of immunoreactive corticotropin-releasing factor secretion into the hypophysical-portal circulation by delayed glucocorticoid feedback. Endocrinology 119:1126–1130, 1986

Punnen S, Willette R, Krieger AJ, et al: Cardiovascular response to injections of enkephalin in the pressor area of the ventrolateral medulla. Neuropharmacology 23:939–946, 1984

Rasmussen K, Aghajanian GK: Failure to block responses of locus coeruleus neurons to somatosensory stimuli by destruction of two major afferent nuclei. Synapse 4:162–164, 1989a

Rasmussen K, Aghajanian GK: Withdrawal-induced activation of locus coeruleus neurons in opiate-dependent rats: attenuation by lesions of the nucleus paragigantocellularis. Brain Res 505:346–350, 1989b

Rasmussen K, Morilak DA, Jacobs BL: Single unit activity of locus coeruleus neurons in the freely moving cat, I: during naturalistic behaviors and in response to simple and complex stimuli. Brain Res 371:324–334, 1986

Reiner PB: Correlational analysis of central noradrenergic neuronal activity and sympathetic tone in behaving cats. Brain Res 378:86–96, 1986

Rivier C, Vale W: Influence of corticotropin-releasing factor on reproductive function in the rat. Endocrinology 114:914–922, 1984

Ross CA, Armstrong DA, Ruggiero DA, et al: Adrenaline neurons in the rostral ventrolateral medulla innervate thoracic spinal cord: a combined immunocytochemical and retrograde transport demonstration. Neurosci Lett 25:257–262, 1981

Ross CA, Ruggiero DA, Park DH, et al: Tonic vasomotor control by the rostral ventrolateral medulla: effect of electrical or chemical stimulation of the area containing C1 adrenaline neurons on arterial pressure, heart rate, and plasma catecholamines and vasopressin. J Neurosci 4:474–494, 1984

Ruggiero DA, Cravo SL, Arango V, et al: Central control of the circulation by the rostral ventrolateral reticular nucleus: anatomical substrates, in Progress in Brain Research. Edited by Ciriello J, Caverson MM, Polosa C. New York, Elsevier, 1989, pp 49–79

Ruggiero DA, Giuliano R, Anwar M, et al: Anatomical substrates of cholinergic-autonomic regulation in the rat. J Comp Neurol 292:1–53, 1990

Sakanaka M, Shibasaki T, Lederis K: Corticotropin releasing factor–like immunoreactivity in the rat brain as revealed by a modified cobalt-glucose oxidase-diaminobenzidine method. J Comp Neurol 260:256–298, 1987

Satoh M, Akaike A, Takagi H: Excitation by morphine and enkephalin of single neurons of nucleus reticularis paragigantocellularis in the rat: a probable mechanism of analgesic action of opiods. Brain Res 169:406–410, 1979

Schulte H, Chrousos G, Gold P, et al: Continuous administration of synthetic ovine corticotropin-releasing factor in man: physiological and pathophysiological implications. J Clin Invest 75:1781–1785, 1985

Segal M, Bloom FE: The action of norepinephrine in the rat hippocampus, I: iontophoretic studies. Brain Res 72:79–97, 1974

Segal M, Bloom FE: The action of norepinephrine in the rat hippocampus, IV: the effects of locus coeruleus stimulation on evoked hippocampal unit activity. Brain Res 107:513–525, 1976

Shiekhattar R, Aston-Jones G: NMDA-receptor–mediated responses of brain noradrenergic neurones are suppressed by in vivo concentrations of extracellular magnesium. Synapse 10:103–109, 1992

Stokes P, Sikes C: Hypothalamic-pituitary-adrenal axis in affective disorders. Psychopharmacology (Berlin) 92:589–607, 1987

Sun M, Guyenet PG: Effect of clonidine and gamma-aminobutyric acid on the discharges of medullo-spinal sympathoexcitatory neurons in the rat. Brain Res 368:1–17, 1986

Sutton R, Koob G, LeMoal M, et al: Corticotropin-releasing factor produces behavioral activation in rats. Nature 297:331–333, 1982

Svensson TH: Peripheral, autonomic regulation of locus coeruleus noradrenergic neurons in brain: putative implications for psychiatry and psychopharmacology. Psychopharmacology (Berlin) 92:1–7, 1987

Svensson TH, Engberg G: Effect of nicotine on single cell activity in the noradrenergic nucleus locus coeruleus. Acta Physiol Scand Suppl 479(31):31–34, 1980

Svensson TH, Thorén P: Brain noradrenergic neurons in the locus coeruleus: inhibition by blood volume through vagal afferents. Brain Res 172:174–178, 1979

Svensson TH, Engberg G, Tung CS, et al: Pacemaker-like firing of noradrenergic locus coeruleus neurons in vivo induced by the excitatory amino acid antagonist kynurenate in the rat. Acta Physiol Scand 135:421–422, 1989

Swanson LW, Connelly MA, Hartman BK: Ultrastructural evidence for central monoaminergic innervation of blood vessels in the paraventricular nucleus of the hypothalamus. Brain Res 136:166–173, 1977

Swanson LW, Sawchenko PE, Rivier J, et al: Organization of ovine corticotropin-releasing factor immunoreactive cells and fibers in the rat brain: an immunohistochemical study. Neuroendocrinology 36:165–186, 1983

Swerdlow N, Geyer M, Vale W, et al: Corticotropin-releasing factor potentiates acoustic startle in rats: blockade by chlordiazepoxide. Psychopharmacology (Berlin) 88:142–152, 1986

Tache Y, Gotto Y, Gunion M, et al: Inhibition of gastric acid secretion in rats by intracerebral injection of corticotropin-releasing factor (CRF). Science 222:935–937, 1983

Tazi A, Dantzer R, LeMoal M, et al: Corticotropin-releasing factor antagonist blocks stress-induced fighting in rats. Regul Pept 18:37–42, 1987

Tung CS, Ugedo L, Grenhoff J, et al: Peripheral induction of burst firing in locus coeruleus neurons by nicotine mediated via excitatory amino acids. Synapse 4:313–318, 1989

Ungestedt U: Sterotaxic mapping of the monoamine pathways in the rat brain. Acta Physiol Scand Suppl 367:1–48, 1971

Vale W, Spiess J, Rivier C, et al: Characterization of 41-residue ovine hypothalamic peptide that stimulates secretion of corticotropin and ß-endorphin. Science 213:1394–1397, 1981

Valentino R: Corticotropin-releasing factor: putative neurotransmitter in the noradrenergic nucleus locus coeruleus. Psychopharmacol Bull 25:306–311, 1989

Valentino RJ, Foote SL: Corticotropin-releasing factor disrupts sensory responses of brain noradrenergic neurons. Neuroendocrinology 45:28–36, 1987

Valentino RJ, Foote SL: Corticotropin-releasing hormone increases tonic but not sensory-evoked activity of noradrenergic locus coeruleus neurons in unanesthetized rats. J Neurosci 8:1016–1025, 1988

Valentino RJ, Wehby RG: Corticotropin-releasing factor: evidence for a neurotransmitter role in the locus coeruleus during hemodynamic stress. Neuroendocrinology 48:674–677, 1988

Valentino RJ, Foote SL, Aston-Jones G: Corticotropin-releasing factor activates noradrenergic neurons of the locus coeruleus. Brain Res 270:363–367, 1983

Valentino RJ, Bockstaele EJV, Aston-Jones G: Corticotropin-releasing factor immunoreactive (CRF-IR) neurons are localized in nuclei which project to the locus coeruleus. Society for Neuroscience Abstracts 16:519, 1990

Valentino RJ, Page ME, Curtis AL: Activation of noradrenergic locus coeruleus neurons by hemodynamic stress is due to local release of corticotropin releasing factor. Brain Res 555:25–34, 1991

Valentino RJ, Page M, Van Bockstaele EJ, et al: Corticotropin-releasing factor–immunoreactive cells and fibers in the locus coeruleus region: distribution and sources of input. Neuroscience 48:689–705, 1992

Van Bockstaele EJ, Pieribone VA, Aston-Jones G: Diverse afferents converge on the nucleus paragigantocellularis in the rat ventrolateral medulla: retrograde and anterograde tracing studies. J Comp Neurol 290:561–584, 1989

Waterhouse BD, Woodward DJ: Interaction of norepinephrine with cerebrocortical activity evoked by stimulation of somatosensory afferent pathways in the rat. Exp Neurol 67:11–34, 1980

Waterhouse BD, Moises HC, Woodward DJ: Noradrenergic modulation of somatosensory cortical neuronal responses to iontophoretically applied putative neurotransmitters. Exp Neurol 69:30–49, 1980

Waterhouse BD, Moises HC, Yeh HH, et al: Comparison of norepinephrine- and benzodiazepine-induced augmentation of Purkinje cell responses to gamma-aminobutyric acid (GABA). J Pharmacol Exp Ther 228:257–267, 1984

Chapter 3

Altered Electrophysiology of the Locus Coeruleus Following Uncontrollable Stress: Relationship to Anxiety and Anxiolytic Action

Peter E. Simson, Ph.D.
Jay M. Weiss, Ph.D.

I n this chapter we describe the effects of exposure to uncontrollable stress in rats on electrophysiological activity of neurons of the brain-stem nucleus locus coeruleus (LC), and then relate these effects to the actions of anxiolytics on electrophysiological activity of LC neurons.

A brief description of early neurochemical studies is presented, showing that exposure of rats to uncontrollable stress 1) produces behavioral symptoms characteristic of depression and anxiety, and 2) results in decreased levels of norepinephrine in the brain-stem nucleus LC. Pharmacological studies are then presented which suggest that the behavioral effects of exposure to uncontrollable stress are mediated by decreased stimulation of alpha$_2$-adrenergic (α_2) receptors in the LC.

Electrophysiological investigations into the effects of decreased pharmacological stimulation of α_2 receptors on LC neuronal activity are then described. These studies provide evidence that α_2 receptors regulate the responsiveness of LC neurons to

Preparation of this manuscript was supported by Public Health Service Grant MH42637 to the authors.

excitatory stimulation by demonstrating that blockade of α_2 receptors augments the responsiveness of LC neurons to excitatory stimulation.

Exposure to uncontrollable stress is next shown in electrophysiological studies to be associated with alterations in neuronal activity of the LC. These alterations are shown to be consistent with decreased stimulation of α_2 receptors in the LC. Specifically, LC neurons exhibit augmented responsiveness to excitatory stimulation following exposure to uncontrollable stress. These electrophysiological studies, in conjunction with the earlier neurochemical studies, support the notion that exposure to uncontrollable stress is associated with a "functional blockade" of α_2 receptors in the LC, resulting in a hyperresponsiveness of LC neurons to excitatory stimuli.

Finally, studies are described which demonstrate that anxiolytics of the benzodiazepine class have effects on LC electrophysiological activity opposite to those produced by exposure to uncontrollable stress. The significance of this finding in relation to an "anxious component" of the effects of exposure to uncontrollable stress is discussed.

NEUROCHEMISTRY OF EXPOSURE TO UNCONTROLLABLE STRESS

Exposing rats to an uncontrollable stressor produces behavioral and vegetative changes that bear remarkable similarity to changes associated with human depression (see Weiss et al. 1982 for review). These behavioral changes include weight loss and decreased intake of food and water, decreased ability to produce active behavior in numerous situations, decreased ability to compete with other animals and loss of normal aggressiveness, decreased grooming and play activity, decreased responding for appetitive rewards, decreased responding for rewarding brain stimulation (see Zacharko, Chapter 5, this volume), deficits in ability to make correct choices in an attentional situation, and decreased sleep behavior marked especially by early morning waking. Additionally, rats exposed to uncontrollable stress display symptoms reminiscent of anxiety (Weiss and Simson 1985;

Weiss et al. 1982, 1985), a condition that is often seen in conjunction with clinical depression (Redmond et al. 1986; Roy et al. 1986; Stavrakaki and Vargo 1986). Throughout this chapter, rats displaying the aforementioned symptoms following some form of exposure to uncontrollable stress will be referred to as *behaviorally depressed.*

One of the earliest and still most prominent hypotheses linking clinical depression to a biochemical disturbance in the brain proposes that depression is associated with altered availability of biogenic amines, most notably norepinephrine, in the central nervous system (CNS) (Bunney and Davis 1965; Schildkraut 1965; Schildkraut and Kety 1967). Consequently, much research has been carried out attempting to determine whether changes in CNS norepinephrine are responsible for behavioral depression produced by uncontrollable shock in experimental animals (i.e., rats). In support of this notion, several neurochemical studies have indicated that such stress-induced depression is correlated with depletion of norepinephrine in the brain, and in particular, with depletion of norepinephrine in the brain-stem nucleus LC. These studies indicate that large depletion of norepinephrine in the LC region accompanies depression of active behavior following exposure to uncontrollable shock, being present when behavioral depression is observed and being absent when it is not observed (Hughes et al. 1984; Lehnert et al. 1984; Weiss et al. 1981).

Behavioral Depression May Be Mediated by a "Functional Blockade" of Alpha$_2$ Receptors in the Locus Coeruleus

In the rat, the LC is a small pontine nucleus located underneath the fourth ventricle. The LC contains the largest cluster of norepinephrine-containing neurons in the CNS and gives rise, through its diffuse projection system, to more than 50% of all norepinephrine-containing nerve terminals in the CNS (Dahlström and Fuxe 1964; Huang et al. 1975; Nygren and Olson 1977). The correlation described above between norepinephrine levels in the LC and behavioral depression raises the intriguing possibility that variations in norepinephrine levels in the LC are causally related to behavioral depression—that is, that decreased norepinephrine levels in the LC *mediate* behavioral depression.

To explain how exposure to uncontrollable stress could decrease norepinephrine levels in the LC, thereby mediating behavioral depression, the following mechanism has been proposed (Weiss et al. 1981, 1982). Under conditions of uncontrollable stress, norepinephrine terminals in the LC region depolarize more frequently, causing more norepinephrine to be released into the synapse than under normal conditions. Eventually, norepinephrine concentrations in the LC region decrease as norepinephrine release and degradation exceed synthesis, presumably because of a "bottleneck" imposed by the rate-limiting step in norepinephrine synthesis, tyrosine hydroxylase (Bliss et al. 1968). Because norepinephrine normally stimulates α_2 receptors in the LC (Cedarbaum and Aghajanian 1977), the result of exposure to uncontrollable stress is decreased stimulation, or a "functional blockade," of α_2 receptors. Thus, such blockade of α_2 receptors in the LC has been proposed as a mediating step in the development of behavioral depression (Weiss et al. 1981, 1982).

Testing the Functional Blockade Hypothesis

If this hypothetical mechanism is correct—that is, that behavioral depression is mediated by decreased stimulation of α_2 receptors in the LC—then one should be able not only to mimic exposure to uncontrollable stress by pharmacologically blocking α_2 receptors in the LC region but also to reverse behavioral depression by stimulating α_2 receptors in the LC. Indeed, studies have shown that 1) pharmacological blockade of α_2 receptors in the LC region produces behavioral depression in unstressed animals (Weiss et al. 1986), and 2) stimulation of α_2 receptors specifically in the LC region after exposure to stressful conditions eliminates behavioral depression (Simson et al. 1986b). Moreover, selective elimination (by pharmacological treatment) of norepinephrine depletion in the LC region after exposure to stressful conditions eliminates behavioral depression (Simson et al. 1986a). Taken as a whole, these experiments support the notion that behavioral depression is mediated by a functional blockade of α_2 receptors in the LC.

ELECTROPHYSIOLOGY OF THE LOCUS COERULEUS

The neurochemical and neuropharmacological studies described above, which link the behavioral effects of exposure to uncontrollable stress with alterations in LC neurochemistry, prompted our laboratory to investigate the effects of uncontrollable stress on LC electrophysiology. Although the ultimate objective of these studies was to describe the relationship between behavioral depression and the electrophysiological activity of LC neurons, we began these series of experiments by investigating the role of α_2 receptors in regulating LC neuronal activity in the normal animal. Specifically, given the pharmacological evidence that a functional blockade of α_2 receptors in the LC mediates behavioral depression, we first examined the consequence of decreased stimulation of LC α_2 receptors, through pharmacological means, on the electrophysiology of LC neurons.

Alpha$_2$ Receptors Regulate Responsiveness of Locus Coeruleus Neurons

Alpha$_2$ receptors are found in high density in the LC and have a strong inhibitory influence on LC firing (Svensson et al. 1975; Young and Kuhar 1980). To explain the role played by α_2 receptors in inhibiting LC firing, Aghajanian and colleagues offered an elegant hypothesis (Aghajanian et al. 1977). This hypothesis was based on the observation that the response of LC neurons to excitatory stimulation consists of a burst of impulses followed by a period of quiescence, or poststimulation inhibition (PSI). Together with anatomic data showing collateral branching of LC axons (Shimizu and Imamoto 1970; Swanson 1976), Aghajanian and his colleagues proposed that the LC is inhibited by transmitter released from LC collaterals onto α_2 receptors, and it is this stimulation of α_2 receptors that produces PSI (Aghajanian et al. 1977). Thus, the LC was thought to fire in a burst and then inhibit its own subsequent firing by releasing its transmitter (i.e., norepinephrine) onto α_2 receptors in the LC. In support of this hypothesis, it was shown that blockade of α_2 receptors in the LC reduced PSI that followed activation of the LC by orthodromic (i.e., in the direction of normal neural impulse propagation [Cedarbaum and Aghajanian 1978]) or antidromic (i.e., in the direction opposite to normal neural impulse propagation [Aghajanian et al. 1977]) stimulation.

Subsequent findings, however, cast doubt on the notion that α_2 receptors are responsible for PSI. Instead, this same group of investigators proposed, based on intracellular in vivo and in vitro LC recordings, that a calcium-dependent change in potassium conductance arising directly from depolarization produces PSI (Aghajanian et al. 1983; Andrade and Aghajanian 1984). In that membrane changes in ion conductance arising directly from depolarization are now thought to be responsible for the quiescent period following bursts of LC activity, the role of α_2 receptors in regulating LC activity became unclear.

Two observations previously made by other investigators suggested to us that α_2 receptors might influence a different aspect of LC activity than had been studied heretofore. The first observation was that the magnitude of the neuronal response of LC neurons to both simple stimuli (e.g., tone, light flash, touch) and complex stimuli (e.g., food, novel objects) varies positively with the vigilance of the animal (Aston-Jones and Bloom 1981b; Foote et al. 1980): the more vigilant the state of the animal, the greater the magnitude of the neuronal response. This finding suggested to us that the *initial* response of LC neurons to stimulation was a particularly important aspect of LC activity. The second observation was that doses of the highly selective α_2-adrenergic antagonist idazoxan required to elevate spontaneous LC activity were much higher than doses of the same drug required to reverse (or block) the inhibitory effects of the α_2 agonist clonidine on spontaneous LC activity (Freedman and Aghajanian 1984). Thus, a low dose of an adrenergic antagonist that appeared to be affecting α_2 receptors so as to block the action of an adrenergic agonist had no effect on spontaneous activity of the LC. This finding suggested that the antagonist could be affecting α_2 receptors in some way that was not apparent from examining spontaneous LC firing. Putting these two observations together suggested to us that one should consider, first, whether α_2 receptors might influence the response of the LC to sensory input rather than just spontaneous firing of the LC, and, second, whether α_2 blocking agents might affect this LC response to stimulation at doses below those required to elevate spontaneous firing of the unstimulated LC. We therefore examined, in a series of experiments, whether α_2 receptors modulate the responsiveness of LC neurons to excitatory stimuli.

Augmentation of Locus Coeruleus
Responsiveness by Blockade of Alpha$_2$ Receptors

In the first of a series of pharmacological investigations into the role of α_2 receptors in regulating LC activity, various doses of the α_2 antagonist idazoxan were administered peripherally to rats and the effects observed on both spontaneous LC firing rates and the responsiveness of LC neurons to an excitatory stimulus (i.e., compression of the hind paw). The results of this study (Simson and Weiss 1987) demonstrated that blockade of α_2 receptors with idazoxan markedly augments the responsiveness of LC neurons to hind paw compression at doses of α_2 antagonist far below those that increase spontaneous activity (Figure 3–1). Because the responsiveness of LC neurons to stimulation was far more sensitive to blockade of α_2 receptors than was spontaneous LC activity, this result suggests that α_2 receptors primarily regulate LC responsiveness. However, this experiment did not rule out the possibility that the observed increase in LC responsiveness was due to an increase in excitatory input to the LC resulting from blockade of α_2 receptors outside the LC, rather than an increase in the excitability of LC neurons.

To test this possibility, we performed an additional experiment in which we infused small quantities of idazoxan directly into the LC. When blockade of α_2 receptors was restricted to the LC region in this way, the responsiveness of LC neurons to stimulation was still markedly augmented at doses of α_2 blocker well below those that increased spontaneous firing rates (Simson and Weiss 1987). Additionally, we have shown that the augmentation of LC responsiveness resulting from α_2 blockade is not restricted to a specific α_2 antagonist or to a specific type of excitatory stimulus. For example, we have demonstrated that another α_2 antagonist, yohimbine, also augments LC responsiveness, and that, following α_2 blockade, LC neurons are hyperresponsive to the excitatory stimulus of injections of nicotine (Simson and Weiss 1987).

The major finding of these initial electrophysiological studies is that blockade of α_2 receptors in the LC markedly elevates the responsiveness of LC neurons to excitatory stimulation at doses far below those required to increase spontaneous LC activity. This finding suggests that α_2 receptors in the LC play a particularly important role in modulating the magnitude of the initial response of LC neurons to stimulation.

LC firing rate (% of baseline)

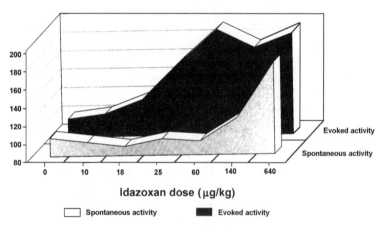

Idazoxan dose (μg/kg)

☐ Spontaneous activity   ■ Evoked activity

Figure 3–1. Pharmacological blockade of alpha$_2$ (α_2) receptors with idazoxan augments sensory-evoked locus coeruleus (LC) activity at doses of idazoxan well below those that increase spontaneous LC firing rates. Spontaneous activity is the ongoing rate of LC firing in anesthetized animals; evoked activity is the rate recorded during 1-second compressions of the paw contralateral to the LC in which recording is being made. The measure presented above is the change in LC rate from what is observed when no drug is given (i.e., "0" dose of idazoxan). Augmented sensory-evoked LC activity was observed with a variety of α_2 antagonists, whether applied systemically or locally (Simson and Weiss 1987). Increased responsiveness of LC neurons following α_2 blockade has also been observed to injections of nicotine (Simson and Weiss 1987), as well as to microiontophoretically applied glutamate (unpublished observations).

Possible Uniqueness of Alpha$_2$ Receptors Among Inhibitory Locus Coeruleus Receptors in Regulating Locus Coeruleus Responsiveness

Locus coeruleus neurons are inhibited by stimulation of a variety of receptor types in addition to α_2 receptors. For example, stimulation of opiate receptors potently depresses the spontaneous activity of LC neurons (Bird and Kuhar 1977; Korf et al. 1974). Additionally, stimulation of GABA$_A$ receptors (Cedarbaum and Aghajanian 1976) and serotonin (5-hydroxytryptamine [5-HT]) receptors (Segal 1979) reduces LC firing rates. Consistent with these electrophysiological findings are autoradiographic and immunocytochemical studies revealing that the LC contains a high density of opiate receptors (Atweh and Kuhar 1977). Furthermore, the LC receives a rich serotonergic innervation (Leger and Descarries 1978), and LC neurons stain positively for glutamic acid decarboxylase (Fuxe et al. 1978).

Because other receptors in the LC besides α_2 receptors inhibit LC activity, the question arose as to whether or not regulation of LC responsiveness is unique to α_2 receptors. Thus, we tested the effects of blockade of opiate, serotonin, and GABA$_A$ receptors on LC responsiveness. The results of this experiment were that the GABA$_A$ antagonists bicuculline and picrotoxin failed to augment the responsiveness of LC neurons to excitatory stimulation throughout a wide range of doses (Simson and Weiss 1989). Similarly, the 5-HT antagonists cyproheptadine, methysergide, and LY 53857 failed to augment the responsiveness of LC neurons to excitatory stimulation throughout a wide range of doses (Simson and Weiss 1989). Finally, administration of the opiate receptor antagonist naloxone also failed to augment the responsiveness of LC neurons to excitatory stimulation throughout a wide range of doses (Simson and Weiss 1989).

These data suggest that α_2 receptors may be unique among inhibitory receptors in regulating the responsiveness of LC neurons to excitatory stimulation independently of spontaneous firing rate. This is evidenced by the fact that blockade of α_2 receptors produces a large increase in LC responsiveness at doses of an α_2 blocker both above and below those necessary to augment spontaneous activity, whereas blockade of a number of other inhibitory receptors—namely GABA$_A$, 5-HT, and opiate receptors—fails to augment LC responsiveness even when blockade of these receptors augments spontaneous activity of LC neurons.

Summary of Electrophysiological Studies in Normal Animals

The electrophysiological results presented thus far suggest that α$_2$ receptors may be uniquely capable, at least among inhibitory receptors in the LC, of modulating the responsiveness of LC neurons to excitational influences. Blockade of α$_2$ receptors, but not blockade of any other inhibitory LC receptor tested to date, augments the responsiveness of LC neurons to stimulation. Further, these results point to the possibility that modulation of LC responsiveness occurs through a type of α$_2$ receptor distinct from that regulating spontaneous activity of LC neurons. The evidence for this is threefold: 1) the magnitude of the response of LC neurons to stimulation is independent of spontaneous firing rate, 2) α$_2$ receptor blockers augment LC responsiveness at doses markedly below those that augment spontaneous activity, and 3) opiate receptor blockade augments spontaneous LC activity without augmenting LC responsiveness, even though opiate receptors share a common second messenger with α$_2$ receptors that affect spontaneous activity (Andrade and Aghajanian 1985).

ELECTROPHYSIOLOGY OF THE LOCUS COERULEUS FOLLOWING UNCONTROLLABLE STRESS

As stated earlier, clinical depression was first linked to a disturbance of noradrenergic activity in the brain more than two decades ago (Bunney and Davis 1965; Schildkraut 1965; Schildkraut and Kety 1967). Since that time, studies of LC activity and function have provided "tantalizing but inconclusive evidence for a causal relationship between disease processes and NE [norepinephrine]–LC function" (Aston-Jones et al. 1984, p. 106). Unfortunately, examining the role of LC cells in depression has not been possible because of the inability to assess the activity of this nucleus in individuals who are depressed. In the experiment to be described, we measured electrophysiological activity of the LC in conjunction with depression in an animal model.

Alteration of Locus Coeruleus Neuronal Activity Following Uncontrollable Stress

It has been proposed that large norepinephrine depletions in the LC give rise to behavioral depression in the following way. Norepinephrine depletions of large magnitude result in decreased norepinephrine release from terminals in the LC, thereby leading to decreased stimulation of adrenergic receptors in this region. The principal adrenergic receptors that respond to norepinephrine release in the LC region are α_2 receptors. Thus, symptoms of depression following uncontrollable stress are thought to result from decreased stimulation, or "functional blockade," of α_2 receptors in the LC region.

Our previous electrophysiological studies indicated that α_2 receptors appear to play an important role in determining the responsiveness of LC cells to excitatory inputs. Consequently, we measured electrophysiological activity of LC neurons to determine whether activity of these cells was altered in animals showing behavioral depression following uncontrollable stress. If decreased active behavior following uncontrollable stress results from decreased stimulation, or "functional blockade," of α_2 receptors in the LC region, then LC neurons in such animals should be disinhibited. In view of recent studies showing the important influence of α_2 receptors on responsiveness of LC neurons, we wished to determine if this disinhibition would particularly appear as increased responsiveness of LC cells to excitatory input as has been found to occur with α_2 blockade.

The results of this experiment (Simson and Weiss 1988) were as follows. First, LC neurons of animals exposed to uncontrollable stress showed a greater response to an excitatory stimulus than did LC neurons of control animals (Figure 3–2). Although exposure to stress had a more pronounced effect on the responsiveness of LC neurons to stimulation, spontaneous LC activity was nevertheless significantly elevated in behaviorally depressed animals. Second, by measuring behavioral depression prior to electrophysiological measurement in some animals, it was possible to correlate behavioral activity with LC electrophysiological activity in these animals. The correlation between the depression of active behavior (measured in a swim test) and the augmentation of LC firing (i.e., increase from spontaneous firing rate) produced by excitatory stimulation (paw compression) was 0.70. Thus, the extent to which the LC cells showed an increased response to an excitatory stimulus during the single-unit recording procedure was highly correlated with the amount of depressed activity that animals showed during a poststress behavioral test given just prior to electrophysiological measurement.

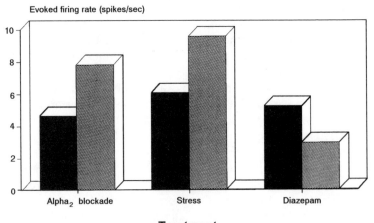

Figure 3–2. Firing rate of locus coeruleus (LC) cells (spikes per second) in response to a sensory stimulus (paw compression) as affected by pharmacological blockade of alpha (α_2) receptors, uncontrollable stress, and peripheral benzodiazapine administration. Similar to what is seen when α_2 receptor antagonists are given (shown above is α_2 blockade by idazoxan at a dose of 25 μg/kg), exposure to uncontrollable stress markedly augments sensory-evoked activity of LC neurons (adapted from Simson and Weiss 1988). In contrast to the effects of α_2 antagonists and exposure to uncontrollable stress, anxiolytics of the benzodiazepine class, including diazepam (shown above at a dose of 0.25 μg/kg), alprazolam, and chlordiazepoxide, potently suppress sensory-evoked LC activity. Adapted from Simson and Weiss 1989.

In addition to differences in spontaneous and evoked LC activity between behaviorally depressed and control animals, aberrations in the pattern of spontaneous activity were observed in some of the behaviorally depressed animals. These proved to be the subjects that displayed the largest amount of behavioral depression. In contrast to the steady LC firing rate typically observed in an anesthetized rat, LC cells in these animals showed cyclical changes in their spontaneous rate of firing. In addition, spontaneous activity of LC cells in these animals was marked by bursts of firing followed by periods of quiescence. This pattern of spontaneous activity in these animals bore remarkable resemblance to the evoked activity (i.e., response to paw compression) of a typical LC neuron.

The elevated responsiveness of LC neurons that was observed in animals showing behavioral depression (Simson and Weiss 1988) was similar to what was seen in normal animals when their α_2 receptors in the LC region were blocked pharmacologically (Figure 3–2) (Simson and Weiss 1987). Clearly, the elevated responsiveness seen in animals exposed to uncontrollable stress is consistent with the hypothesis that behavioral depression following uncontrollable stress is mediated by reduced stimulation of α_2 receptors in the LC. To further test for the possibility of functional blockade of LC α_2 receptors in this model of depression, we examined the consequences of pharmacological blockade of α_2 receptors on LC activity in behaviorally depressed and control (i.e., nonstressed) animals (Simson and Weiss 1988). If α_2 receptors in behaviorally depressed animals are functionally blocked as a result of exposure to the stressful condition, additional pharmacological blockade of α_2 receptors should, in these subjects, have less effect on responsiveness of LC cells than would occur in control animals. Indeed, administration of the α_2 blocker idazoxan was ineffective in augmenting the responsiveness of LC cells in animals exposed to uncontrollable stress, whereas this drug produced the usual significant increase in responsiveness of LC cells in control animals. That pharmacological blockade of α_2 receptors could not elevate responsiveness of the LC in behaviorally depressed animals provides further support for the notion that a functional blockade of α_2 receptors in the LC is present following exposure to an uncontrollable stressor.

Implications of Altered Locus Coeruleus
Electrophysiology Following Uncontrollable Stress

The results of the study just described, showing that electrophysiological activity of LC neurons is increased in animals showing depression of active behavior, are consistent with a number of observations that have been made concerning clinical depression. First, in showing that a lack of normal inhibition of LC neurons occurs in conjunction with depression of active behavior, the results point to increased noradrenergic activity of the dorsal noradrenergic bundle in the brain as a mediator of this behavioral disturbance. Several studies have found evidence of increased noradrenergic activity in depressed individuals (Koslow et al. 1983; Roy et al. 1985). Further, the present results are consistent with the most commonly noted action of antidepressant medication—that is, the downregulation of postsynaptic beta receptors (Frazer and Lucki 1982; Stone 1979; Sulser 1979, 1982; Vetulani et al. 1976)—because downregulation of postsynaptic receptors would counteract the higher-than-normal norepinephrine release resulting from a hyperactive noradrenergic system.

In addition, the present results indicate that subnormal activation of α_2 receptors appears to be importantly involved in producing the increased activity of LC neurons that was observed in animals exposed to uncontrollable stress. Other research has suggested that subnormal activation of α_2 receptors is found in depression (Annseau et al. 1984; Charney et al. 1982; Checkley et al. 1981; Matussek et al. 1980; Siever et al. 1982, 1984). Subnormal activity of α_2 receptors has also been associated with anxiety (Charney et al. 1987), a condition often seen in conjunction with depression (Redmond et al. 1986; Roy et al. 1986; Stavrakaki and Vargo 1986) and also seen in the animal model described in this chapter (Weiss and Simson 1985; Weiss et al. 1982, 1985). Thus, although it seems safe to assume that different forms of depression will involve different physiological mechanisms, some of which may be fundamentally quite different, the present results suggest that abnormalities of the dorsal noradrenergic bundle of the brain accompany some forms of depression and related behavioral disorders.

INDIRECT ATTENUATION OF RESPONSIVENESS OF LOCUS COERULEUS NEURONS BY ANXIOLYTICS

As should now be clear from the aforementioned electrophysiological studies, the bursting response of LC neurons to sensory stimulation appears to be a neural event of considerable significance for behavior. This is evidenced, for example, by the findings that 1) the magnitude of the bursting response of LC neurons to sensory stimulation is correlated with the state of vigilance of the animal (Aston-Jones and Bloom 1981a), and 2) not only is the bursting response of the LC to sensory stimulation augmented following uncontrollable stress, but the degree to which the bursting response of LC neurons increases is correlated with the magnitude of behavioral depression (Simson and Weiss 1988). As described earlier, the magnitude of the bursting response of LC neurons to stimulation is regulated by α_2 receptors (Simson and Weiss 1987), which are found in high density in the LC (Young and Kuhar 1980). Further, evidence has been provided that α_2 receptors are unique, at least among inhibitory receptors in the LC, in regulating the bursting response of LC neurons to stimulation (Simson and Weiss 1989).

Benzodiazepine receptors are also found in the LC (Young and Kuhar 1980), and systemic administration of benzodiazepines has been reported to suppress both the bursting response of LC neurons to sensory stimulation (Rasmussen and Jacobs 1986) and spontaneous LC firing rates (Grant et al. 1980). Indeed, activation of LC neurons in primates has been reported to be anxiogenic (Redmond and Huang 1979). Inhibition of LC spontaneous activity has been proposed as a possible mechanism for the anxiolytic action of benzodiazepines (Grant et al. 1980). However, the above-mentioned pharmacological studies do not make clear whether the decreases in spontaneous LC activity and LC responsiveness following benzodiazepine administration result from stimulation of benzodiazepine receptors in the LC or from stimulation of benzodiazepine receptors at other central, or perhaps even peripheral, sites.

We compared the effects of systemic, intracerebroventricular, and local administration of benzodiazepines on LC activity in an attempt to determine whether benzodiazepine receptors in the LC regulate spontaneous and/or sensory-evoked LC activity. When administered systemically throughout a wide range of behaviorally relevant doses, diazepam, chlordiazepoxide, and alprazolam had similar effects on the electrophysiological activity of LC neurons (Figure 3–2). Although all three benzodiazepines reduced spontaneous LC activity, they attenuated the responsiveness of LC neurons to excitatory stimulation to a far greater extent (Simson and Weiss 1989). To determine whether the decrease in spontaneous LC activity and LC responsiveness observed following systemic administration of benzodiazepines was due to stimulation of benzodiazepine receptors in the LC, we next infused small quantities of benzodiazepines into the LC region. When infused into the LC, diazepam, chlordiazepoxide, and alprazolam had effects on spontaneous firing rates comparable to those observed when these drugs were administered systemically. However, no attenuation of LC responsiveness accompanied this reduction in spontaneous LC firing rates (Simson and Weiss 1989). When the animals infused with diazepam into the LC were subsequently administered diazepam systemically (0.5 mg/kg iv), sensory-evoked LC activity fell to the same rate seen when the drug was administered systemically without prior microinfusion, with no further reduction in spontaneous activity observed.

The fact that infusion of a wide range of doses of benzodiazepines into the LC region failed to attenuate evoked LC activity suggests that benzodiazepines attenuate evoked LC activity either through action at brain sites other than the LC or through action at peripheral sites. To attempt to distinguish between these two possibilities, benzodiazepines were next infused into the ventricular system, as intraventricular administration would stimulate benzodiazepine receptors at brain sites accessible to the ventricular system without affecting peripheral benzodiazepine receptor sites.

Intracerebroventricular administration of chlordiazepoxide and diazepam had effects on LC activity similar to those seen following microinfusion of these drugs into the LC. That is, both drugs significantly depressed spontaneous LC firing rates without affecting evoked LC activity (Simson and Weiss 1989). Following intracerebroventricular administration, no changes in LC responsiveness were observed for as long as recordings from neurons could be maintained (approximately 30 minutes). Yet, when diazepam was subsequently administered systemically, sensory-evoked LC activity was markedly reduced, whereas spontaneous LC activity remained constant.

The results of this experiment suggest that benzodiazepines suppress spontaneous LC firing rates through stimulation of benzodiazepine receptors in the LC, whereas benzodiazepines attenuate sensory-evoked LC activity through stimulation of benzodiazepine receptors that are neither in the LC nor at brain sites accessible to the ventricular system. Thus, benzodiazepine receptors in the LC appear to regulate spontaneous LC activity, but not responsiveness of LC neurons to excitatory stimulation.

These findings (Simson and Weiss 1989) also suggest that the primary effect of systemically administered benzodiazepines on LC firing is on sensory-evoked, rather than spontaneous, LC activity. The evidence for this is twofold. First, systemically administered benzodiazepines decreased the responsiveness of LC neurons to stimulation more than twice as much as they decreased spontaneous LC activity. Second, the attenuation of LC responsiveness occurred at doses of benzodiazepines below those that decreased spontaneous LC activity. Thus, when benzodiazepines are given by the systemic route, their primary effect on LC neurons appears to be an attenuation of evoked LC activity. The present findings extend those of Rasmussen and Jacobs (1986) by indicating that benzodiazepines attenuate the responsiveness of LC neurons to sensory stimulation through stimulation of benzodiazepine receptors that are neither in the LC nor at sites accessible to benzodiazepines introduced into the ventricular system. It is therefore likely that benzodiazepines attenuate sensory-evoked LC activity by stimulating benzodiazepine receptors at peripheral sites, which presumably disrupts sensory input to the LC.

The Locus Coeruleus and Anxiety

Activation of the LC has been suggested to play a role in the production of anxiety (Redmond and Huang 1979). The present

results, demonstrating a profound inhibitory effect of benzodiazepines on sensory-evoked LC activity, are consistent with the
notion that LC neurons are activated in anxiety and that this
activation is particularly characterized by heightened responsiveness of LC neurons to stimulation. Further support for this
view comes from the finding that the magnitude of the response
of LC neurons to sensory stimuli is positively correlated with
increases in vigilance (Foote et al. 1980). Moreover, the anxiogenic drug yohimbine (Charney et al. 1987) augments sensory-
evoked LC activity at doses well below those that augment
spontaneous LC activity (Simson and Weiss 1987). Thus, attenuation of sensory input to LC neurons through stimulation of peripheral benzodiazepine receptors may be a mechanism for at
least some of the anxiolytic action of benzodiazepines.

In this regard, it is of interest that symptoms of anxiety have
been reported to be associated with behavioral depression in the
uncontrollable shock model of depression (Weiss et al. 1982,
1985). The fact that hyperresponsiveness of LC neurons to sensory stimulation also occurs in this model (Simson and Weiss
1988) suggests that augmented LC responsiveness may play a
role in producing an "anxious component" to behavioral depression.

An additional comment can be made about the selective, and
opposite, actions of α_2 antagonists and benzodiazepines on the
responsiveness of LC neurons to stimulation. As has been stated,
α_2 receptors in the LC regulate the responsiveness of LC neurons
to stimulation; that is, when α_2 receptors in the LC are blocked,
the magnitude of the response of LC neurons to stimulation is
markedly augmented (Simson and Weiss 1987). Moreover, drugs
that block α_2 receptors are highly selective for augmenting LC
responsiveness, as opposed to affecting spontaneous LC activity,
up to very high doses (Simson and Weiss 1987). The present
study shows that benzodiazepines have the intriguing capacity
to produce changes in LC activity that are essentially the mirror
image of changes observed following administration of α_2 blockers; that is, when administered systemically, benzodiazepines
potently suppress LC responsiveness while having relatively
minor effects on spontaneous LC activity (Table 3–1). The present
results make clear that although α_2 antagonists and benzodiaze-

pines have relatively selective, opposite effects on the responsiveness of LC neurons to stimulation, these effects apparently derive from influences on receptors in different anatomic locations.

SUMMARY

In this chapter, neurochemical, pharmacological, and behavioral data have been described supporting the notion that behavioral changes following exposure to uncontrollable stress are mediated by decreased stimulation of α_2-adrenergic receptors in the brain-stem nucleus locus coeruleus. This decreased stimulation, or "functional blockade," of α_2 receptors in the LC is particularly characterized by a heightened responsiveness of LC neurons to excitatory stimulation. Moreover, benzodiazepines, when administered by the normal systemic route, potently attenuate LC responsiveness, although this action apparently occurs through effects on receptors outside the LC. Thus, suppression of LC

Table 3–1. Capabilities of various pharmacological agents to alter sensory-evoked activity of locus coeruleus (LC) neurons without concomitant changes in spontaneous LC activity

Drug	Class	Alter evoked activity? (direction of evoked change)
Idazoxan	Alpha₂ antagonist	Yes (increase)
Yohimbine	Alpha₂ antagonist	Yes (increase)
Diazepam	Benzodiazepine agonist	Yes (decrease)
Chlordiazepoxide	Benzodiazepine agonist	Yes (decrease)
Alprazolam	Benzodiazepine agonist	Yes (decrease)
Cyproheptadine	5-HT antagonist	No
Methysergide	5-HT antagonist	No
LY 53857	5-HT antagonist	No
Naloxone	Opiate antagonist	No
Bicuculline	GABA antagonist	No

Note. 5-HT = serotonin (5-hydroxytryptamine); GABA = gamma-aminobutyric acid.

responsiveness may be at least one mechanism by which benzo-diazepines produce anxiolysis. Together, these findings suggest that the symptoms of anxiety and depression observed following exposure to uncontrollable stress may be inextricably linked.

REFERENCES

Aghajanian GK, Cedarbaum JM, Wang RY: Evidence for norepineph-rine-mediated inhibition of locus coeruleus neurons. Brain Res 136:570–577, 1977

Aghajanian GK, Vandermaelen CP, Andrade R: Intracellular studies on the role of calcium in regulating activity and reactivity of locus coeruleus neurons in vivo. Brain Res 273:237–243, 1983

Andrade R, Aghajanian GK: Locus coeruleus activity in vitro: intrinsic regulation by a calcium-dependent potassium conductance but not alpha-2 adrenoreceptors. J Neurosci 4:161–170, 1984

Andrade R, Aghajanian GK: Opiate- and alpha-2-adrenoreceptor-induced hyperpolarizations of locus coeruleus neurons in brain slices: reversal by cyclic adenosine 3′,5′-monophosphate analogues. J Neurosci 5:2159–2164, 1985

Annseau M, Scheyvaert M, Doumont A: Concurrent use of REM latency, dexamethasone suppression, clonidine and apomorphine tests as a biological marker of endogenous depression: a pilot study. Psychiatry Res 12:261–272, 1984

Aston-Jones G, Bloom FE: Activity of norepinephrine-containing locus coeruleus neurons in behaving rats anticipates fluctuations in the sleep-waking cycle. J Neurosci 1:876–886, 1981a

Aston-Jones G, Bloom FE: Norepinephrine-containing locus coeruleus neurons in behaving rats exhibit pronounced responses to non-noxious environmental stimuli. J Neurosci 1:877–900, 1981b

Aston-Jones G, Foote SL, Bloom FE: Anatomy and physiology of locus coeruleus neurons: functional implications, in Norepinephrine (Frontiers of Clinical Neuroscience). Edited by Zeigler M, Lake CR. Baltimore, MD, Williams & Wilkins, 1984, pp 92–116

Atweh SF, Kuhar MJ: Autoradiographic localization of opiate receptors in rat brain, II: the brain stem. Brain Res 129:1–12, 1977

Bird SJ, Kuhar MJ: Iontophoretic application of opiates to the locus coeruleus. Brain Res 122:523–533, 1977

Bliss EL, Ailion J, Zwanziger J: Metabolism of norepinephrine, serotonin and dopamine in rat brain with stress. J Pharmacol Exp Ther 164:122–134, 1968

Bunney WE Jr, Davis JM: Norepinephrine in depressive reactions. Am J Psychiatry 13:483–494, 1965

Cedarbaum JM, Aghajanian GK: Noradrenergic neurons of the locus coeruleus: inhibition by epinephrine and activation by the alpha-antagonist piperoxane. Brain Res 112:413–419, 1976

Cedarbaum JM, Aghajanian GK: Catecholamine receptors on locus coeruleus neurons: pharmacological characterization. Eur J Pharmacol 44:375–385, 1977

Cedarbaum JM, Aghajanian GK: Activation of locus coeruleus neurons by peripheral stimuli: modulation by collateral inhibitory mechanism. Life Sci 23:1383–1392, 1978

Charney DS, Heninger GR, Sternberg DE, et al: Adrenergic receptor sensitivity in depression: effects of clonidine in depressed and healthy patients. Arch Gen Psychiatry 39:290–294, 1982

Charney DS, Woods SW, Goodman WK, et al: Neurobiological mechanisms of panic anxiety: biochemical and behavioral correlates of yohimbine-induced panic attacks. Am J Psychiatry 144:1030–1036, 1987

Checkley SA, Slade AP, Shur E: Growth hormone and other responses to clonidine in patients with endogenous depression. Br J Psychiatry 138:51–55, 1981

Dahlström A, Fuxe K: Evidence for the existence of monoamine-containing neurons in the central nervous system, I: demonstration of monoamines in the cell bodies of brain stem neurons. Acta Physiol Scand Suppl 62:1–55, 1964

Foote SL, Aston-Jones G, Bloom FE: Impulse activity of locus coeruleus neurons in awake rats and monkeys is a function of sensory stimulation and arousal. Proc Natl Acad Sci U S A 77:3033–3037, 1980

Frazer A, Lucki I: Effects of beta-adrenergic and serotonergic receptors, in Typical and Atypical Antidepressants: Molecular Mechanisms. Edited by Costa E, Racagni C. New York, Raven, 1982, pp 69–90

Freedman JE, Aghajanian GK: Idazoxan (RX 781094) selectively antagonizes alpha-2 adrenoreceptors on rat central neurons. Eur J Pharmacol 105:265–272, 1984

Fuxe K, Hokfelt T, Agnati LF, et al: Mapping out central catecholamine neurons: immunohistochemical studies on catecholamine-synthesizing enzymes, in Psychopharmacology: A Generation of Progress. Edited by Lipton MA, DiMascio A, Killam K. New York, Raven, 1978, pp 67–95

Grant SJ, Huang YH, Redmond DE Jr: Benzodiazepines attenuate single unit activity in the locus coeruleus. Life Sci 27:2231–2237, 1980

Huang YH, Redmond DE Jr, Snyder DR, et al: Behavioral effects of stimulation of the nucleus locus coeruleus in the stumptailed monkey (*Macaca arctoides*). Brain Res 100:157–162, 1975

Hughes CW, Kent TA, Campbell J, et al: Cerebral blood flow and cerebrovascular permeability in an inescapable shock (learned helplessness) animal model of depression. Biochem Behav 21:891–894, 1984

Korf J, Bunney BS, Aghajanian GK: Noradrenergic neurons: morphine inhibition of spontaneous activity. Eur J Pharmacol 25:165–169, 1974

Koslow SH, Maas JW, Bowden CL, et al: CSF and urinary amines and metabolites in depression and mania. Arch Gen Psychiatry 40:999–1010, 1983

Leger L, Descarries L: Serotonin nerve terminals in the locus coeruleus of adult rat: a radioautographic study. Brain Res 145:1–13, 1978

Lehnert H, Reinstein DK, Stowbridge BW, et al: Neurochemical and behavioral consequences of acute, uncontrollable stress: effects of dietary tyrosine. Brain Res 303:215–223, 1984

Matussek N, Ackenheil M, Hippius H, et al: Effect of clonidine on growth hormone release in psychiatric patients and controls. Psychiatry Res 2:25–36, 1980

Nygren LG, Olson L: Intracisternal neurotoxins and monoamine neurons innervating the spinal cord: acute and chronic effects on cell and axon counts and nerve terminal densities. Histochemistry 52:281–306, 1977

Rasmussen K, Jacobs BL: Single unit activity of locus coeruleus neurons in the freely moving cat, II: conditioning and pharmacological studies. Brain Res 371:335–344, 1986

Redmond DE Jr, Huang YH: New evidence for a locus coeruleus–norepinephrine connection with anxiety. Life Sci 25:2149–2182, 1979

Redmond DE Jr, Katz MM, Maas JW, et al: Cerebrospinal fluid amines metabolites. Arch Gen Psychiatry 43:938–947, 1986

Roy A, Pickar D, Linnoila M, et al: Plasma norepinephrine level in affective disorders. Arch Gen Psychiatry 42:1181–1185, 1985

Roy A, Jimerson DC, Pickar D: Plasma MHPG in depressive disorders and relationship to the dexamethasone suppression test. Am J Psychiatry 143:846–850, 1986

Schildkraut JJ: The catecholamine hypothesis of affective disorders: a review of supporting evidence. Am J Psychiatry 122:509–522, 1965

Schildkraut JJ, Kety S: Biogenic amines and emotion. Science 156:21–30, 1967

Segal M: Serotonergic innervation of the locus coeruleus from the dorsal raphe and its action on responses to noxious stimuli. J Physiol (Lond) 286:401–415, 1979

Shimizu N, Imamoto K: Fine structure of the locus coeruleus in the rat. Archivum Histologicum Japonicum 31:229–246, 1970

Siever LJ, Uhde TW, Silberman EK, et al: Growth hormone response to clonidine as a probe of noradrenergic receptor responsiveness in affective disorder patients and controls. Psychiatry Res 6:171–183, 1982

Siever LJ, Uhde TW, Jimerson DC, et al: Differential inhibitory noradrenergic responses to clonidine in 25 depressed patients and 25 normal control subjects. Am J Psychiatry 141:733–741, 1984

Simson PE, Weiss JM: Alpha-2 receptor blockade increases responsiveness of locus coeruleus neurons. J Neurosci 7:1732–1740, 1987

Simson PE, Weiss JM: Altered activity of the locus coeruleus in an animal model of depression. Neuropsychopharmacology 1:287–295, 1988

Simson PE, Weiss JM: Peripheral, but not local or intracerebroventricular, administration of benzodiazepines attenuates evoked activity of locus coeruleus neurons. Brain Res 490:236–242, 1989

Simson PE, Weiss JM: Responsiveness of locus coeruleus neurons is regulated by alpha-2 receptors, but not GABA, 5-HT, or opiate receptors. Neuropharmacology 28:651–660, 1989

Simson PG, Weiss JM, Ambrose MJ, et al: Infusion of a monoamine oxidase inhibitor into the locus coeruleus can prevent stress-induced behavioral depression. Biol Psychiatry 21:724–734, 1986a

Simson PG, Weiss JM, Hoffman LJ, et al: Reversal of behavioral depression by infusion of an alpha-2 agonist into the locus coeruleus. Neuropharmacology 25:385–389, 1986b

Stavrakaki C, Vargo B: The relationship of anxiety and depression: a review of the literature. Br J Psychiatry 149:7–16, 1986

Stone EA: Subsensitivity to norepinephrine as a link between adaptation to stress and antidepressant therapy: an hypothesis. Research Communications in Psychology, Psychiatry and Behavior 3:241–255, 1979

Sulser F: New perspectives on the mode of action of antidepressant drugs. Trends Pharmacol Sci 1:92–94, 1979

Sulser F: Antidepressant drug research: its impact on neurobiology and psychobiology, in Typical and Atypical Antidepressants: Molecular Mechanisms. Edited by Costa E, Racagni G. New York, Raven, 1982, pp 1–20

Svensson TH, Bunney BS, Aghajanian GK: Inhibition of both noradrenergic and serotonergic neurons in brain by the alpha-adrenergic agonist clonidine. Brain Res 92:291–306, 1975

Swanson LW: The locus coeruleus: a cytoarchitectonic, Golgi and immunocytochemical study in the albino rat. Brain Res 110:39–56, 1976

Vetulani J, Stawarz RJ, Dingell JV, et al: A possible mechanism of action of antidepressant treatments: reduction in the sensitivity of the noradrenergic cyclic AMP generating system in the rat limbic forebrain. Naunyn-Schmiedeberg's Arch Pharmacol 293:109–114, 1976

Weiss JM, Simson PG: Neurochemical basis of depression. Psychopharmacol Bull 21:447–457, 1985

Weiss JM, Goodman PA, Losito BG, et al: Behavioral depression produced by an uncontrollable stressor: relationship to norepinephrine, dopamine, and serotonin levels in various regions of rat brain. Brain Res Rev 3:167–205, 1981

Weiss JM, Bailey WH, Goodman PA, et al: A model for neurochemical study of depression, in Behavioral Models and the Analysis of Drug Action. Edited by Spiegelstein MY, Levy A. Amsterdam, Elsevier. 1982, pp 195–223

Weiss JM, Simson PG, Ambrose MJ, et al: Neurochemical basis of behavioral depression, in Advances in Behavioral Medicine, Vol 1. Edited by Katkin E, Manuck S. Greenwich, CT, JAI Press, 1985, pp 233–275

Weiss JM, Simson PG, Hoffman LJ, et al: Infusion of adrenergic receptor agonists and antagonists into the locus coeruleus and ventricular system of the brain: effects on swim-motivated and spontaneous motor activity. Neuropharmacology 25:367–389, 1986

Young WS III, Kuhar MJ: Noradrenergic alpha-1 and alpha-2 receptors: light microscopic autoradiographic localization. Proc Natl Acad Sci U S A 77:1696–1700, 1980

Chapter 4

Time-Dependent Change Following Acute Stress: Relevance to the Chronic and Delayed Aspects of PTSD

Seymour M. Antelman, Ph.D.
Rachel Yehuda, Ph.D.

I n recent years, several animal models of stress effects have been proposed as simulating various aspects of the clinical syndrome of posttraumatic stress disorder (PTSD). Some of these models are summarized elsewhere in this volume (see Aston-Jones et al., Chapter 2; Simson and Weiss, Chapter 3; Charney et al., Chapter 6).

In this chapter we describe the phenomenon of time-dependent change (TDC) and explore the potential relevance of this model to PTSD. TDC refers to the fact that a single exposure to a physical or psychological stressor can induce an extremely long-lasting alteration in the behavioral and or physiological responsiveness of the organism to a subsequent stressor, and that this changed responsiveness strengthens with the passage of time following the stressful event. As such, the model of TDC may specifically address aspects of the clinical syndrome of PTSD that are not clearly accounted for in other animal models of stress.

It is now well documented that exposure of humans to a

Support of this work was provided by National Institute on Alcohol Abuse and Alcoholism Grant P50AA08746 (SMA), and National Institute of Mental Health Grants MH24114 (SMA), MH49536-01 (RY), and MH49555-01(RY).

traumatic event can trigger long-term alterations in responsiveness to subsequent stressful situations even when the immediate response to stress may be relatively short-lasting. This point is well illustrated in a study of PTSD among Israeli Defense Forces by Solomon et al. (1987), who note that

> traumatic experiences scar the traumatized individuals, weakening their resilience to future stress. Furthermore, even when individuals seem to have resolved their reaction to trauma, heightened vulnerability that is easily reawakened often ensues. . . . It appears that even when combat-related posttraumatic stress disorder remits or, on the other hand, persists and evolves into a more stable form, the afflicted person may become highly sensitized to stress in general. He is permanently altered, harboring the potential for a future response on reexposure to threatening stimuli. (p. 54)

These remarks quite clearly define the phenomenon of TDC, as will now be described.

BRIEF DESCRIPTION OF TIME-DEPENDENT CHANGE

Time-dependent change describes the observation that a stressful experience induces an alteration of the responsiveness of an animal that develops with the passage of time. The changes that occur as a result of stress exposure appear to be quite permanent and show a progressive intensification: animals who have been stressed in the laboratory will thereafter show markedly different responses to stressors imposed on them even several months later. In other words, the longer the delay between the initial and subsequent stressors, the greater the magnitude of the alteration. Thus, in studies where more than one interval between the inducing and recall stimuli have been measured, it has been shown that the influence of the first stressor strengthens entirely as a function of the increased passage of time since the first stressor (Antelman 1988).

To systematically study the phenomenon of TDC, laboratory animals are typically subjected to an inducing stressor and, at different times thereafter, are challenged with the same or another recall stressor. Physiological and behavioral responsiveness to the second stressor is then measured in animals previously exposed, and compared with those receiving the stressor(s) at different intervals or for the first time. The "inducing" stressor may be very brief and relatively mild, such as insertion of an empty standard gauge syringe needle or an injection of isotonic saline, or it may be prolonged and severe, such as a 48-hour period of food deprivation. The "recall" stressor might also be relatively mild or severe (e.g., injection of a pharmacological agent, or exposure to a shock) and may be administered several hours, days, weeks, or months following the inducing stressor.

One of the most interesting features of the TDC phenomenon is that both low-intensity and high-intensity "stimuli" (i.e., stressors) will cause a time-dependent change in the organism's response to subsequent stress. Not all changes that occur are regarded as those leading to "pathological states." Thus, the model of TDC has the potential of explaining both "adaptive" and "maladaptive" manifestations in response to stress. In TDC, the nature of the change that occurs—that is, sensitization or "immunization" to subsequent stressors—appears to vary depending on the severity of the "inducing" stressor, thereby providing at least one potential insight into the heterogeneity of the stress response. Specifically, as will be discussed below, "lower"-intensity stressors have been associated with a progressive "enhancement" of behavioral changes, whereas "higher"-intensity stressors have been associated with more inhibitory biological and behavioral changes (i.e., decreased biological activity and behaviors). Therefore, the "changes" that occur following an inducing stressor can be more specifically described: time-dependent *sensitization* (TDS) refers to a time-dependent change in which subsequent biobehavioral alterations in response to stress are increased or excitatory, while time-dependent *decrement* (TDD) refers to biobehavioral changes that are decreased or become progressively more inhibitory with the passage of time.

As will be more fully described below, time-dependent effects on behavioral and physiological systems appear to be ubiquitous. Alterations have been found in indices of several different neurotransmitter systems, including dopamine, norepinephrine, serotonin, and gamma-aminobutyric acid (GABA) (Antelman et al. 1980, 1986, 1987, 1988); endocrine systems, including cortico-sterone and ACTH (Antelman et al. 1991a; Caggiula et al. 1989); the immune system (Antelman et al. 1990); the cardiovascular system (Antelman et al. 1989a); and carbohydrate metabolism (Antelman et al. 1991b). Before describing some of the specific biological and behavioral alterations that have been observed, we first outline the clinical aspects of PTSD that seem to be particularly well simulated by this animal model.

PHENOMENOLOGICAL ASPECTS OF PTSD THAT ARE ADDRESSED BY TIME-DEPENDENT CHANGE

In many cases, symptoms of PTSD—particularly intrusive recollections of the inducing event—may be quite chronic in nature and/or may be delayed for periods of months to years after the trauma. Moreover, even symptoms that begin immediately following the trauma may intensify with time. These points are well illustrated in a study by Archibald and Tuddenham (1965) of 62 World War II veterans, 20 years after the end of the war. Although only 6% of the group had appeared at the clinic by 1950, another 60% presented within the next 10 years, and symptom frequency of individual patients increased with time since the combat experience. The phenomenon of TDC may parallel these and other specific aspects of PTSD as follows:

1. The paradigm of TDC demonstrates the presence of *long-lasting* changes following exposure to a stressor and is therefore quite different from many other paradigms of stress that have been proposed as modeling PTSD. In most animal models of stress, the biobehavioral abnormalities return to normal within several hours—or, at the very least, a few days—following the termination of the stressor. In studies of learned helplessness, for example, most data have shown that behavioral and biological alterations are no longer present 3 days following the inescapable shock exposure. The long-lasting changes observed in TDS speak directly to the issue of chronicity in PTSD.

2. In TDC, the biological and behavioral changes following the stressor actually grow more pronounced as time passes. Thus, not only are the changes following the initial stressor long-lasting, but they actually *strengthen* entirely as a function of time. Given the fact that PTSD is often manifest as a chronic or delayed syndrome even after a single traumatic event, any realistic model of this disorder should be able to demonstrate that responses to acute presentation of experimental stressors similarly persist and/or actually grow with the passage of time. It has now been well documented that PTSD can occur months—or even years—after a traumatic event. The paradigm of TDC, therefore, offers an opportunity to explore this particular aspect of PTSD in an animal model of the effects of stress.

3. The biological and behavioral alterations that can be observed in animals undergoing this paradigm occur regardless of the type of actual stress that has been utilized in either the inducing or the recall stress. TDC has been studied in response to both acute and chronic stressors, controllable and uncontrollable stressors, and relatively mild and unusually severe stressors. Unlike most paradigms of stress in the animal literature, in which biological and behavioral changes alter as a function of the type of stressor itself (i.e., inescapable shock vs. escapable shock, uncontrollable vs. controllable stress, acute vs. chronic stress), in TDC what is being studied seems to relate to the very fact of undergoing stress rather than reflect the aftermath of specific stressors. Because PTSD in humans can occur in response to many different traumas, brief or chronic (e.g., rape vs. war, etc.), this model may be relevant to more global aspects of acquiring stress response disorders. Furthermore, because the intensity of stressors utilized influences the direction of change of a particular system, the model of TDC offers an opportunity to explore biological and behavioral differences that may occur in response to degrees of stressor as well as commonalities of the basic stress response.

4. The biological and behavioral effects of TDC can be either excitatory or inhibitory (Antelman et al. 1991b). As mentioned above, it has very recently been found that the behavioral effects of a lower-intensity stressor are progressively en-

hanced, whereas those of a higher-intensity stressor are progressively inhibited with the passage of time. Thus, TDC results in symptoms that show bipolarity and as such may mimic aspects of the "clinical" bipolarity observed in PTSD (i.e., alternating intrusive/reexperiencing vs. avoidance symptoms). Even more importantly, the concept of "bipolarity" can be extended to ultimately explain why some individuals do not show PTSD symptoms following a trauma.

We now provide several illustrations of the phenomenon of TDC in laboratory animals.

PERSISTENT EFFECTS OF EXPOSURE TO STRESS

Earlier Studies Describing This Effect

In one of the initial studies of this phenomenon, the influence of electroconvulsive shock (ECS) on midbrain dopamine autoreceptor sensitivity was examined (Chiodo and Antelman 1980). A single exposure to a very brief ECS (0.7 seconds in duration) was administered to rats. Seven days later, rats were injected with an autoreceptor-specific dose of the dopamine agonist apomorphine. At the dose used, apomorphine normally inhibits the firing of dopamine neurons. However, in animals that had been given the ECS 7 days earlier, the response to apomorphine was markedly attenuated. When apomorphine was administered 1 hour following the brief exposure to ECS, there were no differences in the rate of dopamine firing in stressed versus unstressed animals. Thus, the influence of ECS on apomorphine-induced firing of dopamine neurons became evident only over time. It was not observed immediately following the initial stressor. A similar instance of dopamine-neuronal sensitization occurring with the passage of time was observed when a 4-hour immobilization stress was substituted for the ECS (Antelman 1988). That is, the effects of immobilization stress on apomorphine-induced inhibition of dopamine firing were not demonstrable in animals studied 1 hour following the immobilization, but could be observed in animals studied 1 week or 10 days later.

Time-Dependent Change in Other Biological Systems

The phenomenon of TDS can be observed in many biological systems, not just the dopaminergic system. In one study, a single intraperitoneal insertion of a standard 26-gauge syringe needle prevented diazepam-induced alterations of plasma corticosterone levels following administration of an anxiogenic and convulsant stimulant (i.e., pentylenetetrazole). In the absence of the needle jab, diazepam enhanced pentylenetetrazole-induced increases in plasma corticosterone. The "antagonistic" effect of the needle jab on the action of diazepam on pentylenetetrazole grew significantly with the passage of time (Antelman 1988).

Time-Dependent Changes and Behavioral Responses

Time-dependent changes can be observed in behavioral responses as well as biochemical changes. For example in one study, the effect of food deprivation on electrical self-stimulation of the nucleus accumbens was explored (Antelman and Chiodo 1983). The inducing stressor was a 72-hour period of food deprivation, and the recall stressor was the electrical self-stimulation paradigm. Self-stimulation refers to a paradigm in which animals are placed in a chamber where they may press a bar and receive an electrical current to the brain that they experience as reinforcing. Although self-stimulation is generally thought of as the prototypical reward behavior, it also produces the same hormonal concomitants as recognized stressors, and was therefore used as the recall stressor. Bar-press rates were greatly elevated not only during the period of food deprivation, but even for the remainder of the 23-day experiment, long after the resumption of food intake and recovery of normal body weight. Indeed, the stress-induced enhancement in self-stimulation continued to intensify during this period of time.

Effect of Prior Treatment With Pharmacological Agents on Subsequent Stressors

Prior treatment with pharmacological agents has the same effect on subsequent stressors as do prior nonpharmacological stressors. In one study, the effect of amphetamine on stress-induced eating was examined. A single exposure to amphetamine was able to sensitize stressor-induced eating up to at least 30 days later (Antelman et al. 1980). Similarly, one treatment with the anxiogenic and convulsant stimulant pentylenetetrazole sensitized the hypokinetic influence of the alpha$_2$ agonist clonidine up to at least 2 weeks later (Antelman et al. 1989). It should be noted that, in addition to their pharmacological actions, virtually all drugs are foreign and are therefore stressful substances to the organism that is experiencing them for the first time, or following a hiatus.

Time-Dependent Change and Severity of Stressor

The effect of TDC can occur even if the inducing stressor appears to be quite mild (compared, for example, with electric shock or immobilization stress). We have already described the persistent influence of one jab with an empty syringe needle. In another study, a single injection of isotonic saline 1 month earlier substantially interfered with the ability of diazepam to antagonize pentylenetetrazole-induced increases in dopamine levels in several brain regions (Antelman et al. 1989b). The same results were seen when a 2-hour period of immobilization was substituted for the saline injection (Antelman et al. 1988).

It is important to note that although administering a single jab with an empty syringe needle or one injection of saline might typically be considered low-intensity stressors to a rat, the impact of such stressors on the organism could, in fact, be considerable, depending on the animal's baseline stress level. For example, to a laboratory rat reared under extremely controlled conditions in which background stressors are kept to a minimum, such perturbations might be quite stressful. Indeed, under such circumstances such perturbations can induce significant and substantial elevations in plasma corticosterone. Obviously, in individuals whose background "stress" level is higher, the impact of such perturbations would be considered negligible.

To best maximize the utility of the TDC paradigm, it is prudent to conceptualize "stressors" as events producing a marked difference from the animal's baseline experiences. This may be what is in fact implied in DSM-III-R (American Psychiatric Association 1987) in the definition of trauma as "an event that is outside the range of usual human experiences" (p. 250). An understanding of this point allows for a more critical analysis of the impact of potentially "traumatic" events in animals, and a more sophisticated ability to make comparisons to human trauma.

Intensity of Inducing Stressor and Direction of Change in Biological Systems

The direction of change in a specific biological system may vary depending on the intensity of the inducing stressor. In one recent study (Antelman et al. 1991b), it was found that a single exposure to a "higher intensity" stressor (e.g., 1 hour of immobilization or a high dose of 2-deoxy-D-glucose or ethanol) 2 weeks earlier significantly reduced the ability of haloperidol to induce catalepsy. Injection of haloperidol 2 hours following either immobilization or high-dose ethanol had no effect on catalepsy. Interestingly, one preexposure to a milder stressor (i.e., a jab with an empty syringe needle or "lower intensity" doses of 2-deoxy-D-glucose or ethanol) potentiated, rather than antagonized, the cataleptic effect of haloperidol 2 weeks, but not 2 hours, later. The consistent finding that changes in haloperidol-induced catalepsy depended on the intensity of the inducing stressor demonstrated the "bipolarity" of TDC as a function of the severity of the stressor. This example provides a basis of comparison for the sensitizing impact of acute experimental stressors in animals and PTSD in humans. Just as the intensity of the trauma can influence the severity of later symptoms, so too can the degree of initial stress determine the manifestations of later time-dependent sensitization.

This particular example may provide a striking insight into the factors relevant to sensitization versus immunization to future trauma. It may be that exposure to certain types of stressors elicits strong coping responses that actually "protect" the organism from subsequent stressors. It is intuitive that such stressors would be "higher intensity" stimuli. On the other hand, "lower intensity" stressors may not be provocative enough to initiate such responses and may therefore render organisms more vulnerable to subsequent stress. Interestingly, neonatal animals that receive the stress of chronic handling (which might be considered a high-intensity stress in rats at this age) react to subsequent stress by showing attenuated corticosterone responses. Such formulations can be further tested empirically using the model of TDC and may have considerable relevance for understanding why some individuals develop PTSD in response to a particular traumatic event, while others do not.

CONCLUSIONS

Data have been briefly reviewed suggesting that the persistent sensitizing influence of exposure to stressful stimuli may provide a good animal model of PTSD. Although there are many other examples of the effect of TDC in the animal stress literature, emphasis has been placed on modeling the typically long-term nature of PTSD as well as the fact that symptoms are often delayed and/or intensify with the passage of time. The further use of this paradigm to raise hypotheses concerning biological alterations in PTSD is clearly warranted.

Interestingly, the heuristic value of TDC research for PTSD may have already been demonstrated. Antelman (1988), based on his TDC findings, predicted dopamine impairments in PTSD. It has recently been reported that increased urinary dopamine excretion may be present in individuals with chronic PTSD (Yehuda et al. 1992). Although this volume is devoted to discussing the role of catecholamines in PTSD, it should be noted that stress undoubtedly affects every cell in the body. In this regard, it bears repeating that TDC is demonstrable in noncatecholamine transmitter systems as well as in the immune and cardiovascular systems (Antelman et al. 1990) and in carbohydrate metabolism (Antelman et al. 1989a). Given the ubiquitous effects of stress, animal models such as TDC may afford us the opportunity to characterize further the many systems that stress alters and then to make predictions about what may be occurring in patients with PTSD.

REFERENCES

American Psychiatric Association: Diagnostic and Statistical Manual of Mental Disorders, 3rd Edition, Revised. Washington, DC, American Psychiatric Association, 1987

Antelman SM: Time-dependent sensitization as the cornerstone for a new approach to pharmacotherapy: drugs as foreign/stressful stimuli. Drug Development Research 14:1–30, 1988

Antelman SM, Chiodo LA: Amphetamine as a stressor, in Stimulants: Neurochemical, Behavioral and Clinical Perspectives. Edited by Creese I. New York, Raven, 1983, pp 269–299

Antelman SM, Eichler AJ, Black CA, et al: Interchangeability of stress and amphetamine in sensitization. Science 207:329–331, 1980

Antelman SM, Kocan D, Edwards DJ, et al: Behavioral effects of a single neuropeptic treatment grow with the passage of time. Brain Res 385:58–67, 1986

Antelman SM, Kocan D, Edwards DJ, et al: A single injection of diazepam induces long-lasting sensitization. Psychopharmacol Bull 23:430–434, 1987

Antelman SM, Knopf S, Kocan D, et al: One stressful event blocks multiple actions of diazepam for up to at least a month. Brain Res 445:380–385, 1988

Antelman SM, DeGiovanni LA, Kocan D: A single exposure to cocaine or immobilization stress provides extremely longlasting selective protection against sudden cardiac test from tetracaine. Life Sci 44:201–207, 1989a

Antelman SM, Kocan D, Edwards DJ, et al: Anticonvulsants and other effects of diazepam grow with the time after a single treatment: Pharmacol Biochem Behav 33:31–39, 1989b

Antelman SM, Sunnick JE, Lysle DT, et al: Immobilization 12 days (but not 1 hour earlier) enhanced 2-deoxy-d-glucose-induced immunosuppression: evidence for stressor-induced time-dependent sensitization of the immune system. Prog Neuropsychopharmacol Biol Psychiatry 14:579–590, 1990

Antelman SM, Caggiula AR, Knopf S, et al: Exposing rats to a single brief stressor two weeks earlier modifies the response of plasma ACTH and glucose to ethanol. Neuroscience Abstracts 17:494–496, 1991a

Antelman SM, Caggiula AR, Kocan D, et al: One experience with "lower" or "higher" intensity stressors, respectively, enhances or diminishes responsiveness to haloperidol weeks later: implications for understanding drug variability. Brain Res 566:276–183, 1991b

Archibald HC, Tuddenham RO: Persistent stress reaction after combat: a twenty-year follow up. Arch Gen Psychiatry 12:475–481, 1965

Caggiula AR, Antelman SM, Aul E, et al: Prior stress attenuates the analgesic response but sensitizes the corticosterone and cortical dopamine responses to stress 10 days later. Psychopharmacology (Berlin) 99:233–237, 1989

Chiodo LA, Antelman SM: Electroconvulsive shock: progressive dopamine autoreceptor subsensitivity independent of repeated treatment. Science 210:799–801, 1980

Solomon Z, Garb R, Bleich A, et al: Reactivation of combat-related posttraumatic stress disorder. Am J Psychiatry 144:51–55, 1987

Yehuda R, Southwick SM, Ma X, et al: Urinary catecholamine excretion and severity of PTSD. J Nerv Ment Dis 180:321–325, 1992

Chapter 5

Stressors, the Mesocorticolimbic System, and Anhedonia: Implications for PTSD

Robert M. Zacharko, Ph.D.

S tressful life events in humans have been associated with the induction or exacerbation of a number of disorders, including depression (Akiskal and McKinney 1973; Anisman and Zacharko 1982). Because of certain behavioral similarities between human depression and the response to stressors (particularly uncontrollable stressors) among infrahuman (i.e., animal) subjects (Zacharko and Anisman 1989; see also Simson and Weiss, Chapter 3; Charney et al., Chapter 6, this volume), uncontrollable stressor paradigms have been investigated as potential models of depression. Indeed, some biological changes may be similar in the two conditions (Zacharko and Anisman 1989). However, human depression is a heterogeneous disorder. Even within the universe of patients meeting the criteria for major depression, variability of symptoms, of biological profile, and of

This work was supported by grants from the Department of Graduate Studies and Research, Carleton University (GR-5), the Medical Research Council of Canada (MA8130), the Natural Sciences and Engineering Research Council of Canada (A1087), and the Gustavus and Louis Pfeiffer Research Foundation. I would also like to thank various members of my laboratory, including Glenda MacNeil, Marilyn Kasian, Jerry LaLonde, Bill Gilmore, Rachel Dickson, Cindy Wolfe, Chris Dean, and Kevin Keough, for their efforts. I would also like to extend my appreciation to Dr. Michele Murburg for her invitation to contribute to this very interesting volume.

response to therapeutic agents has been well documented (Janowsky and Risch 1987; Jimerson 1987; Meltzer and Lowy 1987; Rush 1986). Moreover, symptoms of depression often accompany other disorders, and symptoms of other disorders may overlap with those of depression. For instance, attentional disturbance and anhedonia have been noted in patients with posttraumatic stress disorder (PTSD). It is likely that the spectrum of human depression is associated with disturbances in the function of, and interactions between, a number of central nervous system (CNS) pathways.

In animals, the behavioral and biochemical effects of stressors differ depending on a number of variables (Zacharko and Anisman 1989). The possibility has been raised that some animal stressor paradigms may prove to be viable models for human PTSD. Although no one paradigm can provide a parallel for all the symptoms of PTSD, specific paradigms may prove to be useful models for specific symptoms. For example, the description of the startle circuit in animals has clear implications for research into the mechanisms of exaggerated startle response seen in PTSD (see Charney et al., Chapter 6; Rausch et al., Chapter 14, this volume). Similarly, studies of the biological mechanisms of motivation and reward may have relevance to the loss of interest seen in patients with PTSD and depression (Dinan et al. 1990).

The present chapter reviews animal studies that have investigated the effects of stressors on motivational processes as revealed by responding for rewarding brain stimulation (i.e., intracranial self-stimulation [ICSS]). In this paradigm, brain stimulation is delivered to a discrete brain region via a chronically implanted electrode. Animals emit a response to obtain such brain stimulation, and response profiles are plotted with respect to a specific current intensity or a range of current intensities available to the animal. Variations in such an index of reward are employed to assess motivational/reward shifts following experimental manipulation. Although dopamine may contribute to the rewarding effects of ICSS, other known or putative neurotransmitters may also influence reward processes (Wise and Rompre 1989). Similarly, stressor-induced alterations of ICSS may stem from alterations in both dopaminergic and nondopaminergic systems (Zacharko and Anisman 1991b). Genetic differences in ICSS following stressor application may parallel to some extent the interindividual differences in symptoms of mood disorders in humans. The effects of specific antidepressants and neuropeptides in ameliorating the effects of stressors on ICSS are also reviewed here.

STRESSOR EFFECTS ON CENTRAL DOPAMINE TURNOVER

Stressful events influence turnover of central neurotransmitters, including norepinephrine, dopamine, and serotonin (5-hydroxytryptamine [5-HT]). The conditions that result in norepinephrine and 5-HT activation have been evaluated extensively (Abercrombie and Jacobs 1988; Anisman and Zacharko 1982; Glavin 1985; Weiss et al. 1981; see also Aston-Jones et al., Chapter 2; Simson and Weiss, Chapter 3; Charney et al., Chapter 6, this volume) and will not be reiterated. Rather, the present review will focus on dopamine turnover elicited by stressors and the conditions that lend themselves to the expression of such effects.

The effects of stressors on dopamine activation were initially reported for the arcuate nucleus (Kvetnansky et al. 1976) and the lateral septum (Saavedra 1982), and subsequently extended to include the mesocorticolimbic system (Bannon and Roth 1983; Blanc et al. 1980; Thierry et al. 1979). Stressors exert prominent dopamine neuron activation of the anteromedial dopaminergic pathway that arises from the medial tegmental (A10) area. Footshock provokes a significant elevation of the dopamine metabolite 3,4-dihydroxyphenylacetic acid (DOPAC) in both the nucleus accumbens and, especially, the medial prefrontal cortex (mPFC) (Dantzer et al. 1984; Deutch et al. 1985; Fadda et al. 1978; Laveille et al. 1978; Thierry et al. 1979). Nevertheless, Mantz et al. (1989) reported that the unit response of mPFC neurons to a stressor was not uniform: the majority of neurons responded with increased activation, but some neurons were inhibited. Similarly, Deutch et al. (1985) reported that midbrain tegmental (A10) dopamine neurons were also differentially affected by stressors.

It should be emphasized that although stressors increased

DOPAC accumulation in both the mPFC and the nucleus accumbens, the time course of the metabolite changes differed between these sites (Roth et al. 1988). Increased DOPAC accumulation in the mPFC was evident within 10 minutes of immobilization, peaked within 20 minutes, and declined thereafter. In the nucleus accumbens the accumulation of DOPAC first appeared after 30 minutes of immobilization, and metabolite levels remained elevated for the remainder of the 120-minute stressor session. These data suggest that the mPFC and the nucleus accumbens not only are differentially sensitive to stressor exposure but also are subject to differential rates of adaptation. Accordingly, analysis of biological and behavioral effects of stressors should consider not only which brain regions are influenced by the stressor but also the nature and duration of the response to aversive treatment.

The nature and duration of the stressor employed may also be important determinants of biochemical and behavioral outcomes following stressor exposure. A number of reports have indicated that striatal dopamine turnover is relatively insensitive to a number of stressors (Anisman and Zacharko 1986; Bowers et al. 1987). Nevertheless, specific stressors may in fact influence striatal dopamine turnover. For example, a combination of cold exposure and restraint reduced dopamine levels and increased the DOPAC/dopamine ratio in the striatum, the nucleus accumbens, and—most prominently—the mPFC (Dunn and File 1983). A subsequent report indicated that exercise stress significantly elevated striatal levels of dopamine and its metabolites, DOPAC and homovanillic acid (HVA) (Heyes et al. 1988). Thus, a stressor that imposes stringent motoric requirements may affect dopamine turnover in the nigrostriatal system.

Using in vivo microdialysis, Abercrombie et al. (1989) observed that dopamine release was more pronounced in the mPFC than in the nucleus accumbens, in which the level of dopamine release in turn exceeded that in the striatum, during the course of a 30-minute tailshock session. Interestingly, within 15 minutes of stressor termination, a significant increase in extracellular dopamine was evident in the striatum. Although these data are consistent with previously described regional variations in dopamine release associated with a stressor (mPFC > nucleus accumbens > striatum), they also suggest that an aversive experience may, in fact, influence striatal dopamine levels. It remains to be determined, however, whether the alterations of striatal dopamine turnover are related to the stressor per se or are secondary to the motoric behaviors induced by the aversive experience.

The effects of a stressor on dopamine activity within the anteromedial system may be affected by sensitization or conditioning. For example, stressor-induced increase of dopamine turnover within the mPFC and the ventral tegmental area (VTA) was reinduced by cues previously associated with uncontrollable footshock (Deutch et al. 1985; Herman et al. 1982). This effect was not apparent in the nucleus accumbens and several other brain regions (e.g., amygdala, olfactory tubercle). An acute stressor may thus influence brain response to a subsequently applied stimulus, and when analyzing the behavioral effects of environmental insults, one needs to consider not only the immediate effects of the stressor per se but also effects that may be elicited by subsequent stressor-related cues.

Alterations in central norepinephrine functions are more readily induced by uncontrollable than by controllable stressors. Limited data are available, however, regarding the effects of stressor controllability on dopamine turnover. In some cases, controllable and uncontrollable footshock appear to be equally effective in altering dopamine and DOPAC concentrations (Anisman and Zacharko 1986). However, recent investigations have demonstrated that stressor controllability influences dopamine turnover in the mPFC of female but not male rats (Heinsbroek et al. 1990, 1991). The possibility that some aspects of coping may be sex related is interesting and clearly deserves further consideration.

In contrast to the reduction in mesocortical dopamine seen following an acute stressor, altered dopamine concentrations in this region may not be evident following a chronic stressor regimen. While increased norepinephrine levels associated with repeated stressor exposure are due to enhanced norepinephrine synthesis (Irwin et al. 1986a, 1986b), dopamine adaptation is determined, at least in part, by moderation of excessive dopamine utilization. For example, DOPAC accumulation following chronic stressor exposure is less pronounced than after an acute stressor (Anisman and Zacharko 1986; Herman et al. 1982), and a chronic stressor may increase dopamine synthesis (Kramarcy et al. 1984).

It has been suggested that stressor-induced variations in dopamine turnover may be associated with the anxiety or arousal provoked by the stressor rather than by the aversive stimulus per se. Indeed, anxiolytic administration prevents stressor-induced increases in DOPAC accumulation in the mPFC (Fadda et al. 1978; Ida et al. 1989; Laveille et al. 1978), and this effect can be reinstated by benzodiazepine antagonists (Roth et al. 1988). The mechanism through which benzodiazepines attenuate stressor-provoked dopamine turnover in the mesocorticolimbic system remains to be elucidated. However, the use of anxiogenic agents has been useful in simulating the effects of stressors on dopamine turnover in the mesocorticolimbic system. Roth et al. (1988) and Knorr et al. (1989) have demonstrated that methyl-ß-carboline-3-carboxyamide (FG 7142) increased dopamine synthesis and utilization in the mPFC and the VTA but not in the nucleus accumbens or the nigrostriatal system. Benzodiazepines and anxiogenics may exert their effects through a presynaptic (terminal-field) mechanism, although the possibility of direct actions in the VTA is reinforced by the demonstration of benzodiazepine receptors in the VTA of the human brain (Knorr et al. 1989).

STRESSORS AND BEHAVIOR

Uncontrollable stressors provoke a wide array of behavioral changes (Zacharko and Anisman 1991b). It has been suggested that the behavioral deficits associated with stressor exposure may stem from alterations in motivation (Maier and Seligman 1976); however, few paradigms adequately address this issue. In the shuttle escape paradigm, assessment of motivational change may be compromised by motoric disturbances induced by the stressor (Zacharko and Anisman 1984). In appetitive tasks, disturbances in acquiring response-outcome associations may be due to associative or nonassociative learning factors. Furthermore, carrying out studies under conditions of food deprivation in the latter paradigm may introduce a further chronic stressor as a confounding factor. Some investigators have attempted to circumvent these problems by assessing the effects of stressors on saccharin consumption (Katz 1982). Although stressors reduce saccharin intake, central neurochemical concomitants of such behavioral alterations have not been investigated, and the implication for reward alteration is speculative at best.

Research conducted in my laboratory has focused on the potential effects of stressors on motivational/reward processes by assessing ICSS from various dopamine-containing brain regions. The advantages of this technique include the immediacy of brain stimulation and neuroanatomic specificity. The immediacy of brain stimulation, the precision of electrode placement in discrete CNS sites, and the effectiveness of stressors in inducing selective dopamine turnover in the mesocorticolimbic system have been instrumental in demonstrating the anhedonic effects of stressors (Danysz et al. 1985).

It has been demonstrated that stressors influence ICSS performance in rate-dependent and rate-independent paradigms. Such effects are dependent on stressor controllability and are region-specific. In particular, escapable footshock did not affect ICSS in mice, whereas an identical amount of uncontrollable footshock (applied in a yoked paradigm) produced appreciable reductions of ICSS. These effects were initially demonstrated when stimulation electrodes were positioned in the nucleus accumbens and the medial forebrain bundle (along the edges of the internal capsule to ensure activation of the rostrally coursing dopaminergic pathways) (Zacharko et al. 1983a). These disturbances of ICSS were relatively long-lasting, being as marked 1 week after footshock as in the interval immediately after the stressor (Figure 5–1). In contrast, ICSS from the nigrostriatal system (i.e., substantia nigra) was unaffected by inescapable shock. In effect, altered rates of responding for brain stimulation 1) are evident in the mesocorticolimbic system, where uncontrollable stressors influence dopamine turnover; and 2) are ineffective in inducing anhedonia from those central sites (e.g., nigrostriatal system) where stressors do not typically provoke neurochemical change.

The long-term ICSS performance deficits from either the medial forebrain bundle or the nucleus accumbens were evident in animals that had been tested immediately after inescapable shock and then retested at subsequent intervals. However, if animals were exposed to inescapable shock and the immediate post-stressor ICSS session was delayed for 168 hours, reductions in ICSS rates were not apparent. Accordingly, the long-term deficits in ICSS induced by a stressor are dependent on the pairing of the stressor (or perhaps the transient neurochemical changes associated with the stressor) with the perception of reward associated with brain stimulation (Zacharko et al. 1983a).

Recent data collected in my laboratory revealed that uncontrollable stressors also influence ICSS from the mPFC. Depressed ICSS rates were apparent from the mPFC in the interval immediately following uncontrollable footshock, although there were intersubject differences in the duration of the performance impairments. In some animals, ICSS deficits were persistent, whereas in other animals the reward alterations were transient and response reductions were not apparent at more protracted intervals (Wolfe and Zacharko 1991). These stressor-induced ICSS profiles may be related to the position of the stimulating electrode in the mPFC, but a more extensive anatomic analysis must be undertaken before firm conclusions can be drawn.

Consistent with the observation that uncontrollable stressors provoke alterations in ICSS from both the mPFC and the nucleus accumbens, reductions in ICSS have also been reported from the VTA (Kamata et al. 1986; Kasian and Zacharko 1989; Kasian et al. 1987; Zacharko et al. 1990b). However, we have also reported

Figure 5–1. *(at right)* Mean (± SEM) rates of responding for brain stimulation (i.e., intracranial self-stimulation [ICSS]) from either the medial forebrain bundle, the nucleus accumbens, or the substantia nigra. Following the establishment of baseline ICSS rates, mice received either escapable shock, yoked inescapable shock, or no shock, and were tested in the self-stimulation task immediately thereafter and again 24 and 168 hours poststressor. Note that performance deficits in ICSS appeared only from the nucleus accumbens and the medial forebrain bundle. Nigrostriatal ICSS was unaffected by the uncontrollable stressor. Reprinted from Zacharko RM, Bowers WJ, Kokkinidis L, et al: "Region- Specific Reductions of Intracranial Self-Stimulation After Uncontrollable Stress: Possible Effects on Reward Processes." *Behavior and Brain Research* 9:129–141, 1983. Copyright 1983, Elsevier Science Publishers. Used with permission.

that the ICSS alterations varied with the position of the stimulating electrode in the midbrain tegmental field (Kasian et al. 1987; Zacharko et al. 1990a). Following exposure to inescapable shock,

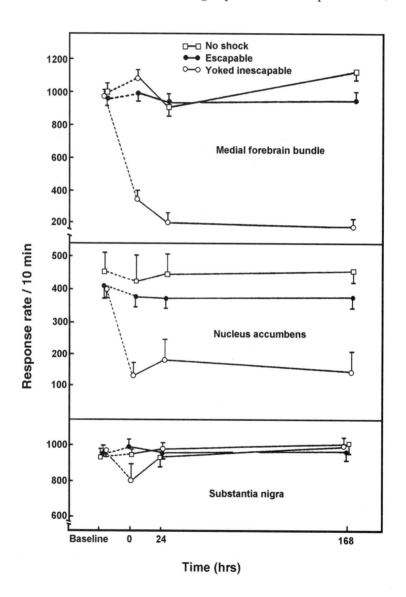

ICSS from the dorsal VTA was reduced appreciably, whereas ICSS from the ventral VTA was unaffected, despite the fact that comparable baseline ICSS rates were evident from these regions. These data indicate a functional differentiation of neurons within the VTA and are consistent with the neurochemical/electrophysiological descriptions of the A10 area provided by Deutch et al. (1985) and Mantz et al. (1989) that indicate that the midbrain tegmental area (A10 region) is not uniformly affected by stressors.

It is unlikely that the impairments in responding for ICSS from mesolimbic/mesocortical sites are peculiar to the stimulation parameters employed. Bowers et al. (1987) demonstrated that inescapable footshock reduced ICSS rates from the nucleus accumbens across a range of brain stimulation intensities. Only with the lower stimulation parameters, which ordinarily yielded low ICSS rates, was the stressor ineffective in affecting performance. As previously observed, responding for ICSS from the substantia nigra was unaffected by the stressor at any of the currents examined. Employing this current intensity paradigm, Kasian et al. (1987) subsequently reported that uncontrollable footshock also disrupted ICSS performance from the dorsal, but not the ventral, aspects of the A10 region (Figure 5–2). These results are consistent with previous data collected in this laboratory. Self-stimulation performance from the substantia nigra was unaffected by uncontrollable stressors in this procedure.

Taken together, these data suggest that stressors reduce the rewarding value of ICSS from the mesocorticolimbic system at the point of origin of this pathway (i.e., the VTA), as well as its terminal sites (i.e., nucleus accumbens, mPFC). In some cases the time course for such reward alteration was dependent on the brain region in which the stimulating electrode was positioned (e.g., dorsal versus ventral A10 region). Moreover, the emergence of the ICSS disturbances, at least within the medial forebrain bundle and the nucleus accumbens, was dependent on stressor controllability. In contrast to the effects of stressor application on mesolimbic ICSS, the stressor hardly affected ICSS from the substantia nigra. Because stressors do not ordinarily influence nigrostriatal dopamine activity, these data provide evidence that stressor-provoked dopamine alterations in the mesocorticolimbic system contribute to the alterations of ICSS.

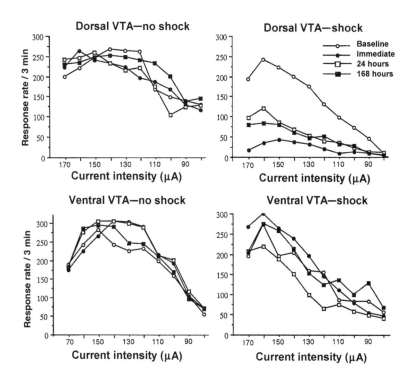

Figure 5–2. Mean rate of responding for electrical brain stimulation (i.e., ICSS) from either the ventral or dorsal aspects of the ventral tegmental area (VTA). Baseline ICSS rates are provided, as well as self-stimulation performance at each of three intervals (0, 24, and 168 hours) following exposure to either inescapable footshock or no shock. Mice were tested in a descending (170–80 µA) current intensity paradigm in which animals were permitted to respond for 3 minutes at each current intensity, decreasing in 10-µA steps over the course of the 30-minute test session. Reprinted from Zacharko RM, Kasian M, MacNeil G, et al: "Stressor-Induced Alterations in Intracranial Self-Stimulation From the Ventral Tegmental Area: Evidence for Regional Variations." *Brain Research Bulletin* 25:617–621, 1990. Copyright 1990, Pergamon Press. Used with permission.

STRESSOR-INDUCED BEHAVIORAL
IMPAIRMENTS AND ANTIDEPRESSANTS

Some of the behavioral deficits induced by uncontrollable stressors may be ameliorated by chronic but not acute antidepressant administration. The therapeutic effects of such antidepressants may be related to the norepinephrine and 5-HT receptor changes following repeated treatment (Anisman and Zacharko 1982; Stone 1987), as well as to increased amine availability. Similarly, chronic stressor exposure may provoke postsynaptic ß-noradrenergic receptor downregulation, which may prevent development of pathology (Stone 1987). Organismic or experiential variables that interfere with, or delay appearance of, altered receptor sensitivity may favor development of illness; pharmacological intervention may then be necessary to provoke receptor alterations that are conducive to behavioral recovery (Molina et al. 1990). At least some of these receptor changes may be functionally interdependent (i.e., norepinephrine and 5-HT), and the interactive or cascading influence of the dopaminergic system on other neurotransmitter systems remains to be elucidated (Zacharko and Anisman 1989). It has been proposed that some antidepressant agents may exert their therapeutic effects by altering central dopamine neurotransmission. In fact, chronic antidepressant administration can induce a subsensitivity of dopamine autoreceptors (Antelman and Chiodo 1981; Serra et al. 1980), and chronic administration of a variety of clinically effective antidepressant treatments, including monoamine oxidase inhibitors (MAOIs) or electroconvulsive therapy (ECT), produces a pattern of behavioral, neurochemical, and electrophysiological data consistent with the dopamine subsensitivity hypothesis of chronic antidepressant action (Jimerson 1987).

Repeated administration of antidepressants has also been shown to influence some of the behavioral effects of stressors (Weiss and Goodman 1984; Zacharko and Anisman 1989). Chronic treatment with desipramine has been found to lower the threshold for ICSS from the VTA (Fibiger and Phillips 1981) and the medial forebrain bundle (McCarter and Kokkinidis 1988). In our laboratory, chronic desipramine administration prior to uncontrollable footshock attenuated ICSS deficits from the nucleus accumbens (Zacharko et al. 1984) (Figure 5–3). The magnitude of the ICSS response reduction from the nucleus accumbens was reduced immediately following stressor presentation, and the ICSS rates were comparable to those of control animals 24 and 168 hours following initial stressor presentation.

In addition to its prophylactic effects, chronic desipramine treatment also eliminated the disturbances of ICSS from the nucleus accumbens induced by a previously applied stressor (Zacharko et al. 1984). However, some variability was detected in the behavioral effects of antidepressant treatment. In particular,

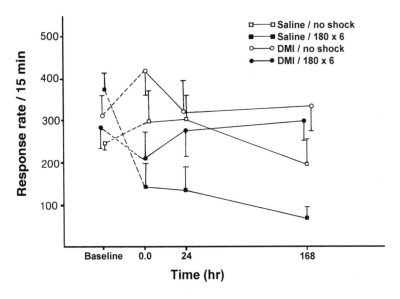

Figure 5–3. Mean (± SEM) number of responses for electrical brain stimulation (i.e., ICSS) from the nucleus accumbens over a 15-minute period among CD1 mice that were exposed to 180 shocks (150 μA, 180 x 6 seconds) or no shock. Mice had received treatment with either desipramine (DMI), 5 mg/kg twice a day for 15 days, or saline prior to uncontrollable footshock. Mice were tested for ICSS immediately (0), and again at 24 and 168 hours, after the stressor treatment. Reprinted from Zacharko RM, Bowers WJ, Kelley MS, et al.: "Prevention of stressor-induced disturbances of self-stimulation by desmethylimipramine." *Brain Research* 321:175–179, 1984. Copyright 1984, Elsevier Science Publishers. Used with permission.

although chronic desipramine administration was effective in ameliorating stressor-induced deficits in ICSS in the majority of animals, performance in some animals was unaffected by desipramine administration, whereas other animals showed an initial recovery followed by a reduction in ICSS rates. A similar response profile following chronic desipramine treatment has been detected in mice with electrodes positioned in the mPFC (Figure 5–4). Accordingly, it would appear that although desipramine is

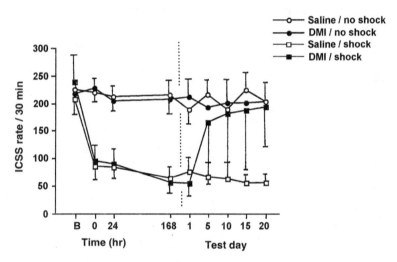

Figure 5–4. Mean (± SEM) rate of responding for electrical brain stimulation (i.e., ICSS) from the frontal cortex in CD-1 mice exposed to no shock and mice in which reduced ICSS rates were evident 168 hours following stressor exposure. Half the animals of the shock and no-shock treatment groups were subdivided and administered either saline or desipramine (5 mg/kg x 2) intraperitoneally for 20 consecutive days following the 168-hour ICSS test. ICSS rates were assessed on day 1 of the chronic drug regimen and thereafter at 5-day intervals for the duration of the 20-day treatment period. Note the variability in the therapeutic efficacy of DMI among mice previously exposed to uncontrollable footshock. Reprinted from *Brain Research Bulletin*, Vol. 27, Wolfe CL, Zacharko RM: "Desmethylimipramine Promotes Recovery of Self-Stimulation From the Prefrontal Cortex Following Footshock," pp. 601–604, Copyright 1991, with permission from Pergamon Press Ltd., Headington Hill Hall, Oxford 0X3 0BW, UK.

generally effective in reversing the stressor-induced reward alterations from the mesolimbic system, the therapeutic efficacy of desipramine is subject to considerable interindividual variability (Zacharko et al. 1983b).

Some of the interindividual variability in the response to therapeutic agents may be related to individual differences in the patterns of adaptation to a chronic stressor. For example, it has been reported by many investigators that a chronic stressor regimen reverses the reductions in CNS dopamine and norepinephrine concentrations ordinarily associated with acute stressor exposure. In a like fashion, the disturbances of ICSS that are ordinarily evident from the nucleus accumbens after an acute stressor session were found to be absent in mice receiving chronic footshock (Zacharko and Anisman 1989; Zacharko et al. 1984). It has been suggested that although adaptive changes ordinarily occur in response to a repeated stressor, pathology may ensue when these adaptive changes do not develop owing to organismic or experiential factors. We found that when behavioral adaptation was not evident following a repeated stressor, chronic treatment with desipramine ameliorated the behavioral impairment. However, when the repeated stressor treatment was associated with an amelioration of the behavioral response to an acute stressor, then treatment with desipramine disrupted responding for ICSS from the nucleus accumbens (Zacharko et al. 1984). Thus, the efficacy of desipramine was dependent on the presence or absence of adaptation to the chronic stressor.

OPIOIDS AND CHANGES IN CENTRAL DOPAMINE ACTIVITY

Neuropeptides, including endogenous opioids, may also modulate both stressor-induced amine turnover (Kalivas et al. 1988) and ICSS. Immunocytochemical analyses have shown anatomic proximity of dopamine and neuropeptides in the VTA (Johnson et al. 1980; Uhl et al. 1979). Intracerebral administration of the enkephalin D-Ala^2-Met^5-enkephalinamide (DALA) into the VTA produced a dose-dependent enhancement of conditioned place preference and ICSS (Broekkamp et al. 1979; Phillips and LePiane

1980). Pharmacological manipulations that prevented neuropeptide release in the A10 region attenuated both the enhanced dopamine turnover within the nucleus accumbens and the mPFC, and the behavioral consequences of the applied stressor (Zacharko and Anisman 1991a, 1991b).

Conditioning/sensitization of mesocortical dopamine turnover has been reported among animals reexposed to a mild stressor or to cues previously associated with a stressor (see Antelman and Yehuda, Chapter 4; Charney et al., Chapter 6; Rausch et al., Chapter 14, this volume). Such dopaminergic neurochemical conditioning might also be influenced by endogenous opioids. Kalivas (1985) and Kalivas and Duffy (1987) reported a progressive increase in behavioral output and increased dopamine turnover in the VTA, the nucleus accumbens, and the mPFC following repeated challenge doses of opioids. Moreover, behavioral and neurochemical cross-sensitization between animals subjected to daily footshock or intra-VTA DALA administration has been reported (Kalivas et al. 1986).

We have recently reported that opioid manipulations influenced the disruption of responding for ICSS from the dorsal VTA ordinarily induced by inescapable footshock (Wolfe and Zacharko 1990). Acute intraventricular administration of DALA antagonized the marked reductions of ICSS from the dorsal VTA induced by uncontrollable footshock (Figure 5–5). However, while postshock administration of DALA eliminated the disruption of ICSS immediately after inescapable shock, the performance deficits were again evident when animals were tested 24 and 168 hours later (in the nondrug state). Thus, DALA administered therapeutically had only a transient effect on the disruption of ICSS induced by inescapable shock. When DALA was administered prior to uncontrollable footshock, however, an attenuation of the stressor-induced alterations on ICSS was apparent, and such performance alterations were no longer apparent 168 hours following initial stressor exposure (Figure 5–6). In effect, prophylactic administration of this neuropeptide was effective in blunting the immediate impact of the stressor on reward processing from the VTA, and the anhedonic effects of the stressor were eliminated at protracted intervals (Maddeaux and Zacharko 1992).

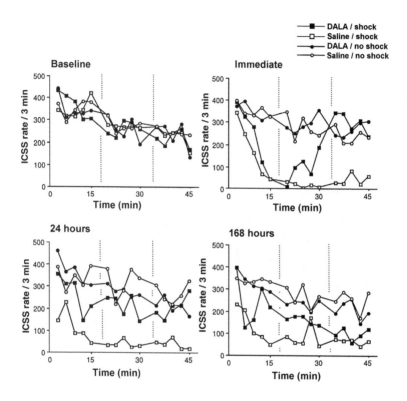

Figure 5–5. Mean rate of responding for electrical brain stimulation (i.e., ICSS) from the dorsal VTA among mice exposed to either inescapable footshock or no shock. Self-stimulation rates were assessed during baseline and at three poststressor intervals (immediate [0], and again at 24 and 168 hours). Mice received an acute intraventricular infusion of either D-Ala^2-Met^5-enkephalinamide (DALA) (1.0 μg in a 1 μl volume) or vehicle 15 minutes after commencement of the "Immediate" ICSS test session. Reprinted from *Brain Research Bulletin,* Vol. 28, Maddeaux C, Zacharko RM: "Intraventricular Administration of D-Ala^2-Met^5-enkephalinamide Induces Rapid Recovery of Responding for Electrical Brain Stimulation From the Ventral Tegmental Area Following Uncontrollable Footshock," pp. 337–341, Copyright 1992, with permission from Pergamon Press Ltd., Headington Hill Hall, Oxford 0X3 0BW, UK.

STRAIN-SPECIFIC EFFECTS OF STRESSORS

Strain-dependent variations in response to stressors have been reported in several paradigms (Zacharko and Anisman 1991a, 1991b). In contrast to the results reported thus far in this chapter, which were obtained for the non-inbred CD-1 mouse strain, ICSS performance among inbred mouse strains was not entirely pre-

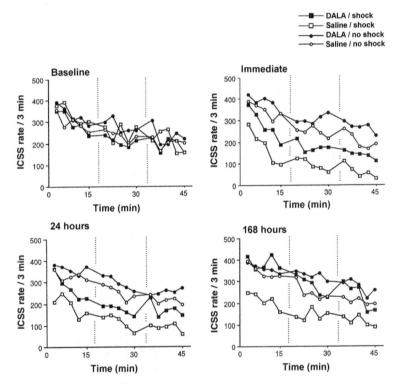

Figure 5–6. Mean rate of responding for electrical brain stimulation (ICSS) from the dorsal VTA among mice exposed to either uncontrollable footshock or no-shock condition. Self-stimulation rates were assessed during baseline training and at three poststressor test intervals (immediate [0], and again at 24 and 168 hours). Mice received an acute intraventricular infusion of either D-Ala^2-Met^5- enkephalina- mide (DALA) (1.0 µg in a volume of 1 µl) or vehicle 15 minutes prior to the stressor session. Data from Wolfe and Zacharko 1990.

dictable. For example, the effect of uncontrollable footshock on ICSS from the nucleus accumbens varied with the strain of mouse employed (Figure 5–7). In particular, responding for ICSS in C57BL/6J mice was unaffected by uncontrollable footshock at any of the poststressor intervals examined. In contrast, BALB/cByJ mice actually increased responding for ICSS immediately following exposure to the stressor, whereas DBA/2J mice exhibited marked reductions in ICSS (Zacharko et al. 1987).

The stressor-elicited disturbances of ICSS not only vary across strains of mice but also are dependent on the brain region supporting ICSS. The strain-dependent ICSS response profiles evident in the nucleus accumbens following uncontrollable footshock are fundamentally different when the comparison is extended to the mPFC and the VTA. We observed (Zacharko et al. 1990a) that uncontrollable footshock provoked a marked depression in ICSS from the mPFC of BALB/cByJ and DBA/2J mice, whereas alterations of ICSS rates were not apparent among C57BL/6J mice (Figure 5–8). Moreover, whereas the ICSS response depressions induced by the stressor were marked and persistent among the DBA/2J mice, the impairment of ICSS among the BALB/cByJ mice was apparent only during the interval immediately following stressor presentation. In contrast, when ICSS from the VTA was assessed, ICSS rates were *augmented* in both the BALB/cByJ and DBA/2J strains of mice, whereas ICSS was *disrupted* in the C57BL/6J strain (Kasian and Zacharko 1989). Evidently interstrain alterations of ICSS provoked by uncontrollable footshock within the mesocorticolimbic system are not uniform, and it remains to be determined whether these variations of ICSS represent different types of reward. These data suggest that the appearance of behavioral deficits in these strains is not simply related to variations in the vulnerability of these animals to the impact of stressors. If a strain were particularly sensitive to a stressor or vulnerable to its effects, then it might be expected that performance deficits would be evident in a specific strain irrespective of the brain region examined. Moreover, the strain-specific alterations of performance are task-specific (Zacharko and Anisman 1989).

The effectiveness of some antidepressants in ameliorating reward alterations induced by a stressor was also dependent on the

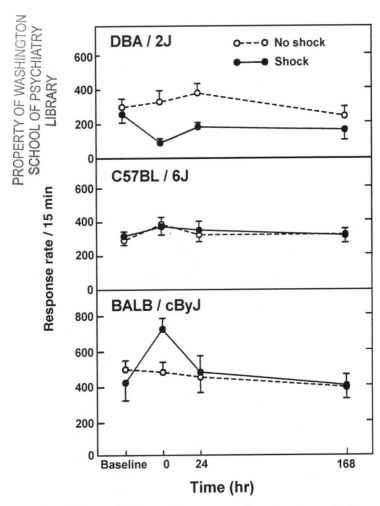

Figure 5–7. Mean (± SEM) rate of responding for electrical brain stimulation (i.e., ICSS) from the nucleus accumbens in three strains of mice. Animals received a 15-minute test session prior to treatment (Baseline) and again immediately (0), 24, and 168 hours after exposure to either inescapable footshock (360 shocks of 150 μA of 2-second duration) or no shock. Reprinted from Zacharko RM, Lalonde GT, Kasian M, et al: "Strain-Specific Effects of Inescapable Shock on Intracranial Self-Stimulation From the Nucleus Accumbens." *Brain Research* 426:164–168, 1987. Copyright 1987, Elsevier Science Publishers. Used with permission.

strain of mouse examined as well as the specific task in which mice were tested following exposure to inescapable shock (Zacharko and Anisman 1991a, 1991b). In CD-1 mice, chronic desipramine eliminated the stressor-provoked ICSS deficits from the nucleus accumbens (Zacharko et al. 1984). In contrast to the CD-1 mice, the stressor-induced disruption of ICSS from either the nucleus accumbens or the mPFC in DBA/2J mice was not affected by repeated desipramine or amitriptyline treatment. We have some preliminary data to suggest that chronic desipramine followed by chronic amitriptyline can reinstate ICSS performance (Baillie et al. 1988). Several tentative conclusions can be drawn from these data. The therapeutic effectiveness of antidepressants may be specific to some of the behavioral changes (symptoms) elicited by inescapable shock but may not alleviate the entire constellation of disturbances induced by a stressor. The neurochemical basis of particular behavioral alterations induced by stressors may be variable across strains of animals and consequently would be differentially responsive to specific pharmacological interventions.

The provisional effectiveness of a desipramine-amitriptyline regimen in reversing reward alteration in DBA/2J mice suggests that perhaps the amelioration of particular behavioral deficits may, in some instances, be a prerequisite to the alleviation of anhedonia induced by stressors. Indeed, it should be emphasized that uncontrollable stressors induce a variety of behavioral (and neurochemical) changes acting in concert. It is tempting to speculate, for example, that perception of improved sleep and appetitive patterns in human subjects might be conducive to the "lifting" of depressed mood. Moreover, cognitive appraisal of such improved vegetative functioning in depressed humans might potentially permit more effective pharmacological treatment of anhedonia. Although speculative, such an interpretation deserves some consideration.

Several investigators have reported that stressor-provoked alterations of catecholamine activity vary across strains of mice (e.g., Cabib et al. 1988). We have observed that the effectiveness of stressors in influencing amine turnover varies not only with the strain of mouse examined but also with the brain region under consideration. For instance, although inescapable footshock increased DOPAC accumulation in the nucleus accumbens in C57BL/6J and DBA/2J mice, such metabolite changes were not associated with significant dopamine reductions. BALB/cByJ mice, in contrast, exhibited a significant dopamine depletion in the nucleus accumbens in the absence of accompanying alterations of DOPAC levels. When the mPFC was considered, a different strain profile emerged. Once again, significant dopamine reductions were evident in BALB/cByJ mice, but DOPAC accumulation was unaffected. In CD-1 mice, DOPAC levels were found to be enhanced significantly by the stressor, whereas dopamine concentrations were not altered. Finally, in the VTA the strain pattern was different from that of either the mPFC or the nucleus accumbens. Pronounced reductions of dopamine were apparent in the CD-1, DBA/2J, and BALB/cByJ mice, but only in CD-1 mice was there an appreciable increase of DOPAC (Zacharko and Anisman 1991b).

Clearly, although a stressor may promote significant dopamine turnover in some strains of mice, such an effect may be restricted to only some brain regions. Moreover, a stressor in one strain may promote dopamine turnover in one brain region but not another, whereas in a second strain an opposite pattern may be apparent. If variations in dopamine turnover were solely responsible for the alterations of ICSS described earlier, then it would have been expected that alterations of ICSS across the different strains and brain regions would parallel such neurochemical change. It would appear that variations of dopamine

Figure 5–8. *(at right)* Mean (± SEM) rate of responding for electrical brain stimulation (i.e., ICSS) from the mesocortex in each of three strains of mice (DBA/2J, BALB/cByJ, C57BL/6J). Mice received a 30-minute ICSS test session 24 hours prior to treatment, and again immediately (0), 24, and 168 hours after exposure to uncontrollable shock (360 shocks of 150 µA of 2-second duration) or no shock. Reprinted from Zacharko RM, Gilmore E, MacNeil G, et al: "Stressor-Induced Variations of Intracranial Self-Stimulation From the Mesocortex in Several Strains of Mice." *Brain Research* 530:353–357, 1990. Copyright 1990, Elsevier Science Publishers. Used with permission.

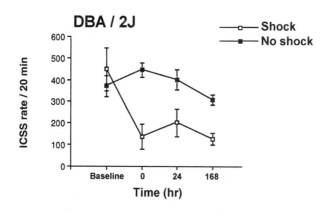

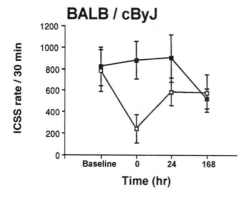

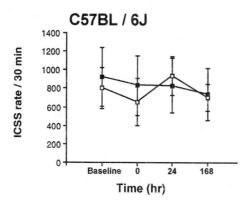

activity represent only one of several neurochemical effects that are influenced by stressor presentation. The resultant effects on behavior presumably reflect the conjoint and interactive effects of several transmitter systems and the neuromodulatory role of specific neuropeptides.

CONCLUSIONS

It has been demonstrated that exposure to uncontrollable stressors in nonhuman species may induce behavioral disturbances. Most notably, animals exposed to uncontrollable footshock exhibit a marked and long-lasting anhedonia as gauged by disturbances of responding for ICSS from the mesocorticolimbic system. Although behavioral pathology following a stressor has typically been associated with alterations of norepinephrine and 5-HT turnover and/or receptor sensitivity, stressor-induced alterations in dopamine function may also contribute to the behavioral profile seen in animals. In addition, the stressor-induced alterations in dopamine turnover may be affected by the neuromodulatory influence of endogenous neuropeptides.

The data summarized in this chapter suggest that reward and motivation involve neurochemical activity in the mesocorticolimbic system and are affected by stressors that activate the A10 region. The vulnerability of animals to reward alteration following stressor exposure appears to depend, at least in part, on the release of endogenous neuropeptides that modulate dopamine activity in the A10 area, a focal point in central reward neurocircuitry. However, it will also be recalled that stressors do not influence the VTA or the mPFC, the principal projection site of the A10 cell grouping, uniformly. Our data suggest that specific regions within the midbrain tegmental area, notably the dorsal A10 region, appear to be particularly vulnerable to uncontrollable footshock, which produces severe anhedonia. This effect can be attenuated by prophylactic, and ameliorated following therapeutic, neuropeptide administration.

The findings preserved here also indicate that the effectiveness of pharmacological treatment is dependent on the prior stressor history of the organism and appears to be related in part to the interactive influence of dopamine and opioid activity. It would appear, at least at face value, that such findings may have relevance to the phenomenology and treatment of motivational loss in PTSD. It should be underscored, however, that the etiologic stressors in PTSD are, by definition, severe. The stressors provoking reward alteration in the mesocorticolimbic system (i.e., anhedonia) among infrahuman species are, on the other hand, mild. Indeed, it has been demonstrated that mild but not severe stressors (which actually provoke neurochemical adaptation) promote dopamine turnover in the mesocorticolimbic system (see, e.g., Roth et al. 1988).

Any attempt to evaluate the effects of stressors on motivation must also consider that the distribution of opioid receptors in the VTA is heterogeneous. Mu, delta, and kappa receptors and their respective endogenous ligands have been identified (Met- and Leu-enkephalin as well as dynorphin). Preliminary data collected in this laboratory have revealed that the nature of the opioid receptor interface with dopamine activity in the A10 region can influence the expression of stressor-induced reward. In like fashion, the anxiogenic properties of stressors and their interaction with the locus coeruleus and reward may be similarly modulated (see, e.g., Deutch et al. 1986). While some of these observations are speculative in nature, these variables clearly deserve further consideration.

In summary, it would seem appropriate to emphasize that the appearance of stressor-induced behavioral disturbances may be dependent on a number of experiential and organismic variables, including genetic factors. Thus, the symptom profile elicited by a stressor in one strain of mouse may be very different from that evoked in a second strain. Likewise, the neurochemical consequences of a stressor may vary with the brain region being examined, and it seems that the therapeutic efficacy of antidepressants or neuropeptides will be dependent on the specific symptoms elicited by the stressor in particular genetic strains. It is suggested that the symptoms induced by a stressor may be dependent on the nature of the neurochemical alterations that are provoked and the brain regions in which these occur. Individual (or interstrain) differences exist that influence vulnerability to these neurochemical disturbances, and might account for the diverse behavioral profiles evident among animals exposed to aversive stimulation. Consideration of such variables may prove to be appropriate in the assessment of PTSD.

Finally, the clinical literature on PTSD has raised a number of issues that require comment. First, it should be emphasized that no one animal model can be deemed to be representative or descriptive of the entire constellation of symptoms of PTSD, and any attempts to oversimplify this reality are likely to be counter-productive at best. Second, it is not particularly surprising that victims of a traumatic life event(s) experience considerable and protracted anxiety and agitation when exposed to cues reminis-cent of the original traumatic event(s). However, it should also be considered that there is very little information currently available (but see Sierles et al. 1983) that describes the premorbid history of individuals suffering from PTSD. The contribution of premorbid variables to the persistence and severity of at least some of the symptoms of this disorder should be considered. Taken together, a comprehensive assessment of PTSD and the potential develop-ment of animal models simulating this disorder must consider not only the empirical evidence suggesting potential neural mechanisms subserving the disorder but also the influence of variables that can sustain or exacerbate the illness.

REFERENCES

Abercrombie ED, Jacobs BL: Systemic naloxone administration potenti-ates locus coeruleus noradrenergic neuronal activity under stressful but not non-stressful conditions. Brain Res 441:362–366, 1988

Abercrombie ED, Keefe KA, DiFrischia DS, et al: Differential effects of stress on in vivo dopamine release in striatum, nucleus accumbens and medial frontal cortex. J Neurochem 52:1655–1658, 1989

Akiskal HS, McKinney WT: Depressive disorders: towards a unified hypothesis. Science 182:20–29, 1973

Anisman H, Zacharko RM: Depression: the predisposing influence of stress. Behavioral and Brain Sciences 5:89–137, 1982

Anisman H, Zacharko RM: Behavioral and neurochemical consequences associated with stressors. Ann N Y Acad Sci 467:205–225, 1986

Antelman SM, Chiodo LA: Dopamine autoreceptor subsensitivity: a mechanism common to the treatment of depression and the induc-tion of amphetamine psychosis. Biol Psychiatry 16:717–724, 1981

Baillie P, Wolfe C, MacNeil G, et al: Antidepressant specificity in the reversal of performance deficits in intracranial self-stimulation from mesolimbic and mesocortical sites in the DBA/2J mouse strain. Society for Neuroscience Abstracts 14:45, 1988

Bannon MJ, Roth RH: Pharmacology of mesocortical dopamine neurons. Pharmacol Rev 35:53–68, 1983

Blanc G, Herve D, Simon H, et al: Response to stress of mesocortico-frontal dopaminergic neurons in rats after long-term isolation. Nature 284:265–267, 1980

Bowers MB, Bannon MJ, Hoffman FJ: Activation of forebrain dopamine systems by phencyclidine and footshock stress: evidence for distinct mechanisms. Psychopharmacology (Berlin) 93:133–135, 1987

Bowers WJ, Zacharko RM, Anisman H: Evaluation of stressor effects on intracranial self-stimulation from the nucleus accumbens and the substantia nigra in a current intensity paradigm. Behav Brain Res 23:85–93, 1987

Broekkamp CL, Phillips AG, Cools AR: Facilitation of self-stimulation behavior following intracerebral microinjections of opioids into the ventral tegmental area. Pharmacol Biochem Behav 11:289–295, 1979

Cabib S, Kempf E, Schleef C, et al: Effects of immobilization stress on dopamine and its metabolites in different brain regions of the mouse: role of genotype and stress duration. Brain Res 441:153–160, 1988

Dantzer R, Guilloneau D, Mormede P, et al: Influence of shock-induced fighting and social factors on dopamine turnover in cortical and limbic areas in the rat. Pharmacol Biochem Behav 20:331–335, 1984

Danysz W, Fowler CJ, Archer T: Electrical intra-cranial self-stimulation: a potentially valid model for antidepressant action. Trends Pharmacol Sci 7:278–279, 1985

Deutch AY, Tam S-Y, Roth RH: Footshock and conditioned stress increase 3,4-dihydroxyphenylacetic acid (DOPAC) in the ventral tegmental area but not substantia nigra. Brain Res 333:143–146, 1985

Deutch AY, Goldstein M, Roth RH: Activation of the locus coeruleus induced by selective stimulation of the ventral tegmental area. Brain Res 363:307–314, 1986

Dinan TG, Barry S, Yatham LN, et al: A pilot study of a neuroendocrine test battery in posttraumatic stress disorder. Biol Psychiatry 28:665–672, 1990

Dunn AJ, File SA: Cold restraint alters dopamine metabolism in frontal cortex, nucleus accumbens and striatum. Physiol Rev 31:511–513, 1983

Fadda F, Argiolas A, Melis M, et al: Stress induced increase in 3,4-dihydroxyphenylacetic acid (DOPAC) levels in the cerebral cortex but not in the nucleus accumbens: reversal by diazepam. Life Sci 23:2219–2224, 1978

Fibiger HC, Phillips AG: Increased intracranial self-stimulation in rats after long-term administration of desipramine. Science 124:683–684, 1981

Glavin GB: Stress and brain noradrenaline: a review. Neurosci Biobehav Rev 9:233–243, 1985

Heinsbroek RPW, van Haaren F, Feenstra MGP, et al: Sex differences in the effects of inescapable footshock on central catecholaminergic and serotonergic activity. Pharmacol Biochem Behav 37:539–550, 1990

Heinsbroek RPW, van Haaren F, Feenstra MGP, et al: Controllable and uncontrollable footshock and monoaminergic activity in the frontal cortex of male and female rats. Brain Res 551:247–255, 1991

Herman JP, Guillonneau R, Dantzer R, et al: Differential effects of inescapable footshocks and of stimuli previously paired with inescapable footshocks on dopamine turnover in cortical and limbic areas of the rat. Life Sci 30:2207–2214, 1982

Heyes MP, Garnett ES, Coates G: Nigrostriatal dopaminergic activity is increased during exhaustive exercise stress in rats. Life Sci 42:1537–1542, 1988

Ida Y, Tsuda A, Sueyoshi K, et al: Blockade by diazepam of conditioned fear-induced activation of rat mesoprefrontal dopamine neurons. Pharmacol Biochem Behav 33:477–479, 1989

Irwin J, Ahluwalia P, Anisman H: Sensitization of norepinephrine activity following acute and chronic footshock. Brain Res 379:98–103, 1986a

Irwin J, Ahluwalia P, Zacharko RM, et al: Central norepinephrine and plasma corticosterone following acute and chronic footshock. Brain Res 376:98–103, 1986b

Janowsky DS, Risch SC: Role of acetylcholine mechanisms in the affective disorders, in Psychopharmacology: The Third Generation of Progress. Edited by Meltzer HY. New York, Raven, 1987, pp 527–534

Jimerson DC: Role of dopamine mechanisms in the affective disorders, in Psychopharmacology: The Third Generation of Progress. Edited by Meltzer HY. New York, Raven, 1987, pp 505–512

Johnson RP, Sar M, Stumpf W: A topographic localization of enkephalin on the dopamine neurons of the rat substantia nigra and ventral tegmental area demonstrated by combined histofluorescence-immunocytochemistry. Brain Res 194:566–571, 1980

Kalivas PW: Sensitization to repeated enkephalin administration into the ventral tegmental area of the rat, II: involvement of the mesolimbic dopamine system. J Pharmacol Exp Ther 235:544–550, 1985

Kalivas PW, Richardson-Carlson R, Van Orden G: Cross sensitization between foot shock stress and enkephalin-induced motor activity. Biol Psychiatry 21:939–950, 1986

Kalivas PW, Duffy P: Sensitization to repeated morphine injection in the rat: possible involvement of A10 dopamine neurons. J Pharmacol Exp Ther 241:204–212, 1987

Kalivas PW, Duffy P, Dilts R, et al: Enkephalin modulation of A10 dopamine neurons: a role in dopamine sensitization. Ann N Y Acad Sci 537;405–414, 1988

Kamata K, Yoshida S, Kameyama T: Antagonism of footshock stress-induced inhibition of intracranial self-stimulation by naloxone or methamphetamine. Brain Res 371:197–200, 1986

Kasian M, Zacharko RM: Strain differences in responding for self-stimulation from the ventral tegmentum following acute and chronic shock. Society for Neuroscience Abstracts 15:1135, 1989

Kasian M, Zacharko RM, Anisman H: Regional variations in stressor provoked alterations of intracranial self-stimulation from the ventral tegmental area. Society for Neuroscience Abstracts 13:1551, 1987

Katz RJ: Animal model of depression: pharmacological sensitivity of a hedonic deficit. Pharmacol Biochem Behav 16:965–968, 1982

Knorr AM, Deutch AY, Roth RH: The anxiogenic-carboline FG-7142 increases in vivo and in vitro tyrosine hydroxylation in the prefrontal cortex. Brain Res 495:355–361, 1989

Kramarcy NR, Delanoy RL, Dunn AJ: Footshock treatment activates catecholamine synthesis in slices of mouse brain regions. Brain Res 290:311–319, 1984

Kvetnansky R, Mitro A, Palkovits M, et al: Catecholamines in individual hypothalamic nuclei in stressed rats, in Catecholamines and Stress. Edited by Usdin E, Kvetnansky R, Kopin IJ. New York, Elsevier, 1976, pp 39–50

Laveille S, Tassin J, Thierry A, et al: Blockade by benzodiazepines of the selective high increase in dopamine turnover induced by stress in mesocortical dopaminergic neurons of the rat. Brain Res 168:585–594, 1978

Maddeaux C, Zacharko RM: Intraventricular administration of D-Ala^2-Met^5-enkephalinamide induces rapid recovery of responding for electrical brain stimulation from the ventral tegmental area following uncontrollable footshock. Brain Res Bull 28:337–341, 1992

Maier SF, Seligman MEP: Learned helplessness: theory and evidence. J Exp Psychol [Gen] 105:3–46, 1976

Mantz J, Thierry AM, Glowinski J: Effect of noxious tail pinch on the discharge rate of mesocortical and mesolimbic dopamine neurons: selective activation of the mesocortical system. Brain Res 476:377–381, 1989

McCarter BD, Kokkinidis L: The effects of long-term administration of antidepressant drugs on intracranial self-stimulation responding in rats. Pharmacol Biochem Behav 31:243–247, 1988

Meltzer HY, Lowy MT: The serotonin hypothesis of depression, in Psychopharmacology: The Third Generation of Progress. Edited by Meltzer HY. New York, Raven Press, 1987, pp 513–526

Molina VA, Volosin M, Cancela L, et al: Effect of chronic variable stress on monoamine receptors: influence of imipramine administration. Pharmacol Biochem Behav 35:335–340, 1990

Phillips AG, LePiane F: Reinforcing effects of morphine microinjection into the ventral tegmental area. Pharmacol Biochem Behav 12:965–968, 1980

Roth RH, Tam S-Y, Ida Y, et al: Stress and mesocorticolimbic dopamine system. Ann N Y Acad Sci 537:138–147, 1988

Rush AJ: Diagnosis of affective disorders, in Depression: Basic Mechanisms, Diagnosis, and Treatment. Edited by Rush AJ, Altshuler KZ. New York, Guilford, 1986, pp 1–31

Saavedra JM: Changes in dopamine, noradrenaline and adrenaline in specific septal and preoptic nuclei after immobilization stress. Neuroendocrinology 35:396–401, 1982

Serra G, Argiolas A, Fadda F, et al: Hyposensitivity of dopamine "autoreceptors" induced by chronic administration of tricyclic antidepressants. Pharmacology Research Communications 12:619–624, 1980

Sierles FS, Chen J-J, McFarland RE, et al: Posttraumatic stress disorder and current psychiatric illnesses: a preliminary report. Am J Psychiatry 140:1177–1179, 1983

Stone EA: Central cyclic-AMP–linked noradrenergic receptors: new findings on properties as related to the actions of stress. Neurosci Biobehav Rev 11:391–398, 1987

Thierry A, Tassin J, Blanc G, et al: Selective activation of the mesocortical dopamine system by stress. Nature 263:242–244, 1979

Uhl GR, Goodman RR, Kuhar MJ, et al: Immunohistochemical mapping of enkephalin containing cell bodies, fibres and nerve terminals in the brain stem of the rat. Brain Res 166:75–94, 1979

Weiss JM, Goodman PA: Neurochemical mechanisms underlying stress-induced depression, in Stress and Coping. Edited by Field T, McCabe P, Schneiderman N. NJ, Lawrence Erlbaum, 1984, pp 93–116

Weiss JM, Goodman PA, Losito BG, et al: Behavioural depression produced by an uncontrollable stressor: relationship to norepinephrine, dopamine and serotonin levels in various regions of rat brain. Brain Res Rev 3:157–205, 1981

Wise RA, Rompre PP: Brain dopamine and reward. Ann Rev Psychol 40:191–225, 1989

Wolfe CL, Zacharko RM: D-Ala^2-Met^5-enkephalinamide attenuates stressor induced alterations in intracranial self-stimulation from the dorsolateral ventral tegmentum. Society for Neuroscience Abstracts 16:444, 1990

Wolfe CL, Zacharko RM: Desmethylimipramine promotes recovery of self-stimulation from the prefrontal cortex following footshock. Brain Res Bull 27:601–604, 1991

Zacharko RM, Anisman H: Motor, motivational and anti-nociceptive consequences of stress: contribution of neurochemical change, in Stress-Induced Analgesia. Edited by Tricklebank MD, Curzon G. London, Wiley, 1984, pp 33–66

Zacharko RM, Anisman H: Pharmacological, biochemical, and behavioral analyses of depression: animal models, in Animal Models of Depression. Edited by Koob GF, Ehlers CL, Kupfer DJ. Boston, MA, Birkhauser, 1989, pp 204–238

Zacharko RM, Anisman H: Stressor induced anhedonia in the mesocorticolimbic system. Neurosci Biobehav Rev 15:391–405, 1991a

Zacharko RM, Anisman H: Stressor-provoked alterations of intracranial self-stimulation in the mesocorticolimbic system: an animal model of depression, in The Mesolimbic Dopamine System: From Motivation to Action. Edited by Willner P, Scheel-Kruger J. London, Wiley, 1991b, pp 409–441

Zacharko RM, Bowers WJ, Anisman H: Stress and desmethylimipramine. Prog Neuropsychopharmacol Biol Psychiatry 8:601–606, 1984

Zacharko RM, Bowers WJ, Kokkinidis L, et al: Region-specific reductions of intracranial self-stimulation after uncontrollable stress: possible effects on reward processes. Behav Brain Res 9:129–141, 1983a

Zacharko RM, Bowers WJ, Prince C, et al: Behavioral alterations following repeated exposure to uncontrollable foot-shock or desmethylimipramine. Society for Neuroscience Abstracts 9:561, 1983b

Zacharko RM, Bowers WJ, Kelley MS, et al: Prevention of stressor induced disturbances of self-stimulation by desmethylimipramine. Brain Res 321:75–179, 1984

Zacharko RM, Lalonde GT, Kasian M, et al: Strain-specific effects of inescapable shock on intracranial self-stimulation from the nucleus accumbens. Brain Res 426:164–168, 1987

Zacharko RM, Gilmore W, MacNeil G, et al: Stressor-induced variations of intracranial self-stimulation from the mesocortex in several strains of mice. Brain Res 530:353-357, 1990a

Zacharko RM, Kasian M, MacNeil G, et al: Stressor-induced alterations in intracranial self-stimulation from the ventral tegmental area: evidence for regional variations. Brain Res Bull 25:617–621, 1990b

Chapter 6

Neurobiological Mechanisms of PTSD

Dennis S. Charney, M.D.
Steven M. Southwick, M.D.
John H. Krystal, M.D.
Ariel Y. Deutch, Ph.D.
M. Michele Murburg, M.D.
Michael Davis, Ph.D.

C urrent data suggest that posttraumatic stress disorder (PTSD) is a disorder of considerable prevalence and morbidity (Browne and Finkelhor 1986; Kulka et al. 1990). Despite the high prevalence of PTSD, comparatively little research has been directed toward understanding the neurobiology of this disorder. The dearth of clinical neurobiological research on PTSD stands in contrast to the large body of investigation of the behavioral, biochemical, and neurophysiological effects of stress in laboratory animals. These studies provide an opportunity to propose certain neural mechanisms and neurochemical alterations that contribute to either the etiology or the persistence of symptoms associated with PTSD.

In this chapter we attempt to synthesize the findings from preclinical investigations of the neurochemical effects of uncontrollable stress, the brain regions mediating responses to stress, and the neural mechanisms that may be responsible for specific

Thanks to Evelyn Testa for excellent manuscript preparation. This work was supported by the Medical Research Service and the National Center for Post Traumatic Stress Disorder of the Department of Veterans Affairs.

PTSD symptoms. This preclinical work logically leads to a set of hypotheses related to the pathogenesis and treatment of PTSD.

NEUROCHEMICAL EFFECTS OF UNCONTROLLABLE STRESS AND THE SPECTRUM OF PTSD SYMPTOMS

Uncontrollable stress produces profound alterations in numerous neurotransmitter and neuropeptide systems that may be responsible for specific PTSD symptoms. The noradrenergic, dopaminergic, gamma-aminobutyric acid (GABA)/benzodiazepine, and hypothalamic-pituitary-adrenal (HPA) systems have been among the best studied.

Noradrenergic System

Uncontrollable stress produces regional increases in norepinephrine turnover in the locus coeruleus (LC), limbic regions (i.e., hypothalamus, hippocampus, amygdala), and cerebral cortex (Glavin 1985; Tsuda and Tanaka 1985). The increase in noradrenergic function in response to uncontrollable stress may relate to activation of LC neurons. The LC firing rate increases in association with fear and anxiety states (Abercrombie and Jacobs 1987; Levine et al. 1990; Redmond 1987), and the limbic and cortical regions innervated by the LC are those involved in the elaboration of adaptive responses to stress (Foote et al. 1983). It appears that uncontrollable stress, in particular, increases the responsiveness of LC neurons to excitatory stimulation. These effects may be due to the development of alpha$_2$ (α_2)–adrenergic autoreceptor subsensivity, because similar changes are produced by α_2 receptor blockade (see Simson and Weiss, Chapter 3, this volume).

Dopaminergic System

The brain dopamine area predominantly involved in the acute stress response is the mesocorticolimbic system. Application of some, but not all, types of acute stressors results in a nonuniform activation of dopamine neurons within this system (see Zachar-ko, Chapter 5, this volume, for review). Biochemical and electro-physiological studies have shown that mesocortical neurons are preferentially activated by stress compared with mesolimbic and striatal dopamine areas (Abercrombie et al. 1989; Deutch and Roth 1990; Roth et al. 1988; Thierry et al. 1976). Further, the mesolimbic dopamine innervation appears to be more sensitive to stress than does the striatum (Abercrombie et al. 1989; Mantz et al. 1989).

Sensitization and conditioning may, however, influence the effects of stressors on dopamine activity. For example, environ-mental cues that have been paired with a stressor increase dopa-mine metabolism in the frontal cortex but not in other regions examined (Deutch et al. 1985; Herman et al. 1982). Chronic effects of stress and repeated cocaine exposure may have similar effects on dopamine neuronal function. Both previous exposure to chronic cocaine administration and repeated stress exposure en-hance the acute stress-induced increase in mesocortical dopa-mine neurotransmission (Kalivas and Duffy 1989). In addition, daily exposure to stress increases subsequent locomotor re-sponses to cocaine and amphetamine (Antelman et al. 1980; Kalivas and Duffy 1989; Maclennan and Maier 1983; Robinson et al. 1985). Functionally, altered dopamine activity in the midbrain tegmental area and its projections to the ventral tegmental area (VTA) and the medial prefrontal cortex (mPFC) may be im-plicated in the motivational alterations observed in stressed ani-mals (see Zacharko, Chapter 5, this volume, for review).

Endogenous Opiate System

Uncontrollable stress produces stress-induced analgesia that is due to actions on endogenous opiate function (Jackson et al. 1979). Stress-induced analgesia is likely to be mediated, in part, by a stress-induced release of endogenous opiates, because levels of opiate peptides are elevated by uncontrollable shock (Amir et al. 1986; Madden et al. 1977). The analgesia is blocked by nal-trexone (Hemingway and Reigle 1987; Hyson et al. 1982; Jackson et al. 1979; Maier 1986; Williams et al. 1984) and shows cross-tol-erance to morphine analgesia (Williams et al. 1984). In addition, uncontrollable, but not controllable, shock decreases the density of mu opiate receptors (Stuckey et al. 1989).

Endogenous Benzodiazepine System

Brain benzodiazepine-GABA receptors may also be linked to the behavioral effects of uncontrollable stress. The behavioral deficits induced by uncontrollable shock are associated with a decrease in GABA receptor–mediated chloride ion flux, depolarization-induced hippocampal release of GABA, and brain benzodiazepine receptor occupancy (Drugan et al. 1989; Petty and Sherman 1981; Weizman et al. 1989). There is also a reduction of the density of low affinity GABA-A receptors and chloride efflux and uptake in the cerebral cortex following uncontrollable stress (Concas et al. 1985, 1987, 1989; Schwartz et al. 1987). Consistent with these data, footshock stress and anxiogenic ß-carbolines increase the binding of ^{35}S-labeled t-butylbicyclophospho-rothionate ([^{35}S]-TBPS) to the picrotoxin recognition site of the benzodiazepine-GABA receptor complex in rat cerebral cortex cells (Concas et al. 1988). The mechanisms responsible for these effects are not known and may involve changes in endogenous modulators of the benzodiazepine-GABA receptor complex and/or molecular events at the receptor level (Biggio et al. 1987; Deutch et al. 1990; Drugan et al. 1989; Majewska 1987; Majewska et al. 1986; Weizman et al. 1989).

Hypothalamic-Pituitary-Adrenal Axis

In laboratory animals, many types of acute stress produce increases in ACTH and corticosterone levels (McEwen et al. 1986). The mechanism responsible for transient stress-induced hyperadrenocorticism and feedback resistance may involve a downregulation of glucocorticoid receptors. Hippocampal Type II glucocorticoid receptors have been suggested to be those brain glucocorticoid receptors most sensitive to the downregulation evoked by elevated glucocorticoid levels (Herman et al. 1984; Sapolsky and Plotsky 1990; Sapolsky et al. 1984a, 1984b).

Both adaptation and sensitization of glucocorticoid activity have been reported in response to chronic stress (Amario et al. 1984; Caggiula et al. 1989; Dallman and Jones 1973; Kant et al.

1985, 1987; Mason 1965). It is not known which factors determine whether adaptation or sensitization of glucocorticoid activity will occur following chronic stress. It is unclear how the effects of uncontrollable stress on the hypothalamic-pituitary-adrenal (HPA) axis may affect behavior. It is possible that the learning deficits produced by uncontrollable stress may be related to neurotoxic effects of elevated glucocorticoid levels on hippocampal neurons.

Two recent investigations in vervet monkeys are important in this regard. Vervet monkeys who died spontaneously after experiencing sustained social stress had marked and preferential hippocampal neuronal degeneration (Uno et al. 1989). In an attempt to identify the mechanism of this effect, high doses of glucocorticoids were administered to vervet monkeys and were found to produce similar damage in terms of cell numbers and morphology in the hippocampus (Sapolsky et al. 1990). The hippocampal cell death seen with acute glucocorticoid exposure is similar to that seen in aging (Elliott and Sapolsky 1991). Given the pivotal role played by the hippocampus in memory processes, it has been hypothesized that hippocampal damage in stressed individuals may relate to memory deficits observed in patients with PTSD (Bremner et al. 1993). The finding of reduced hippocampal volume in PTSD patients is consistent with this hypothesis (Bremner et al. 1992).

In addition to the hippocampal neurotoxicity seen with chronic stress or glucocorticoid administration, enhanced hippocampal neuronal vulnerability to energetic insults is seen with acute glucocorticoid exposure. This "metabolic endangerment" may be mediated by glucocorticoid-induced reduction of hippocampal neuronal and glial glucose transport. This energy depletion then exacerbates or initiates the glutamate/NMDA (N-methyl-D-aspartate)/calcium cascade, with prolonged elevation of intracellular calcium concentration, which activates catabolic enzymes and causes abnormalities in cell structure (Elliott and Sapolsky 1991).

Other evidence for a relationship among uncontrollable stress, HPA axis function, and behavior comes from adrenalectomy experiments. In general, adrenalectomy and the resultant decreased corticosteroid levels increase the frequency of behavioral and learning deficits caused by uncontrollable stress. These deficits are reversed by corticosteroid administration (Edwards et al. 1990). Thus, a certain amount of glucocorticoid activity is necessary for learning and adaptation, but too much activity may result in neurotoxicity.

Corticotropin-Releasing Factor

Corticotropin-releasing factor (CRF) plays an important role in the neuroendocrine, autonomic, and behavioral responses to stress (Chappell et al. 1990; Dunn and Berridge 1990; see also Aston-Jones et al., Chapter 2, this volume). The brain sites mediating the CRF responses to stress include the LC and the amygdala. The data suggesting interactions between CRF and noradrenergic neurons are particularly strong. For example, direct infusion of CRF into the LC is anxiogenic and increases norepinephrine turnover in several forebrain areas such as the amygdala and the hypothalamus (Butler PD et al. 1990). CRF increases in a dose-dependent fashion the firing rate of LC norepinephrine neurons (Valentino and Foote 1988), and stress that activates norepinephrine neurons markedly increases CRF concentrations in the LC (Chappell et al. 1990). These data suggest that CRF and norepinephrine regions, such as the LC, may act in concert as important mediators of the stress response.

NEURAL MECHANISMS RELATED TO THE NEUROBIOLOGY OF PTSD SYMPTOMS

Studies of fear conditioning, extinction, and behavioral sensitization in animals have yielded data that may shed light on the neural mechanisms underlying PTSD symptoms in humans. Some of these mechanisms are presented in Table 6–1.

Fear Conditioning and Associative Memories

Sensory and cognitive stimuli associated with the original trauma may induce a spectrum of symptoms in PTSD patients (Litz and Keane 1989; McNally et al. 1987). Such phenomena may represent

Table 6–1. Theoretical relationships between PTSD symptoms and stress-induced alterations in animals

PTSD symptoms	Possible mechanisms	Related anatomic/neurochemical alterations
Hypervigilance, anxiety, fear; autonomic hyperreactivity to trauma-related stimuli	Enhancement of phasic activation	Locus coeruleus: increased responsiveness to excitatory input
	Sensitization	Amygdala, LC, thalamus: increased norepinephrine turnover Medial prefrontal cortex and VTA: increased dopamine turnover
	Fear conditioning	Central nucleus of the amygdala: norepinephrine, opiate, CRF, and NMDA systems involved
	Unknown	Hippocampus: reduced density of benzodiazepine receptors; reduced release of GABA Cortex: reduced GABA-dependent chloride flux
Intrusive memories	Failure of extinction	Amygdala: increased norepinephrine activity, NMDA receptor blockade
Amnesia, cognitive deficits	Neuronal and receptor damage/ loss	Hippocampus: loss of neurons following chronic exposure to high glucocorticoid levels; acute glucocorticoid-induced energy depletion exacerbates or initiates the glutamate/ NMDA/calcium cascade of cell damage
Stressor-induced analgesia	Sensitization of central opiate mechanisms	Periaqueductal gray: increased endogenous opiate activity
Emotional numbing, loss of interest	Unknown	Midbrain tegmental area (especially A10) and its projections to the VTA and the medial prefrontal cortex: altered neuropeptide and dopamine activity

Note.   LC = locus coeruleus; VTA = ventral tegmental area; NMDA = N-methyl-D-aspartate; GABA = gamma- aminobutyric acid; CRF = corticotropin-releasing factor.

classical conditioning of fear. A neural analysis of fear conditioning in animals, therefore, may suggest mechanisms by which PTSD patients remember and associate specific stimuli with traumatic events. Fear conditioning to visual and auditory stimuli is mediated in large part by subcortical mechanisms involving sensory pathways to the thalamus and amygdala (LeDoux et al. 1990). There is preliminary evidence that emotional memories established via thalamo-amygdala pathways may be very long-lasting (LeDoux et al. 1989).

The fear-potentiated acoustic startle paradigm is useful for illustrating the mechanisms of fear conditioning and for identifying brain sites and neurochemical systems that may be associated with PTSD (Davis 1986). It has recently been shown that PTSD patients exhibit increased startle responses (Butler RW et al. 1990; see also Rausch et al., Chapter 14, this volume). The acoustic startle response is a simple reflex mediated by a defined neural pathway in the brain stem and spinal cord (see Rausch et al., Chapter 14). The response is sensitive to anxiolytic drugs and is disrupted by anatomic lesions that are known to affect conditioned fear (Davis 1986). The central nucleus of the amygdala appears to play a key role in the mechanisms of the fear-potentiated startle response that is regulated by noradrenergic, opiate, and corticotropin-releasing systems (Davis 1986; Hitchcock and Davis 1991; Hitchcock et al. 1989; Rosen et al. 1991). In addition, NMDA antagonists infused into the amygdala antagonize the acquisition of fear-potentiated startle, suggesting that an NMDA receptor–mediated process at the level of the amygdala may be critical for development of fear conditioning (Miserendino et al. 1990). Alterations in noradrenergic neuronal function occur in association with fear conditioning. Neutral stimuli that have been paired with inescapable shock produce increases in brain norepinephrine metabolism and behavioral deficits similar to those elicited by the shock (Cassens et al. 1981). Studies in the freely moving cat reveal that a neutral acoustic stimulus that, upon initial presentation, has no effect on LC firing rate increases LC firing when repeatedly paired with an air puff to the whiskers. (The air puff to the whiskers is aversive to the cat and is associated with increases in LC activity [Rasmussen et al. 1986].) An intact noradrenergic system appears to be necessary for the acquisition of fear-conditioned responses (Cole and Robbins 1987; Rasmussen et al. 1986; Tsaltas et al. 1987).

A Possible Failure of Extinction in PTSD

In PTSD, traumatic memories may remain easily accessible and intrusive for decades. In severe conditions these memories may take the form of flashbacks, that is, dissociative states in which aspects of the original trauma are reenacted. Flashbacks and other forms of intrusive memories are commonly elicited by exposure of the PTSD patient to stimuli that represent the initial trauma. The persistent ability of such conditioned stimuli to elicit intrusive traumatic memories and flashbacks may be due to a failure in the mechanisms of response reduction or extinction. In the experimental setting, extinction is the loss of a previously learned conditioned emotional response following repeated presentations of a conditioned fear stimulus in the absence of a contiguous traumatic event. Extinction is not due to erasure of the original memory, but appears to result from learning a new, perhaps inhibitory, memory that acts to oppose the expression of the original one. This may explain why reexposure to a subsequent stressor, such as the unconditioned stimulus alone (without the conditioned stimulus), can reinstate the effective power of the conditioned stimulus (Rescola and Heth 1975). A failure of extinction may also be related to the common clinical observation that traumatic memories may remain dormant for many years, only to be elicited by a subsequent stressor or unexpectedly by a stimulus long ago associated with the original trauma (Solomon et al. 1987; Van Dyke et al. 1985).

Although cortical structures are not primarily involved in the acquisition of conditioned fear responses, they do appear to be important in the extinction of these responses. Lesions of auditory and visual cortex may block extinction of fear responses (LeDoux et al. 1990; Teich et al. 1989). The amygdala is not only involved in the acquisition and expression of conditioned fear responses, but may also be necessary for extinction. For example, NMDA antagonists infused into the amygdala prevent the extinction of fear-potentiated startle (Falls et al. 1992). How this occurs is not established, but may result from processes within the amygdala itself, or via structures that project to the amygdala (e.g., hippocampus, cortex, septal area) and that have been implicated in extinction in several experimental paradigms. Extinction of conditioned fear responses may represent an active suppression by the cortex of subcortical neural circuits (i.e., thalamus, amygdala) that maintain learned associations over long time periods.

Behavioral Sensitization and Stress Sensitivity in PTSD

Sensitization has been defined as the increase in response magnitude that occurs following repeated administration of a stimulus or shortly following presentation of a different but stronger stimulus. The process of sensitization may be involved in the initiation and maintenance of certain PTSD symptoms and the increased susceptibility of PTSD patients to life stressors in general (Antelman 1988; see also Antelman and Yehuda, Chapter 4, this volume). The best-studied systems in relation to stress-induced behavioral sensitization are the dopaminergic and noradrenergic systems. Single or repeated exposure to a stressor potentiates the capacity of a subsequent stress to increase dopamine function (Caggiula et al. 1989; Kalivas and Duffy 1989) without apparently altering basal dopamine turnover (Kalivas et al. 1990). The development of sensitization in dopaminergic systems is thought to relate to increased somatodendritic dopamine release, which stimulates D_1 dopamine receptors. This increase in dopamine release may be due to intrinsic changes in dopamine cells, or to an alteration in GABA regulation of dopamine cells. The continued expression of behavioral sensitization appears to depend on augmented dopamine release in dopamine terminal fields, or, alternatively, on increased efficacy of dopamine at receptors in these forebrain sites (Kalivas et al. 1990).

Sensitization of certain behaviors may also relate to altered noradrenergic function. Limited shock exposure, which does not alter norepinephrine utilization in naive animals, produces increased norepinephrine utilization that exceeds the rate of synthesis found in animals previously exposed to acute uncontrollable shock (Anisman and Sklar 1978). In chronically shocked animals, reexposure to a shock of lower current than the initial shock produces an increase in turnover reflecting an increase in norepinephrine release and synthesis (Irwin et al. 1986). Recent investigations utilizing in vivo microdialysis observed that rats previously exposed to uncontrollable stress had enhanced synthesis and release of hippocampal (Nisenbaum et al. 1991), hypothalamic (Yokoo et al. 1990), and prefrontal cortical (Kalivas and Duffy 1989) norepinephrine following stress reexposure.

A NEUROBIOLOGICAL MECHANISM FOR TRAUMATIC REMEMBRANCE

The most characteristic feature of PTSD is the pervasive and long-lasting memory of the original trauma. The strength of traumatic memories may relate to the degree to which certain neuromodulatory systems, such as the noradrenergic system, are activated by the traumatic experience. Activation of brain noradrenergic receptors in the amygdala after a learning experience has memory-enhancing effects (McGaugh 1989, 1990). Therefore, activation of the LC-norepinephrine system by acute trauma may facilitate the encoding of traumatic memories.

Simple sensory phenomena circumstantially related to the traumatic event, such as specific smells, sounds, and visions, and stressor exposure can often produce a recrudescence of traumatic memories and flashbacks via the mechanisms involved in fear conditioning and behavioral sensitization. As reviewed above, the brain regions mediating these processes include the amygdala, LC, hippocampus, and sensory cortex. There is considerable evidence that the amygdala may play a pivotal role in the conditioning and extinction of sensory and cognitive associations to the original trauma and subsequent activation of traumatic memories. The amygdala has efferent and afferent projections to and from all of the sensory systems in the cortex (Mishkin and Appenzeller 1987). It is also linked neurophysiologically and neuroanatomically to the LC, which also subserves anxiety and fear behaviors. Thus, the functional interchange between the sensory cortices, where memories of each sense may be stored, and the amygdala may be critical for the ability of specific sensory input to elicit traumatic memories, as well as for the extinction (or failure of extinction) of these conditioned responses. The correlated set of behaviors elicited by these memories may be mediated by the projections from the amygdala to numerous brain structures (Davis 1992).

Recent Clinical Investigations Relevant to the Pathophysiology of PTSD Noradrenergic Systems

Recent clinical investigations suggest that a subgroup of PTSD patients may exhibit abnormalities in noradrenergic function. Combat veterans with PTSD have been shown in some studies to have higher resting mean heart rate and systolic blood pressure, as well as greater increases in heart rate when exposed to combat-related stimuli, than do control subjects (see McFall and Murburg, Chapter 7, this volume, for review). Further, several psychophysiological studies have observed hyperreactive responses to combat-associated stimuli but not to other stressful noncombat-related stimuli (Blanchard et al. 1982, 1986; Kolb 1984; Malloy et al. 1983; McFall et al. 1990; Pallmeyer et al. 1986; Pitman et al. 1987; see also Murburg et al., Chapter 9).

Two of three studies have found significantly elevated 24-hour urine norepinephrine excretion in combat veterans with PTSD compared with healthy subjects or patients with schizophrenia or major depression (Kosten et al. 1987; Yehuda et al. 1992). (However, Pitman and Orr [1990] found no difference between norepinephrine levels in 24-hour urine samples from combat-related PTSD patients and combat-exposed asymptomatic control subjects.) In addition, PTSD patients have a decreased density of platelet α_2-adrenergic receptors that may be reflective of an adaptive downregulation in response to persistently elevated levels of circulating catecholamines (Perry et al. 1987).

Recently, noradrenergic function has been evaluated in PTSD patients by determining the behavioral, biochemical, and cardiovascular responses to the α_2-adrenergic receptor antagonist yohimbine (Charney et al. 1984, 1987). As predicted from the preclinical studies reviewed above, yohimbine induced enhanced behavioral, biochemical, and cardiovascular responses in combat veterans with PTSD compared with healthy subjects. A subgroup of PTSD patients were observed to experience yohimbine-induced panic attacks (14 of 20, or 70%) and flashbacks (8 of 20, or 40%) and had larger yohimbine-induced increases in plasma MHPG, sitting systolic blood pressure, and heart rate (Southwick et al. 1993). These results are very similar to those observed in panic disorder patients using the same paradigm (Charney et al. 1984, 1987, 1992). In contrast, yohimbine rarely induces panic attacks in healthy subjects or in patients with schizophrenia, major depression, generalized anxiety disorder, or obsessive-compulsive disorder. These findings raise the possibility that although the pathophysiological disturbances in PTSD and panic disorder may be similar, the etiologies may be different. Panic disorder is a highly familial disorder, and the disturbances in noradrenergic function may be genetic in origin. In contrast, PTSD may be conceived largely as an environmentally induced disorder. The exposure to trauma or uncontrollable stress may produce abnormalities in noradrenergic function. The treatment implications of these observations remain to be established but suggest that specific PTSD symptoms (e.g., anxiety, panic attacks, flashbacks, autonomic hyperarousal) may be particularly responsive to drugs such as clonidine that reduce noradrenergic function (Kinzie and Leung 1989; Kolb 1986, 1989).

The fact that stress increases noradrenergic activity may account for the choice of drugs of abuse selected by PTSD patients in attempts to relieve their symptoms. Alcohol may be frequently abused by PTSD patients because alcohol reduces stress-induced increases in norepinephrine turnover preferentially in the amygdala and the LC (Shirao et al. 1988). Similarly, opiate drug abuse may be due to the ability of opiates to decrease the LC firing rate and reduce stress-induced increases in norepinephrine release in the amygdala, hippocampus, hypothalamus, thalamus, and midbrain (Redmond 1987; Tanaka et al. 1983). Benzodiazepine drugs also reduce LC activity and stress-induced increases in norepinephrine release in the hypothalamus, hippocampus, cerebral cortex, and the LC region (Ida et al. 1985).

Dopaminergic Systems

The studies of stress-induced effects on dopaminergic systems suggest that activation of mesocortical dopamine neurons may be associated with specific PTSD symptoms. For example, the hypervigilance (which often borders on paranoia) frequently observed in PTSD patients may, based on the hypothesized role of dopamine hyperactivity in psychoses, be related to dopamine neuronal hyperactivity. On the other hand, if excessive responsiveness of dopaminergic systems contributes to the symptoms of PTSD, then drugs that reduce dopamine function would be expected to alleviate the hypervigilance associated with this disorder. However, prospective studies have not been performed to test this possibility. Clinical observation of PTSD patients has revealed that they are very sensitive to the anxiogenic and paranoia-inducing effects of cocaine. This sensitivity may be due to the similar effects of chronic stress and repeated cocaine administration on dopamine function.

Opiate Systems

In Vietnam veterans with PTSD, naloxone has been reported to reverse the analgesia induced by stressful combat films (Pitman et al. 1990). This finding may relate to the reports that wounded combatants during World War II required lower doses of narcotics than did civilians with less severe injuries (Beecher 1946), and is consistent with the notion that acute stress may result in the release of endogenous opiates. It has not been established whether the effects of uncontrollable stress on endogenous opiates are related to the core clinical symptoms associated with PTSD. Opiate drugs do, however, constitute one class of substance preferentially abused by many veterans with PTSD. The use of opiates by traumatized veterans may represent an attempt to self-medicate or to compensate for a more enduring dysregulation of the noradrenergic and/or endogenous opiate systems. If this were the case, they might be using exogenous opiates to accomplish the same physiological effect as the acute stress–induced release of endogenous opioids. Opiate withdrawal, on the other hand, is associated with a deficit in endogenous opiate function and an increase in central norepinephrine activity, as well as an increase in symptoms associated with PTSD (Salloway et al. 1990).

Benzodiazepine Systems

The symptoms of anxiety, fear, insomnia, and nightmares associated with PTSD may involve not only noradrenergic systems but also the benzodiazepine-GABA system (Woods et al. 1991). The therapeutic actions of benzodiazepines and related sedative drugs acting at the GABA-benzodiazepine receptor complex may provide clues to the function of this system in PTSD. In fact, these drugs have had a long history of use in PTSD treatment, particularly for acutely traumatized individuals. In World War II, sodium amytal and sodium pentothal were employed in the treatment of acute "combat exhaustion" and "war neurosis" (Bartemeier 1946). These reports are consistent with the putative beneficial effects of benzodiazepines prescribed in the acute posttraumatic period for anxiolysis and restoration of sleep, as well as the efficacy of benzodiazepines in preventing the behavioral sequelae of inescapable shock in animals. However, the available data suggest that benzodiazepines, while having anxiolytic effects in PTSD patients, are not useful for alleviating core PTSD symptoms (Birkhimer et al. 1985; Braun et al. 1990; Marshall 1975; Reaves et al. 1989; Risse et al. 1990).

Hypothalamic-Pituitary-Adrenal Axis

There is consistent evidence that acute trauma can produce profound increases in glucocorticoid levels (Mason et al. 1990; Rose 1984). However, it is not known if the magnitude of these increases is sufficient to produce hippocampal neuronal cell loss as demonstrated in the nonhuman primate studies. In a recent preliminary magnetic resonance imaging (MRI) study, PTSD patients had a reduced hippocampal volume compared with a carefully matched control group (Bremner et al. 1992, 1993). Furthermore, these patients had marked abnormalities in memory function.

The data on basal urinary cortisol levels in combat veterans with PTSD are conflicting. One research group (Mason et al. 1986; Yehuda et al. 1990), but not another (Pitman and Orr 1990), found reduced urinary free cortisol levels in PTSD patients compared with subjects with other psychiatric disorders and healthy subjects. Consistent with a decrease in urinary free cortisol concentrations is the finding that lymphocyte glucocorticoid receptors may be increased in PTSD (Yehuda et al. 1991b). The HPA system regulatory mechanisms in PTSD have been evaluated by measuring the effects of CRF and dexamethasone. In a small sample of PTSD patients, the ACTH response to CRF was reported to be blunted in the presence of normal plasma cortisol levels (Smith et al. 1989). There is preliminary evidence that some PTSD patients may be overly sensitive to the ability of dexamethasone to suppress cortisol (Yehuda et al. 1991a). Considered together, these results suggest that certain central inhibitory mechanisms suppressing CRF and ACTH function may be increased in chronic PTSD. This finding is consistent with preclinical investigations demonstrating adaptive HPA responses to chronic stress.

Despite the above findings, there is also evidence that substantial cortisol increases can be elicited from PTSD patients in response to intense emotional stimuli and pharmacological agents (Mason et al. 1990; Southwick et al. 1993). Thus, more investigation is needed to elucidate HPA axis function in acute and chronic PTSD in relation to basal activity and regulatory mechanisms involving stimulatory and inhibitory processes.

CONCLUSIONS

Acute Neurobiological Responses to Severe Trauma

Under conditions of acute and severe psychological trauma, the organism mobilizes multiple neurobiological systems for the purpose of survival. The preclinical investigations strongly suggest that trauma may simultaneously activate noradrenergic, benzodiazepine, opiate, dopaminergic, and HPA systems, resulting in a number of behavioral and physiological responses.

Several brain structures, most notably the amygdala, hippocampus, LC, and prefrontal cortex, also appear to become rapidly activated by acute, severe stress. The initial terror, anxiety, and autonomic arousal elicited by the trauma could lead to long-term changes in synaptic transmission in several limbic brain sites. Alterations in the excitability of amygdaloid neurons produced by sensitization or fear conditioning could lead to a persistent state of high arousal, anxiety, and fear, because the amygdala projects directly to a variety of hypothalamic and brain-stem targets that are involved in the somatic and autonomic signs of fear and anxiety (Hitchcock and Davis 1991). The activation of the LC-norepinephrine system will result in increased norepinephrine release at LC projection sites, including the amygdala, hippocampus, and cerebral cortex (Crawley et al. 1980; Ida et al. 1985; Iwata et al. 1987; LeDoux et al. 1988; Redmond 1987). Stress-induced changes in benzodiazepine receptor function or in concentrations of endogenous ligands with affinity for the benzodiazepine receptor will likely occur in many of the same brain regions innervated by the LC, because high densities of benzodiazepine receptors are found in the LC, amygdala, hippocampus, and cerebral cortex. Thus, the noradrenergic and benzodiazepine system modulation of trauma-induced fear and anxiety may be mediated by functional interactions among the LC, amygdala, hippocampus, and cerebral cortex.

Hypervigilance is an adaptive behavioral response to trauma. As mentioned, the stress-induced activation of prefrontal cortex dopamine neurons may be associated with this symptom. Analgesia and blunted emotional responses are also adaptive and frequently associated with physical and psychological trauma (Beecher 1946). These responses may be due to increased release of endogenous opioids and stimulation of opiate receptors following traumatic stress. The behavioral responses produced by the parallel alteration of numerous brain neurochemical systems and structures by psychological and physical trauma represent adaptive responses critical for survival in a dangerous environment. Endogenous norepinephrine, dopamine, and perhaps benzodiazepine receptor ligands appear to mediate fear, autonomic hyperarousal, and hypervigilance, each of which facilitates behavioral reactions to threat. Norepinephrine additionally appears to influence numerous somatic functions including blood pressure, heart rate, and blood clotting. The metabolic activation necessary for sustained physical demands and tissue repair appears to be influenced by trauma-induced cortisol hypersecretion. Secretion of endogenous opiates reduces pain sensitivity, an effect that may be critical for survival. Finally, the encoding of traumatic memories that will facilitate appropriate response to future danger may be facilitated by noradrenergic and opiate systems (McGaugh 1989).

Chronic Maladaptive Neurobiological Sequelae

Although initially of benefit, the acute neurobiological responses to stress have longer-term negative consequences. Stress-induced impairment in long-term potentiation, mediated in part by excitatory amino acid, noradrenergic, and opioid receptor systems, could be responsible for the development of learning deficits postulated or observed in PTSD. Because extinction appears to involve an active learning process, deficits in learning may impair normal extinction in PTSD patients, leading to the abnormal persistence of emotional memories. The effects of fear conditioning may be long-lasting. Patients with PTSD are also highly vulnerable to stress. This vulnerability may be due to the sensitization of dopaminergic and noradrenergic systems, resulting in chronic anxiety, panic attacks, and hyperarousal symptoms. Several clinical observations are consistent with the development of sensitization in these systems. PTSD patients exhibit potentiated behavioral, biochemical, and cardiovascular responses to yohimbine. Most patients with PTSD find cocaine anxiogenic and instead resort to the use of alcohol, benzodiazepines, and opiates to reduce the severity and frequency of anxiety and hyperarousal symptoms and flashbacks.

Implications for Pathophysiological and Treatment Studies of PTSD

Posttraumatic stress disorder can be a devastating, chronic disorder with a wide array of symptoms including the core clusters of reexperiencing, avoidance, and hyperarousal, as well as adjunctive symptoms of paranoia, impulsivity, compulsivity, depression, and panic attacks. In the context of the high prevalence and morbidity of PTSD, far too few carefully designed investigations of the neurobiological consequences of severe trauma have been completed. It is not known to what degree PTSD patients suffer from stress-induced learning disabilities. Clinical studies designed to investigate the neurobiological mechanisms associated with fear conditioning and sensitization are indicated. There needs to be a more comprehensive assessment of neurotransmitter and neuropeptide function at a variety of intervals following different types of severe trauma. The function of identified neurochemical systems and brain regions altered by uncontrollable stress needs to be related to the spectrum of stress-induced clinical symptoms that occur acutely and chronically.

The time has come to apply the increased understanding of the psychobiology of traumatic stress to the development of more effective treatment approaches for PTSD. A particularly important question is to what degree the sequelae of stress-induced brain dysfunctions are reversible by exposure therapies and medication. To date, there is little convincing evidence that direct exposure treatments designed to extinguish conditioned physiological responses to aversive memories are clinically efficacious in reducing physiological responses and the core symptom clusters of PTSD. It has been suggested that the difficulty in eliminating these responses is consistent with the hypothesized neurobiological basis of this behavior (Kolb 1987).

Most drug studies of PTSD have not revealed substantial clinical efficacy for core PTSD symptoms—an observation that is consistent with the concept of PTSD as a multisystem disorder. Drugs are needed that act on selected brain target structures and neurochemical systems mediating specific symptoms associated with PTSD. The proposed relationships between stress-induced alterations in the function of specific brain structures and neurochemical systems and clinical symptoms offer a foundation from which to discover rational, targeted pharmacotherapies for PTSD.

REFERENCES

Abercrombie ED, Jacobs BL: Single-unit response of noradrenergic neurons in the locus coeruleus of freely moving cats, I: acutely presented stressful and nonstressful stimuli. J Neurosci 7:2837–2843, 1987

Abercrombie ED, Keefe KA, DiFrischia DS, et al: Differential effect of stress on in vivo dopamine release in striatum, nucleus accumbens, and medial frontal cortex. J Neurochem 52:1655–1658, 1989

Amario A, Castellanos JM, Balasch J: Adaptation of anterior pituitary hormones to chronic noise stress in male rats. Behav Neural Biol 41:71–76, 1984

Amir S, Brown ZW, Amit Z: The role of endorphins in stress: evidence and speculations. Neurosci Biobehav Rev 4:77–86, 1986

Anisman H, Sklar LS: Catecholamine depletion upon reexposure to stress: mediation of the escape deficits produced by inescapable shock. Journal of Comparative and Physiological Psychology 93:610–625, 1978

Antelman SM: Time-dependent sensitization as the cornerstone for a new approach to pharmacotherapy: drugs as foreign or stressful stimuli. Drug Development Research 14:1–30, 1988

Antelman SM, Eichler AJ, Black CA, et al: Interchangeability of stress and amphetamine in sensitization. Science 207:329–331, 1980

Bartemeier L: Combat exhaustion. J Nerv Ment Dis 144:489–525, 1946

Beecher HK: Pain in the men wounded in battle. Ann Surg 123:96–105, 1946

Biggio G, Concas A, Mele S, et al: Changes in GABA transmission induced by stress, anxiogenic and anxiolytic ß-carbolines. Brain Res Bull 19:301–308, 1987

Birkhimer LJ, DeVane CL, Muniz CE: Posttraumatic stress disorder: characteristics and pharmacological response in the veteran population. Compr Psychiatry 26:304–310, 1985

Blanchard EB, Kolb LC, Pallmeyer TP, et al: A psychophysiological study of posttraumatic stress disorder in Vietnam veterans. Psychiatr Q 54:220–229, 1982

Blanchard EB, Kolb LC, Gerardi RJ, et al: Cardiac response to relevant stimuli as an adjunctive tool for diagnosing post-traumatic stress disorder in Vietnam veterans. Behavior Therapy 17:592–606, 1986

Braun P, Greenberg D, Dasberg H, et al: Core symptoms of posttraumatic stress disorder unimproved by alprazolam treatment. J Clin Psychiatry 51:236–238, 1990

Bremner JD, Seibyl JP, Scott TM, et al: Decreased hippocampal volume in PTSD, in 1992 New Research Program and Abstracts, 145th annual meeting of the American Psychiatric Association, Washington, DC, May 1992, NR 155, p 85

Bremner JD, Scott TM, Delaney RC, et al: Deficits in short-term memory in posttraumatic stress disorder. Am J Psychiatry 150:1015–1019, 1993

Browne A, Finkelhor D: Impact of child sexual abuse: a review of the research. Psychol Bull 99:66–77, 1986

Butler PD, Weiss JM, Stout JC, et al: Corticotropin-releasing factor produces fear-enhancing and behavioral activating effects following infusion into the locus coeruleus. J Neurosci 10:176–183, 1990

Butler RW, Braff DL, Rausch JL, et al: Physiological evidence of exaggerated startle response in a subgroup of Vietnam veterans with combat-related PTSD. Am J Psychiatry 147:1308–1312, 1990

Caggiula AR, Antelman SM, Aul E, et al: Prior stress attenuates the analgesic response but sensitizes the corticosterone and cortical dopamine responses to stress 10 days later. Psychopharmacology (Berlin) 99:233–237, 1989

Cassens G, Kuruc A, Roffman M, et al: Alterations in brain norepinephrine metabolism and behavior induced by environmental stimuli previously paired with inescapable shock. Behav Brain Res 2:387–407, 1981

Chappell PB, Smith MA, Kilts CD, et al: Alterations in corticotropin-releasing factor–like immunoreactivity in discrete rat brain regions after acute and chronic stress. J Neurosci 6:2908–2914, 1990

Charney DS, Heninger GR, Breier A: Noradrenergic function in panic anxiety: effects of yohimbine in healthy subjects and patients with agoraphobia and panic disorder. Arch Gen Psychiatry 41:751–763, 1984

Charney DS, Woods SW, Goodman WK, et al: Neurobiological mechanisms of panic anxiety: biochemical and behavioral correlates of yohimbine-induced panic attacks. Am J Psychiatry 144:1030–1036, 1987

Charney DS, Woods SW, Krystal JH, et al: Noradrenergic neuronal dysregulation in panic disorder: the effects of intravenous yohimbine and clonidine in panic disorder patients. Acta Psychiatrica Scand 86:273–282, 1992

Cole BJ, Robbins TW: Dissociable effects of lesions to dorsal and ventral noradrenergic bundle on the acquisition performance, and extinction of aversive conditioning. Behav Neurosci 101:476–488, 1987

Concas A, Corda MG, Biggio G: Involvement of benzodiazepine recognition sites in the footshock induced decrease of low affinity GABA receptors in the rat cerebral cortex. Brain Res 341:50–56, 1985

Concas A, Mele S, Biggio G: Footshock stress decreases chloride efflux from rat brain synaptoneurosomes. Eur J Pharmacol 135:423–427, 1987

Concas A, Serra M, Atsiggiu T, et al: Footshock stress and anxiogenic ß-carbolines increase t-[^{35}S]butylbicyclo-phosphorothionate binding in the rat cerebral cortex, an effect opposite to anxiolytics and γ-aminobutyric acid mimetics. J Neurochem 51:1868–1876, 1988

Concas A, Serra M, Corda MG, et al: Change of ^{36}CI-flux and ^{35}S-TBPS binding induced by stress and GABAergic drugs, in CI-Channels and Their Modulation by Neurotransmitters and Drugs. Edited by Biggio G, Costa E. New York, Raven, 1989, pp 121–136

Crawley JW, Maas JW, Roth RM: Biochemical evidence for simultaneous activation of multiple locus coeruleus afferents. Life Sci 26:1373–1378, 1980

Dallman MF, Jones MT: Corticosteroid feedback control of ACTH secretion: effect of stress-induced corticosterone secretion on subsequent stress responses in the rat. Endocrinology 92:1367–1375, 1973

Davis M: Pharmacological and anatomical analysis of fear conditioning using the fear-potentiated startle paradigm. Behav Neurosci 100:814–824, 1986

Davis M: The role of the amygdala in fear-potentiated startle: implications for animal models of anxiety. Trends Pharmacol Sci 13:35–40, 1992

Deutch AY, Roth RH: The determinants of stress-induced activation of the prefrontal cortical dopamine system. Prog Brain Res 85:367–402, 1990

Deutch AY, Tain S-Y, Roth RH: Footshock and conditioned stress increase 3,4-dihydroxyphenylacetic acid (DOPAC) in the ventral tegmental area but not substantia nigra. Brain Res 333:143–146, 1985

Deutch Sl, Rosse RB, Huntzinger JA, et al: Profound stress-induced alterations in flurazepam's antiseizure efficacy can be attenuated. Brain Res 520:272–276, 1990

Drugan RC, Morrow AL, Weizman R, et al: Stress-induced behavioral depression in the rat is associated with a decrease in GABA receptor-mediated chloride ion flux and brain benzodiazepine receptor occupancy. Brain Res 487:45–51, 1989

Dunn AJ, Berridge CW: Physiological and behavioral responses to corticotropin-releasing factor administration: is CRF a mediator of anxiety or stress responses? Brain Res Rev 15(2):71–100, 1990

Edwards E, Harkins K, Wright G, et al: Effects of bilateral adrenalectomy on the induction of learned helplessness. Neuropsychopharmacology 3:109, 1990

Elliott E, Sapolsky R: Glucocorticoids, neurotoxicity and calcium regulation, in Neurosteroids and Brain Function. Edited by Costa E, Paul SM. New York, Thieme Medical Publishers, 1991, pp 47–51

Falls WA, Miserendino MJD, Davis M: Excitatory amino acid antagonists infused into the amygdala block extinction of fear-potentiated startle. Society for Neuroscience Abstracts 16:767, 1990

Foote SL, Bloom FE, Aston-Jones G: Nucleus locus coeruleus: new evidence for anatomical and physiological specificity. Physiol Rev 63:844–914, 1983

Glavin GB: Stress and brain noradrenaline: a review. Neurosci Biobehav Rev 9:233–243, 1985

Hemingway RB, Reigle TG: The involvement of endogenous opiate systems in learned and stress-induced analgesia. Psychopharmacology (Berlin) 93:353–357, 1987

Herman JP, Guilloneau PP, Dantzer R, et al: Differential effects of inescapable footshocks and of stimuli previously paired with inescapable footshocks on DA turnover in cortical and limbic areas of the rat. Science 23:1549–1556, 1982

Herman JP, Schafer MKH, Young EA, et al: Evidence for hippocampal regulation of neuroendocrine neurons of the hypothalamus-pituitary-adrenocortical axis. Neuroscience 9:3072–3082, 1984

Hitchcock JM, Davis M: The efferent pathway of the amygdala involved in conditioned fear as measured with the fear-potentiated startle paradigm. Behav Neurosci 105:826–842, 1991

Hitchcock JM, Sananes CB, Davis M: Sensitization of the startle reflex by footshock: blockade by lesions of the central nucleus of the amygdala or its efferent pathway to the brainstem. Behav Neurosci 103:509–518, 1989

Hyson RL, Ashcraft LJ, Drugan RC, et al: Extent and control of shock affects naltrexone sensitivity of stress-induced analgesia and reactivity to morphine. Pharmacol Biochem Behav 17:1019–1025, 1982

Ida Y, Tanaka M, Tsuda A, et al: Attenuating effect of diazepam on stress-induced increases in noradrenaline turnover in specific brain regions of rats: antagonism by Ro 15-1788. Life Sci 37:2491–2498, 1985

Irwin J, Ahluwalia P, Anisman H: Sensitization of norepinephrine activity following acute and chronic footshock. Brain Res 379:98–103, 1986

Iwata J, Chida K, LeDoux JE: Cardiovascular responses elicited by stimulation of neurons in the central amygdaloid nucleus in awake but not anesthetized rats resemble conditioned emotional responses. Brain Res 418:183–188, 1987

Jackson RL, Maier SF, Coon DJ: Long-term analgesic effects of inescapable shock and learned helplessness. Science 206:91–93, 1979

Kalivas PW, Duffy P: Similar effects of daily cocaine and stress on mesocorticolimbic dopamine neurotransmission in the rat. Biol Psychiatry 25:913–928, 1989

Kalivas PW, Duffy P, Abhold R, et al: Sensitization of mesolimbic dopamine neurons by neuropeptides and stress, in Sensitization in the Nervous System. Edited by Kalivas PW, Barnes CD. Caldwell, NJ, Telford Press, 1990, pp 119–124

Kant GJ, Eggleston T, Landman-Roberts L, et al: Habituation to repeated stress in stressor specific. Pharmacol Biochem Behav 22:631–634, 1985

Kant GJ, Leu JR, Anderson SM, et al: Effects of chronic stress on plasma corticosterone, ACTH and prolactin. Physiol Behav 40:775–779, 1987

Kinzie JD, Leung P: Clonidine in Cambodian patients with post traumatic stress disorder. J Nerv Ment Dis 177:546–550, 1989

Kolb LC: The post traumatic stress disorders of combat: a subgroup with a conditioned emotional response. Milit Med 149:237–243, 1984

Kolb LC: A theoretical model for planning treatment of post traumatic stress disorders of combat. Current Psychiatric Therapy 23:119–127, 1986

Kolb LC: A neuropsychological hypothesis explaining post traumatic stress disorders. Am J Psychiatry 144:989–995, 1987

Kolb LC: Chronic post traumatic stress disorder: implications of recent epidemiological and neuropsychological studies. Psychol Med 19:821–824, 1989

Kosten TR, Mason JW, Giller EL, et al: Sustained urinary norepinephrine and epinephrine elevation in posttraumatic stress disorder. Psychoneuroendocrinology 12:13–20, 1987

Kulka RA, Schlenger WE, Fairbank JA, et al: Trauma and the Vietnam War Generation. New York, Brunner/Mazel, 1990

LeDoux JE, Iwata J, Cicchetti P, et al: Different projections of the central amygdaloid nucleus mediate autonomic and behavioral correlates of conditioned fear. J Neurosci 8 (suppl 7):2517–2529, 1988

LeDoux JE, Romanski L, Xagoraris A: Indelibility of subcortical emotional memories. Journal of Cognitive Neuroscience 1:238–243, 1989

LeDoux JE, Cicchetti PO, Xagoris A, et al: The lateral amygdaloid nucleus: sensory interface of the amygdala in fear conditioning. J Neurosci 10:1062–1069, 1990

Levine ES, Litto WJ, Jacobs BL: Activity of cat locus coeruleus noradrenergic neurons during the defense reaction. Brain Res 531:189–195, 1990

Litz BT, Keane TM: Information processing in anxiety disorders: application to the understanding of post-traumatic stress disorder. Clinical Psychology Review 9:243–257, 1989

Maclennan AJ, Maier SF: Coping and stress induced potentiation of stimulant stereotype in the rat. Science 219:1091–1093, 1983

Madden J, Akil H, Patrick RL, et al: Stress-induced parallel changes in central opioid levels and pain responsiveness in the rat. Nature 265:358–360, 1977

Maier SF: Stressor controllability and stress-induced analgesia. Ann N Y Acad Sci 467:55–72, 1986

Majewska MD: Antagonist-type interaction of glucocorticoids with the GABA receptor-coupled chloride channel. Brain Res 418:377–382, 1987

Majewska MD, Harrison Nl Schwartz RD, et al: Steroid metabolites are barbiturate-like modulators of the GABA receptor. Science 232:1004–1007, 1986

Malloy PF, Fairbank JA, Keane TM: Validation of a multimethod assessment of posttraumatic stress disorders in Vietnam veterans. J Consult Clin Psychol 51:488–494, 1983

Mantz J, Thierry AM, Glowinski J: Effect of noxious tail pinch on the discharge rate of mesocortical and mesolimbic dopamine neurons: selective activation of the mesocortical system. Brain Res 476:377–381, 1989

Marshall JR: The treatment of night terrors associated with the posttraumatic syndrome. Am J Psychiatry 132:293–295, 1975

Mason JW: Psychoendocrine approaches in stress research, in Symposium of Medical Aspects of Stress in the Military Climate. Washington, DC, Walter Reed Army Institute of Research, U.S. Government Printing Office, 1965, pp 375–417

Mason JW, Giller EL, Kosten TR, et al: Urinary free cortisol levels in post traumatic stress disorder patients. J Nerv Ment Dis 174:145–149, 1986

Mason JW, Giller EL, Kosten TR, et al: Psychoendocrine approaches to the diagnosis and pathogenesis of posttraumatic stress disorder, in Biological Assessment and Treatment of Posttraumatic Stress Disorder. Edited by Giller E. Washington, DC, American Psychiatric Press, 1990, pp 65–86

McEwen BS, DeKloet ER, Rostene W: Adrenal steroid receptors and actions in the nervous system. Physiol Rev 66:1121–1188, 1986

McFall MF, Murburg MM, Ko GM, et al: Autonomic responses to stress in Vietnam veterans with post traumatic stress disorder. Biol Psychiatry 27:1165–1175, 1990

McGaugh JL: Involvement of hormonal and neuromodulatory systems in the regulation of memory storage. Annu Rev Neurosci 2:255–287, 1989

McGaugh JL: Significance and remembrance: the role of neuromodulatory systems. Psychological Science 1:15–25, 1990

McNally RJ, Luedke DL, Besyner JK, et al: Sensitivity to stress relevant stimuli in post traumatic stress disorder. Journal of Anxiety Disorders 1:105–116, 1987

Miserendino MJD, Sananes CB, Melia KR, et al: Blocking of acquisition but not expression of fear-potentiates startle by NMDA antagonists in the amygdala. Nature 345:716–718, 1990

Mishkin M, Appenzeller T: The anatomy of memory. Sci Am 256:80–89, 1987

Nisenbaum LK, Zigmund MJ, Sved AF, et al: Prior exposure to chronic stress results in enhanced synthesis and release of hippocampal norepinephrine in response to a novel stressor. J Neurosci 11:1478–1484, 1991

Pallmeyer TP, Blanchard EB, Kolb LC: The psychophysiology of combat-induced posttraumatic stress disorder in Vietnam veterans. Behav Res Ther 24:645–652, 1986

Perry BD, Giller EL, Southwick SM: Altered platelet alpha2 adrenergic binding sites in posttraumatic stress disorder. Am J Psychiatry 144:1511–1512, 1987

Petty F, Sherman AD: GABAergic modulation of learned helplessness. Pharmacol Biochem Behav 15:567–570, 1981

Pitman RK, Orr S: Twenty-four hour urinary cortisol and catecholamine excretion in combat-related posttraumatic stress disorder. Biol Psychiatry 27:245–247, 1990

Pitman RK, Orr SP, Forgue DF, et al: Psychophysiologic assessment of post-traumatic stress disorder in Vietnam combat veterans. Arch Gen Psychiatry 44:970–975, 1987

Pitman RK, van der Kolk BA, Orr SP, et al: Naloxone-reversible analgesic response to combat-related stimuli in posttraumatic stress disorder. Arch Gen Psychiatry 47:541–544, 1990

Rasmussen K, Marilak DA, Jacobs BL: Single unit activity of the locus coeruleus in the freely moving cat, I: during naturalistic behaviors and in response to simple and complex stimuli. Brain Res 371:324–334, 1986

Reaves ME, Hansen TE, Whisenand JM: The psychopharmacology of PTSD. VA Practitioner 6:65–72, 1989

Redmond DE Jr: Studies of the nucleus locus coeruleus in monkeys and hypotheses for neuropsychopharmacology, in Psychopharmacology: The Third Generation of Progress. Edited by Melzer HY. New York, Raven, 1987, pp 967–975

Rescola RA, Heth CD: Reinstatement of fear to extinguished conditioned stimulus. J Exp Psychol [Anim Behav] 104:88–96, 1975

Risse SC, Shitters A, Burke J, et al: Severe withdrawal symptoms after discontinuation of alprazolam in eight patients with combat-induced posttraumatic stress disorder. J Clin Psychiatry 51:206–209, 1990

Robinson TE, Angus AL, Becker JB: Sensitization to stress: the enduring effects of prior stress on amphetamine-induced rotational behavior. Life Sci 37:1039–1042, 1985

Rose RM: Overview of endocrinology of stress, in Neuroendocrinology and Psychiatric Disorder. Edited by Brown G. New York, Raven, 1984, pp 95–122

Rosen JB, Hitchcock JM, Sananes CB, et al: A direct projection from the central nucleus of the amygdala to the acoustic startle pathway: anterograde and retrograde tracing studies. Behav Neurosci 105:817–825, 1991

Roth RH, Tam S-Y, Ida Y, et al: Stress and the mesocorticolimbic dopamine systems. Ann N Y Acad Sci 537:138–147, 1988

Salloway S, Southwick S, Sadowsky M: Opiate withdrawal presenting as posttraumatic stress disorder. Hosp Community Psychiatry 41:666–667, 1990

Sapolsky RM, Plotsky PM: Hypercortisolism and its possible neural bases. Biol Psychiatry 27:937–952, 1990

Sapolsky R, Krey L, McEwen BS: Glucocorticoid-sensitive hippocampal neurons are involved in terminating the adrenocortical stress response. Proc Natl Acad Sci U S A 81:6174–6178, 1984a

Sapolsky R, Krey L, McEwen BS: Stress downregulates corticosterone receptors in a site specific manner in the brain. Endocrinology 114:287–293, 1984b

Sapolsky RM, Uno Hideo, Rebert CS, et al: Hippocampal damage associated with prolonged glucocorticoid exposure in primates. J Neurosci 10:2897–2902, 1990

Schwartz RD, Weiss MJ, Labarca R, et al: Acute stress enhances the activity of the GABA receptor–gated chloride inophore ion channel in brain. Brain Res 411:151–155, 1987

Shirao I, Tsuda A, Yoshisshige I, et al: Effect of acute ethanol administration on noradrenaline metabolism in brain regions of stressed and nonstressed rats. Pharmacol Biochem Behav 30:769–773, 1988

Simson PE, Weiss JM: Responsiveness of locus coeruleus neurons to excitatory stimulation is uniquely regulated by alpha-2 receptors. Psychopharmacol Bull 24:349–354, 1988b

Smith MA, Davidson J, Ritchie JC, et al: The corticotropin releasing hormone test in patients with post traumatic stress disorder. Biol Psychiatry 26:349–355, 1989

Solomon Z, Garb R, Bleich A, et al: Reactivation of combat-related posttraumatic stress disorder. Am J Psychiatry 144:51–55, 1987

Southwick SM, Krystal JH, Morgan CA, et al: Abnormal noradrenergic function in posttraumatic stress disorder. Arch Gen Psychiatry 50:266–274, 1993

Stuckey J, Marra S, Minor T, et al: Changes in opiate receptors following inescapable shock. Brain Res 476:167–169, 1989

Tanaka M, Kohnoy, Tsuda A, et al: Differential effects of morphine on noradrenaline release in brain regions of stressed and non-stressed rats. Brain Res 275:105–115, 1983

Teich AH, McCabe PM, Gentile CC, et al: Auditory cortex lesions prevent extinction of Pavlovian differential heart rate conditioning to tonal stimuli in rabbits. Brain Res 480:210–218, 1989

Thierry AM, Tassin JP, Blanc G, et al: Selective activation of the mesocortical DA system by stress. Nature 263:242–243, 1976

Tsaltas E, Gray JA, Fillenz M: Alleviation of response suppression to conditioned aversive stimuli by lesions of the dorsal noradrenergic bundle. Behav Brain Res 13:115–127, 1987

Tsuda A, Tanaka M: Differential changes in noradrenaline turnover in specific regions of rat brain produced by controllable and uncontrollable shocks. Behav Neurosci 99:802–817, 1985

Uno H, Tarara R, Else J, et al: Hippocampal damage associated with prolonged and fatal stress in primates. J Neurosci 9:1705–1711, 1989

Valentino RJ, Foote SL: Corticotropin-releasing hormone increases tonic but not sensory-evoked activity of noradrenergic locus coeruleus neurons in unanesthetized rats. J Neurosci 8:1016–1025, 1988

Van Dyke C, Zilberg NJ, MacKinnon JA: Posttraumatic stress disorder: a thirty-year delay in a World War II Veteran. Am J Psychiatry 142:1070–1073, 1985

Weizman R, Weizman A, Kook KA, et al: Repeated swim stress alters brain benzodiazepine receptors measured in vivo. J Pharmacol Exp Ther 249:701–707, 1989

Williams JL, Drugan RC, Maier SF: Exposure to uncontrollable stress alters withdrawal from morphine. Behav Neurosci 98:836–846, 1984

Woods SW, Charney DS, Silver JM, et al: Behavioral, biochemical and cardiovascular responses to benzodiazepine receptor antagonist flumazenil in panic disorder. Psychiatry Res 36 (suppl 2):115–124, 1991

Yehuda R, Southwick S, Nussbaum G, et al: Low urinary cortisol excretion in patients with post-traumatic stress disorder. J Nerv Ment Dis 178:366–369, 1990

Yehuda R, Lowy MT, Southwick SM, et al: Increased number of glucocorticoid receptors in post-traumatic stress disorder. Am J Psychiatry 144:499–504, 1991b

Yehuda R, Southwick S, Giller EL, et al: Urinary catecholamine excretion and severity of PTSD symptoms in Vietnam combat veterans. J Nerv Ment Dis 180:321–325, 1992

Yehuda R, Southwick SM, Krystal JH, et al: Enhanced suppression of cortisol following dexamethasone administration in posttraumatic stress disorder. Am J Psychiatry 150:83–86, 1993

Yokoo H, Tanaka M, Yoshida M, et al: Direct evidence of conditioned fear-elicited enhancement of noradrenaline release in the rat hypothalamus assessed by intracranial microdialysis. Brain Res 536:305–308, 1990

Section II

Peripheral Autonomic and Catecholamine Function in PTSD

Chapter 7

Psychophysiological Studies of Combat-Related PTSD: An Integrative Review

Miles E. McFall, Ph.D.
M. Michele Murburg, M.D.

There is growing evidence that posttraumatic stress disorder (PTSD) is an anxiety disorder with a unique psychological and physiological profile. Insomnia, irritability, exaggerated startle response, and other characteristics of autonomic hyperarousal have been described in early clinical reports of combat stress reaction in veterans of World War I and World War II (Grinker and Spiegel 1945; Kardiner 1941). Kardiner (1941) was so impressed by the heightened physiological arousal associated with combat-induced stress disorders that he formulated the term "physioneurosis" to describe the disturbance we now refer to as PTSD. Contemporary writers have likewise postulated that PTSD is fundamentally a psychophysiological disorder involving conditioned activation of the sympathetic nervous system (SNS) (Kolb 1987; van der Kolk et al. 1985). Recent research has identified psychophysiological correlates of PTSD symptoms in traumatically stressed veteran populations. In this chapter we review the conditioning model of PTSD and laboratory-based psychophysiological studies of combat veterans with PTSD.

CONDITIONING MODEL OF PTSD

A number of investigators have proposed that the core physiological symptoms of PTSD, such as exaggerated startle reaction, are etiologically based in classical conditioning (Dobbs and Wilson 1960; Gillespie 1942; Kardiner 1941; Kolb 1984). According to this model, unconditioned emotional, behavioral, and physiological responses to traumatically stressful situations become conditioned to otherwise neutral internal and external stimuli so that these conditioned stimuli come to elicit elements of the original "fight-flight" response, including SNS activation.

Keane et al. (1985) extended this formulation of PTSD to a two-factor learning model that invokes principles of both classical and instrumental conditioning. These authors proposed that traumatized individuals first develop a classically conditioned emotional and physiological response to stimuli associated with, or resembling, the original trauma. Through processes of stimulus generalization and higher-order conditioning, stimuli that more distantly resemble the original trauma may come to evoke the same conditioned response. Subsequently, instrumental learning of defensive behaviors takes place when avoidance of conditioned stimuli leads to a reinforcing reduction in anxiety. These avoidant strategies prevent the individual from becoming desensitized to trauma-related conditioned stimuli.

The conditioning theory of PTSD has generated several testable hypotheses. Specifically, it has been hypothesized that individuals with PTSD are more physiologically reactive to reminders of their traumatic experiences than to trauma-unrelated cues. Moreover, research subjects with PTSD would be expected to differ from control subjects in the magnitude and duration of their conditioned responses to memory-evoking stimuli that resemble traumatic events.

PSYCHOPHYSIOLOGICAL STUDIES OF PTSD

A number of controlled experimental investigations have examined the physiological reactivity of PTSD subjects to trauma-related and trauma-unrelated laboratory stressors. These studies have been reviewed in detail elsewhere (see Kolb 1987; McFall et al. 1989; Orr 1990). We present here an updated, integrative summary of 10 published studies that measured psychophysiological responses in combat veterans with PTSD. The data presented have been compiled from the results of the following studies:

Boudewyns and Hyer (1990); Blanchard et al. (1982); Blanchard et al. (1986); Dobbs and Wilson (1960); Gerardi et al. (1989); Malloy et al. (1983); McFall et al. (1990b); Pallmeyer et al. (1986); Pitman et al. (1987); and Pitman et al. (1990).

Heart rate, systolic blood pressure (SBP), and diastolic blood pressure (DBP) were the physiological variables most consistently measured across these investigations. Weighted averages were calculated for these variables by multiplying the mean for the variables in each investigation by the corresponding sample size, and then dividing the sum of these products for these investigations by the total number of subjects. Data were tabulated for three groups of research subjects. The first group, *PTSD subjects,* included veterans with a formal DSM-III/DSM-III-R diagnosis (American Psychiatric Association 1980, 1987) of combat-related PTSD made by structured interviews and psychometric criteria (three studies), structured interviews alone (four studies), and unstructured clinical interview observation (two studies). Also included in this sample was one study (Dobbs and Wilson 1960) of subjects with some symptoms of combat neurosis identified by unspecified psychiatric assessment methods prior to the development of DSM-III. The *"normal"* group refers to subjects who do not have PTSD or other mental disorders.[1] Finally, the *psychiatric* group consists of veterans with various mental disorders other than PTSD.

BASELINE LEVELS OF AROUSAL

Results from the aforementioned studies are pertinent not only to the question of whether PTSD subjects show predicted phasic physiological changes in response to psychologically meaningful stimuli, but also to the question of whether these subjects differ from control subjects in tonic, or resting, levels of autonomic arousal. Correspondingly, weighted means for baseline measurements were calculated from the studies that reported these data and are presented in Table 7–1.

---

[1] It is unknown whether subjects in the group of psychiatric patients without PTSD had been exposed to noncombat forms of traumatic stress.

The PTSD group had notably higher resting heart rate, SBP, and DBP than did the asymptomatic normal control subjects. These differences continued to be evident even when PTSD subjects were compared with the subgroup of normal subjects within the sample who had been exposed to combat stress (combat-exposed normals: heart rate = 69.1 [n = 101]; SBP = 115.3 [n = 19]; DBP = 63.2 [n = 19]). Subjects with PTSD showed only slightly greater elevations in basal heart rate than did psychiatric patients without PTSD. Differences between these patient groups might be expected to be small, because several of the psychiatric group patients had anxiety and affective disorders that share many clinical features in common with PTSD and that are known to be associated with heightened autonomic arousal. Moreover, patients in the psychiatric control group may have been exposed to noncombat forms of trauma or abuse that could have induced subclinical PTSD not detected during subject selection procedures.

When supplemental analyses were performed, PTSD subjects differed substantially from the subgroup of psychiatric control patients who had been exposed to combat (heart rate = 70.1 [n = 14] for psychiatric control subjects). It is unclear why the differences between subjects with PTSD and combat-exposed control subjects, both normal and with psychiatric disorders, were greater for some variables than the differences between PTSD and control subjects not exposed to combat. Methodological differences across settings and the small samples studied to date

Table 7–1.   Baseline physiological arousal

	Measure		
Subject group	Heart rate (beats per minute)	SBP (mmHg)	DBP (mmHg)
PTSD	77.3 (n = 151)	125.0 (n = 39)	72.4 (n = 28)
Normal subjects	68.3 (n = 134)	119.4 (n = 37)	66.3 (n = 26)
Psychiatric subjects (without PTSD)	74.9 (n = 32)	—[a]	—

Note.   SBP = systolic blood pressure; DBP = diastolic blood pressure.
[a]No data are available.

prohibit any definitive statements regarding this finding. It is possible that individuals with lower basal autonomic arousal may be less vulnerable to developing PTSD symptoms after exposure to combat stress. Another possible explanation is that some subjects respond to combat stress by inhibiting or suppressing the usual SNS responses. Differences in the type, duration, and controllability of the stressors may also influence the physiological response pattern, as suggested by animal studies (see Charney et al., Chapter 6; Simson and Weiss, Chapter 3, this volume).

RESPONSE TO TRAUMA-RELATED EXPERIMENTAL STRESSORS

Analog paradigms of stress induction have been employed to test the hypothesis that subjects with PTSD are more reactive than control subjects to psychologically meaningful reminders of combat. In these studies, subjects were exposed to a variety of combat-related stimulus modalities, including sounds of combat, audiovisual film clips of combat, and personalized images of combat experiences presented under experimenter guidance.

The change from baseline scores for PTSD subjects, normal subjects, and psychiatric control subjects is shown in Table 7–2.

Table 7–2. Physiological response during exposure to combat cues: mean change from baseline

	Measure		
Subject group	Heart rate (beats per minute)	SBP (mmHg)	DBP (mmHg)
PTSD	12.9 ($n = 181$)	9.71 ($n = 39$)	4.1 ($n = 10$)
Normal subjects	2.0 ($n = 134$)	−1.5 ($n = 37$)	−1.2 ($n = 8$)
Psychiatric subjects (without PTSD)	1.2 ($n = 27$)	—[a]	—

Note. Values represent mean change from baseline. SBP = systolic blood pressure; DBP = diastolic blood pressure.
[a]No data are available.

Only PTSD subjects showed substantial increases in heart rate, SBP, and DBP in response to trauma-related analog stimuli. Examination of the subgroup of combat-exposed normal subjects ($n = 101$) reveals that they responded only minimally to experimental stressors (changes in heart rate = 2.5; SBP = –1.5; DBP = –1.2). The combat-exposed psychiatric control subgroup ($n = 9$) also showed a comparatively small change from baseline (change in heart rate = 3.0). Thus it appears that PTSD, rather than combat exposure per se, is uniquely associated with increased autonomic response to psychologically meaningful reminders of war stress. It is noteworthy that psychiatric patients without PTSD did not react to these stimuli, despite the fact that they had resting heart rates nearly equivalent to those of PTSD subjects.

RESPONSE TO TRAUMA-UNRELATED EXPERIMENTAL STRESSORS

In many of the studies reviewed, subjects were presented with combat-unrelated forms of experimental stress, such as mental arithmetic, guided imagery of nonmilitary stressful situations (e.g., public speaking), and films of unpleasant, anxiety-provoking situations (e.g., automobile accidents). These experimental conditions were included to determine if PTSD subjects respond specifically to trauma-related reminders, as conditioning theory predicts, or if they are overly reactive to diverse forms of stress, even those unrelated to their traumatic experiences.

The change from baseline in terms of weighted means for the three study groups is shown in Table 7–3. Subjects in all comparison groups reacted to trauma-unrelated stressors with elevated heart rate, SBP, and DBP. However, PTSD subjects did not differ significantly from control subjects in their response to these experimental stressors. Thus, consistent with conditioning models of PTSD, subjects with PTSD did not exhibit a generalized stress reaction to all forms of experimental stress. Rather, the physiological response of PTSD subjects was most pronounced to stimuli of traumatic wartime events specifically, and these subjects were the only experimental group to show substantial increases in autonomic arousal from these stressors. Comparison of Tables

7–2 and 7–3 reveals that PTSD subjects exposed to combat stimuli manifested heart rate and blood pressure changes that were approximately twice as large as those in response to noncombat stressor stimuli.

ADDITIONAL FINDINGS

A number of additional findings were reported in the research reviewed. Keane et al. (1987) noted that multivariate discriminant analyses using physiological variables classify PTSD and non-PTSD criterion groups at high rates of accuracy (80% to 100%). However, many of these results reflect overall "hit rates" that combine classification of PTSD subjects correctly identified as having the disorder (i.e., sensitivity) with control subjects correctly identified as not having the disorder (i.e., specificity). In studies in which specificity and sensitivity data were reported, rather than overall "hit rates" alone, physiological variables were consistently shown to be more accurate in identifying "true negative" cases (specificity) than "true positive" cases (sensitivity). In the six investigations for which this breakdown was available, data for sensitivity and specificity, respectively, were as follows: sensitivity = 61%, 67%, 70%, 71%, 72%, 91%; specificity = 100%, 86%, 88%, 100%, 89%, 100%.

Table 7–3. Psychological response during exposure to noncombat stress: mean change from baseline

	Measure		
Subject group	Heart rate (beats per minute)	SBP (mmHg)	DBP (mmHg)
PTSD	5.0 ($n = 136$)	4.7 ($n = 21$)	2.4 ($n = 28$)
Normal subjects	6.5 ($n = 96$)	6.4 ($n = 18$)	0.9 ($n = 7$)
Psychiatric subjects (without PTSD)	3.8 ($n = 25$)	—[a]	—

Note. Values represent mean change from baseline. SBP = systolic blood pressure; DBP = diastolic blood pressure.
[a]No data are available.

Evaluation of these outcomes should be compared with the probability of correct classification of PTSD versus non-PTSD status resulting from chance alone, which is 50%. The relatively modest sensitivity of physiological variables as diagnostic criteria argues for caution in relying on physiological reactivity measures to diagnose individual cases of PTSD. This caveat is buttressed by the finding of Gerardi et al. (1989) that veterans without PTSD were capable of fabricating a physiological response to combat cues that was similar to the veridical response of actual PTSD subjects.

In a particularly elegant study, Pitman et al. (1987) reported that PTSD subjects were more physiologically aroused by images of individualized traumatic combat experiences than by standardized images of combat events prepared by the investigators. It is interesting to note, however, that the diagnostic sensitivity (61%) and specificity (100%) in classifying PTSD and control subjects using physiological responses to these personalized images were not superior to the classification results obtained in studies that simply used standard combat sounds.

One study reported that PTSD subjects remained physiologically hyperaroused during recovery periods following exposure to combat cues, but not after combat-unrelated stress (McFall et al. 1990b; see also Murburg et al., Chapter 9, this volume). It is possible that PTSD subjects may be distinguished not only by the magnitude of their responses to combat-related stimuli but also by the duration of their responses to such material. One explanation for this result is that exposure to analog combat stimuli activated distressing war-related memories that persisted into the recovery periods. Empirical studies using content analysis are necessary to determine whether subjects have continued intrusive thoughts of trauma-related experiences during poststimulus periods (see Horowitz et al. 1973). Alternatively, it is possible that mechanisms that normally terminate autonomic response to stressors may be impaired in PTSD patients.

Researchers are beginning to examine the correspondence between degree of heightened physiological responsiveness of PTSD subjects and clinical symptomatology of the disorder. Pitman et al. (1987) found moderate correlations between the intrusion subscale of the Impact of Event Scale and heart rate ($r = .47$), skin conductance ($r = .68$), and electromyogram (EMG) ($r = .74$). It has also been reported that increased physiological arousal (heart rate, SBP, DBP, and epinephrine) when subjects were exposed to combat films was accompanied by corresponding increases from baseline in negative mood states as measured by an adjective checklist (McFall et al. 1990b; see also Murburg et al., Chapter 8, this volume). Finally, in a recent study, Orr et al. (1990) used heart rate, skin conductance, and EMG responsiveness (i.e., physiological responsivity) to calculate the probability of subject assignment to a PTSD condition rather than to non-PTSD control groups. This index of physiological responsivity was found to be moderately correlated with various psychometric scales of PTSD symptomatology ($r = .50$ to $.64$). Although causal inferences cannot be made from these correlational findings, such findings are useful in understanding the relationship between physiological changes and associated fluctuations in the subjective and phenomenological aspects of PTSD.

CONCLUSIONS

Excessive SNS activation has been emphasized in formulations of trauma-induced stress disorders throughout modern history. In this chapter we reviewed the evidence to date from psychophysiological studies of PTSD that measured heart rate and blood pressure as indices of autonomic arousal. PTSD subjects show baseline levels of autonomic arousal that are considerably greater than those of normal control subjects, but the former are not clearly distinct from psychiatric patients with mental disorders other than PTSD. Subjects with PTSD, normal subjects, and psychiatric control subjects without PTSD respond similarly when exposed to combat-unrelated laboratory stressors. However, when presented with combat-related experimental cues, only PTSD subjects show a pronounced autonomic response that is specific to these cues. PTSD, rather than combat exposure per se, is the variable associated with heightened tonic and phasic physiological activation. These findings are consistent with the conditioning hypothesis of excessive SNS activation in PTSD. However, it is also possible that suppression of parasympathetic nervous system function contributes to these findings. This research also supports the discriminant and construct validity of the PTSD diagnosis by demonstrating that biological parameters of the disorder respond to experimental manipulations in a predicted manner. Attempts to utilize physiological indices as diagnostic markers for PTSD have been only moderately successful and show greater accuracy in identifying persons who do not have the disorder than in identifying those who do.

The external validity of these findings was supported by their robust replication across diverse experimental settings that employed a variety of stress-induction methodologies and control conditions. However, the results are specific to Vietnam combat veterans (only one study employed veterans from other wars) and require replication with other traumatized populations. From these studies, it is impossible to determine whether the increased autonomic activity of PTSD subjects is a manifestation of their psychiatric disorder, or whether it predated their traumatic experiences and perhaps contributed to the development of PTSD. This question can be answered only by prospective, longitudinal studies that assess autonomic functioning in a population of individuals at risk for exposure to traumatic stress of a specific type and duration.

A number of methodological principles should be considered in future investigations of the psychophysiology of PTSD. Selection of research samples of combat veterans with PTSD is hampered by the high incidence of comorbid diagnoses within this population, particularly depression, substance use disorders, and other anxiety disorders (Kulka et al. 1988). Some of these comorbid disorders are associated with alterations in catecholamine function (Belmaker et al. 1988) and may obscure our ability to attribute the findings of physiological studies to PTSD alone. Because it is difficult, though not impossible, to find cases of PTSD without comorbidity, it is important to match psychiatric comparison groups for the same disorders that are present in PTSD study samples. Only 3 of the 10 studies reviewed here reported what comorbid diagnoses were present in the PTSD samples. In future research, all Axis I mental disorders should be routinely assessed, using structured interviews such as the Structured Clinical Interview for DSM-III-R (SCID; Spitzer et al. 1989).

Psychiatrically normal control groups have been used to provide an absolute standard of comparison to judge "deviant" or "pathological" physiological responses of psychiatrically disordered subjects, including veterans with PTSD. Asymptomatic normal subjects control for the nonspecific, contextual factors associated with having a mental disorder (e.g., the disruption of being hospitalized, the stress of being psychiatrically ill and the associated psychosocial hardship, etc.). However, the inclusion of normal control subjects in experimental designs does not allow us to attribute observed experimental effects specifically to a diagnosis of PTSD as opposed to some other disorder. This interpretive problem underscores the importance of including in study designs psychiatric control subjects who do not have PTSD and who are matched with PTSD subjects for comorbid diagnoses. Matching PTSD and control groups regarding the degree of combat exposure will engender confidence that findings are attributable to PTSD rather than to traumatic stress exposure per se.

Ideally, the method for establishing a diagnosis of PTSD will employ multiple indicators of PTSD symptomatology. Standardized diagnostic interviews such as the SCID can be used to establish a categorical diagnosis of PTSD. Additionally, several psychometric instruments permit assessment of combat trauma and PTSD symptoms on a continuum of severity. The Revised Combat Scale has become a standardly used, well-validated instrument to assess degree of combat exposure (Gallops et al. 1981; Watson et al. 1989). Reliable and valid measures for scaling symptom severity include the Fairbank-Keane MMPI PTSD subscale (Fairbank et al. 1983), the Mississippi Scale for Combat-Related PTSD (Keane et al. 1988; McFall et al. 1990a), and the Impact of Event Scale (Zilberg et al. 1982). These measures correlate moderately with one another and with SCID interview methods of assessment (McFall et al. 1990c). Use of these measurements for selecting study samples of PTSD subjects promotes standardization of procedures across settings and comparability of results. Moreover, the dimensional scaling afforded by these instruments allows for correlational analyses with biological variables of interest.

In psychophysiological studies of PTSD it is important to take into consideration such factors as time of day, body weight, physical activity around the time of the study, and use of substances (prescribed and illicit) that can influence SNS functioning. Of the 10 studies reviewed, only 4 reported that subjects were medication free. In the remaining studies, it was unspecified whether or not subjects were taking medications or were influenced by medication withdrawal effects. It is also important to indicate in research reports whether subjects are lying down or sitting up at the time of assessment, because this variable alters catecholamine output (Henriksen and Skagen 1986) as well as heart rate and blood pressure. Subjects should be drug and alcohol free for at least 2 weeks prior to the study. Abstinence from caffeine and nicotine for 12 hours before the experimental procedure helps standardize the effects of these variables across studies, but persons habitually using more than small amounts of caffeine and nicotine should be excluded from study, because abstinence symptoms attending discontinuation of these substances may influence the variables of interest. Attention to these methodological issues in future psychophysiological research in PTSD should help ensure the validity of findings and minimize interpretative difficulties.

REFERENCES

American Psychiatric Association: Diagnostic and Statistical Manual of Mental Disorders, 3rd Edition. Washington, DC, American Psychiatric Association, 1980

American Psychiatric Association: Diagnostic and Statistical Manual of Mental Disorders, 3rd Edition, Revised. Washington, DC, American Psychiatric Association, 1987

Belmaker RH, Sandler, M, Dahlastrom A: Progress in Catecholamine Research, Part C: Clinical Aspects. New York, AR Liss, 1988

Blanchard EB, Kolb LC., Pallmeyer TP, et al: Psychophysiological study of post traumatic stress disorder in Vietnam veterans. Psychiatr Q 54:220–229, 1982

Blanchard EB, Kolb LC, Gerardi RJ, et al: Cardiac response to relevant stimuli as an adjunctive tool for diagnosing post-traumatic stress disorder in Vietnam veterans. Behavior Therapy 24:645–652, 1986

Boudewyns PA, Hyer L: Physiological response to combat memories and preliminary treatment outcome in Vietnam veteran PTSD patients treated with direct therapeutic exposure. Behavior Therapy 21:63–87, 1990

Dobbs D, Wilson WP: Observations on persistence of war neurosis. Diseases of the Nervous System 21:686–691, 1960

Fairbank JA, Keane TM, Malloy PF: Some preliminary data on the psychological characteristics of Vietnam veterans with post-traumatic stress disorders. J Consult Clin Psychol 51:912–919, 1983

Gallops M, Laufer RS, Yager T: Revised combat scale, in Legacies of Vietnam: Comparative Adjustments of Veterans and Their Peers, Vol 3. Edited by Laufer RS, Yager T, Frey-Wouters E., et al. Washington, DC, U.S. Government Printing Office, 1981, p 125

Gerardi RJ, Blanchard EB, Kolb LC: Ability of Vietnam veterans to dissimulate a psychophysiological assessment for post-traumatic stress disorder. Behavior Therapy 20:229–243, 1989

Gillespie RD: Psychological Effects of War on Citizen and Soldier. New York, WW Norton, 1942

Grinker RR, Spiegel JP: Men Under Stress. Philadelphia, PA, Blakiston, 1945

Henriksen O, Skagen K: Local and central sympathetic vasoconstrictor reflexes in human limbs during orthostatic stress, in The Sympathoadrenal System: Physiology and Pathophysiology. Edited by Christensen JN, Henriksen O, Larsen NA. New York, Raven, 1986, pp 83–94

Horowitz MJ, Becker SS, Malone P: Stress: different effects on patients and nonpatients. J Abnorm Psychol 82:547–551, 1973

Kardiner A: The Taumatic Neuroses of War. New York, Harper & Row, 1941

Keane TM, Zimering RT, Caddell JM: A behavioral formulation of post traumatic stress disorder in Vietnam veterans. Behavior Therapist 8:9–12, 1985

Keane TM, Wolfe J, Taylor KL: Post-traumatic stress disorder: evidence for diagnostic validity and methods of psychological assessment. J Clin Psychol 43:32–43, 1987

Keane TM, Caddell JM, Taylor KL: Mississippi Scale for Combat-Related Post-traumatic Stress Disorder. J Consult Clin Psychol 56:85–90, 1988

Kolb LC: The post traumatic stress disorders of combat: a subgroup with a conditioned emotional response. Milit Med 149:237–243, 1984

Kolb LC: A neuropsychological hypothesis explaining post-traumatic stress disorders. Am J Psychiatry 144:989–995, 1987

Kulka RA, Schlenger WE, Fairbank JA, et al: Contractual report of findings from the National Vietnam Veterans Readjustment Study, Vol I: executive summary, description of findings, and technical appendices. Research Triangle Park, NC, Research Triangle Institute, 1988

Malloy PF, Fairbank JA, Keane TM: Validation of a multimethod assessment of post-traumatic stress disorders in Vietnam veterans. J Consult Clin Psychol 51:488–494, 1983

McFall ME, Murburg MM, Roszell DK, et al: Psychophysiologic and neuroendocrine findings in post-traumatic stress disorder: a review of theory and research. Journal of Anxiety Disorders 3:243–257, 1989

McFall ME, Smith DE, Mackay PW, et al: Reliability and validity of the Mississippi Scale for Combat-Related Post-traumatic Stress Disorder. Psychological Assessment: A Journal of Consulting and Clinical Psychology 2:114–121, 1990a

McFall ME, Murburg MM, Ko GN, et al: Autonomic responses to stress in Vietnam combat veterans with post-traumatic stress disorder. Biol Psychiatry 27:1165–1175, 1990b

McFall ME, Smith DE, Roszell DK, et al: Convergent validity of measures of PTSD in Vietnam combat veterans. Am J Psychiatry 147:645–648, 1990c

Orr SP: Psychophysiologic studies of posttraumatic stress disorder, in Biological Assessment and Treatment of Posttraumatic Stress Disorder. Edited by Giller EL Jr. Washington, DC, American Psychiatric Association, 1990, pp 135–157

Pallmeyer TP, Blanchard EB, Kolb LC: The psychophysiology of combat-induced post-traumatic stress disorder in Vietnam veterans. Behav Res Ther 24:645–652, 1986

Pitman RK, Orr SP, Forgue DF, et al: Psychophysiologic assessment of post-traumatic stress disorder imagery in Vietnam combat veterans. Arch Gen Psychiatry 44:970–975, 1987

Pitman RK, Orr SP, Forgue DF, et al: Psychophysiologic responses to combat imagery of Vietnam veterans with post-traumatic stress disorder versus other anxiety disorders. J Abnorm Psychol 99:49–54, 1990

Spitzer RL, Williams JBW, Gibbon M, et al: Instruction Manual for the Structured Clinical Interview for DSM-III-R (SCID, 5-1-89 Revision). New York, New York State Psychiatric Institute, 1989

van der Kolk BA, Greenberg M, Boyd H, et al: Inescapable shock, neurotransmitters, and addiction to trauma: toward a psychobiology of post traumatic stress. Biol Psychiatry 20:314–325, 1985

Watson CG, Juba MP, Anderson PED: Validities of five combat scales. Psychological Assessment: A Journal of Consulting and Clinical Psychology 1:98–102, 1989

Zilberg JJ, Weiss DS, Horowitz MJ: Impact of Event Scale: a cross-validation study and some empirical evidence supporting a conceptual model of stress response syndromes. J Consult Clin Psychol 50:407–414, 1982

Chapter 8

Basal Sympathoadrenal Function in Patients With PTSD and Depression

M. Michele Murburg, M.D.
Miles E. McFall, Ph.D.
Richard C. Veith, M.D.

Clinical evidence suggests that central and peripheral noradrenergic function, including activity of the sympathetic nervous system (SNS), may be altered in posttraumatic stress disorder (PTSD). Historically, symptoms of anxiety and autonomic instability, including tremor, tachycardia, and elevated blood pressure, have been observed clinically in the veterans of a number of wars (DaCosta 1871; Hartshorne 1863; Wenger 1948). Currently, hypervigilance, exaggerated startle response, difficulty concentrating, irritability, and physiological reactivity to stimuli resembling the trauma are among the DSM-III-R criteria for diagnosing PTSD (American Psychiatric Association 1987).

A number of laboratory findings suggest that SNS activity may be altered in PTSD. Psychophysiological studies have reported increased resting heart rate in patients with PTSD compared with control subjects (Blanchard et al. 1982, 1986; Gerardi

This research was supported by Career Development (MMM) and Merit Review (RCV) Awards from the Department of Veterans Affairs, and by a National Institutes of Health Biomedical Support Grant administered through the University of Washington School of Medicine (MEM). The skillful technical assistance of David Flatness, David Federighi, Nancy Lewis, and Susan Loewen is appreciated.

et al. 1989; Pallmeyer et al. 1986; Pitman et al. 1987) and other patient groups (Pallmeyer et al. 1986). In addition, neuroendocrine studies of traumatized populations and of PTSD patients have found increased catecholamine levels in 24-hour urine collections from these groups (Davidson and Baum 1986; Kosten et al. 1987). Perry et al. (1987) reported a decreased number of alpha$_2$ (α_2)–adrenergic receptor binding sites on platelets of PTSD patients, suggesting increased circulating levels of norepinephrine and/or epinephrine in patients with this disorder. Our group has described a greater release of epinephrine in response to trauma-relevant stressful stimuli than to trauma-irrelevant stressful stimuli in PTSD, and greater and longer-lasting increases in arterialized plasma epinephrine levels after exposure to trauma-relevant stressful stimuli in PTSD patients than in control subjects (McFall et al. 1990; see also Murburg et al., Chapter 9, this volume).

A number of basic neurobiological studies relevant to PTSD also suggest that SNS function may be altered by stress (see Murburg et al. 1990 for review). Animal studies show that acute inescapable stress may increase activity in some central norepinephrine nuclei, including the locus coeruleus (LC), with subsequent norepinephrine depletion, and may produce behaviors similar to those seen in depression (Anisman 1978; Kvetnansky et al. 1977; Lehnert et al. 1984; Nakagawa et al. 1981; Palkovits et al. 1975; Stone 1975; Weiss et al. 1970, 1980; see also Simson and Weiss, Chapter 3, this volume). Similar changes also occur in some central epinephrine nuclei (Kvetnansky et al. 1978; Saavedra et al. 1984). With chronic inescapable stress, synthesis and release of central norepinephrine and epinephrine in many brain areas appear to increase, and the number of ß-adrenergic receptors decreases (Axelrod et al. 1970; Kvetnansky et al. 1977; Musacchio et al. 1969). Peripheral epinephrine and norepinephrine are also released in response to acute stress (Kvetnansky and Mikulaj 1970; Kvetnansky et al. 1977, 1984). With chronic stress, arterial plasma catecholamine levels are high (Kvetnansky et al. 1984), and peripheral norepinephrine turnover rate remains elevated, while norepinephrine reuptake is decreased (see Stone 1975 for review).

Although many of these studies describe alterations in central, as opposed to peripheral, catecholaminergic systems following different types of stress, it has recently been discovered that central and peripheral norepinephrine effector systems may be activated in parallel (see Aston-Jones et al., Chapter 2, this volume). Central (i.e., LC) and peripheral (i.e., SNS) stress-responsive norepinephrine effector systems are coordinately controlled by the nucleus paragigantocellularis (PGi) in the rostral ventral medulla (Aston-Jones and Ennis 1988; Aston-Jones et al. 1990; Chiang and Aston-Jones 1989; Elam et al. 1985, 1986; Reiner 1986; see also Aston-Jones et al., Chapter 2, this volume). Among the neurochemical mediators of this parallel activation may be corticotropin-releasing factor (CRF), a neuropeptide produced by the hypothalamus and other areas of the CNS that is released in response to stress. When centrally applied, CRF increases SNS activity (Brown et al. 1985; Swanson et al. 1983) and increases neuronal firing in the LC (Valentino 1989).

Interpretation of the above-mentioned studies is complicated by a number of factors. First, the applicability of many animal models of stress response to human PTSD is far from straightforward (see Zacharko, Chapter 5; Yehuda and Antelman, Comment, this volume). Second, not all human studies suggest that basal SNS function is altered in PTSD. Some studies have reported no differences in resting heart rate between PTSD patients and control subjects (Dobbs and Wilson 1960; Malloy et al. 1983), and other studies have reported no differences in resting heart rate between PTSD patients and other groups of psychiatric patients (Malloy et al. 1983; Pitman et al. 1990). Neuroendocrine studies of PTSD patients have also included mixed findings: one group of investigators has reported that 24-hour urine levels of catecholamines in PTSD patients were not different from those in combat-exposed control subjects (Pitman and Orr 1990). Third, the measures used in the human studies cited above have some methodological features that limit their interpretation (see Veith and Murburg, Chapter 16, this volume). Heart rate is an indirect indicator of SNS function, because it is influenced so prominently by parasympathetic input. Neuroendocrine studies investigating SNS function in PTSD by measuring urinary catecholamine output (Kosten et al. 1987; Pitman and Orr 1990) have not been specifically designed to detect tonic as opposed to phasic increases in sympathoadrenal activity. Studies that have included patients with comorbid psychiatric conditions in the PTSD group may be confounded by the presence of disorders, such as major depressive disorder, that are known to alter SNS function (Barnes et al. 1983; Louis et al. 1975; Rudorfer et al. 1985; Veith et al. 1988, in press). Thus, the question of whether patients with PTSD have tonically increased levels of sympathoadrenal activity remains unanswered.

The goal of the present study was to evaluate basal sympathoadrenal function in PTSD patients by measuring levels of norepinephrine and epinephrine in arterialized plasma, as well as heart rate and blood pressure, to determine whether basal sympathoadrenal activity in this population differs from that expected of healthy, asymptomatic control subjects. Our hypothesis was that PTSD patients would have increased resting levels of SNS activity, resulting in increased resting pulse rate and blood pressure, as well as increased release of norepinephrine and epinephrine into plasma by sympathetic nerves and the adrenal medulla. As a result, basal plasma levels of norepinephrine and epinephrine were expected to be increased in PTSD patients compared with normal control subjects. Because major depression is a frequent comorbid condition in PTSD, and because increased SNS activity occurs in patients with major depression, particularly in those who are dexamethasone-resistant (presumably those with hyperactivity of the hypothalamic-pituitary-adrenal [HPA] axis) (Barnes et al. 1983; Louis et al. 1975; Rudorfer et al. 1985; Veith et al. 1988, in press), we segregated our patients in this study according to the presence or absence of major depression.

METHODS

Subjects

The sample consisted of 18 Vietnam veterans undergoing treatment for PTSD at the VA Medical Center or the Vietnam Veterans Outreach Center in Seattle. Nine patients were recruited from the Inpatient Psychiatry Service, and the remaining nine were outpatients. Fifteen subjects were white, one was Mexican-American, one was Native American, and one was mixed Eskimo-American. The mean age for the sample was 41.1 years. Control subjects ($n = 16$) were asymptomatic nonpatient volunteers who responded to an advertisement. Fifteen subjects were white, and one was black. Control subjects had an average age of 40.1 years. PTSD subjects and control subjects averaged 116% and 106%, respectively, of ideal body weight, as defined by the 1983 Metropolitan Life Insurance Tables. All subjects were physically healthy, having no diagnosable medical conditions. Participants abstained from alcohol and illicit drug use for at least 2 weeks, and had not taken psychotropic medications or other medications known to alter plasma catecholamine levels for at least 4 weeks prior to the study. Finally, subjects habitually used three or fewer cups of caffeinated beverages per day and abstained entirely from caffeine, nicotine, and food ingestion for 12 hours before the procedure began.

All subjects were screened using the Structured Clinical Interview for DSM-III-R (Patient Version) (SCID; Spitzer et al. 1987). PTSD patients also exceeded published cutoff scores for combat veterans diagnosed with PTSD on the Revised Combat Scale (Gallops et al. 1981), the Mississippi Scale for Combat-Related PTSD (Keane et al. 1988), and the Impact of Event Scale (Zilberg et al. 1982). In order to be included in the study, PTSD subjects had to meet DSM-III-R criteria for PTSD by the SCID, while control subjects could not meet criteria for PTSD or other mental disorder by SCID. Current comorbid diagnoses for the PTSD sample were as follows: major depression ($n = 9$); major depression in partial remission ($n = 3$); dysthymia ($n = 3$); bipolar disorder, depressed ($n = 1$); generalized anxiety disorder ($n = 2$); obsessive-compulsive disorder ($n = 1$); social phobia ($n = 2$); and adjustment disorder ($n = 1$). Ten subjects also had a history of substance use disorder that had been in remission for at least 4 weeks prior to the study.

Procedure

All patients gave written informed consent. Participants remained supine throughout the study. An 18- or 19-gauge intravenous catheter was inserted into a superficial vein on the dorsum of one hand, which was placed in a warming box at 60°C to arterialize the venous blood. Normal saline containing 1,000 U sodium heparin per 500 cc was infused at a rate sufficient to maintain patency of the catheter and to replace blood volume removed.

Subjects rested for 30 minutes after the intravenous catheter was properly operating. After this initial rest period, blood samples were drawn via the catheter, and assessments of vital signs were made at 10-minute intervals over a 30-minute baseline period (at 0, 10, 20, and 30 minutes), beginning at 1:00 P.M. Plasma samples for norepinephrine and epinephrine were collected in prechilled glass tubes containing EGTA and reduced glutathione, and placed on ice until prompt centrifugation at 4°C. Plasma was then stored at −70°C until assay. Heart rate and blood pressure were measured using an automated ultrasonic detector (Dinamap, Critikon, Tampa, Florida).

Circulating levels of norepinephrine and epinephrine were measured in arterialized forearm venous plasma (see Veith and Murburg, Chapter 16, this volume, for a more in-depth discussion of this technique). We have demonstrated in previous studies that forearm venous plasma arterialized by our method contains norepinephrine concentrations that are 94% of simultaneous peripheral arterial concentrations (Veith et al. 1984), thus providing a better indicator of systemic SNS activity than would venous blood, which is more prominently influenced by local factors (Best and Halter 1982, 1985). At each sampling time, a 10-ml sample of arterialized blood was collected in a prechilled glass tube containing EGTA and reduced glutathione, and placed on ice until centrifugation at 4°C. Plasma was then stored at −70°C until assay. Plasma norepinephrine and epinephrine concentrations were measured using a single-isotope enzymatic assay (Evans et al. 1978), and duplicate determinations were made for each sample. The interassay coefficient of variation for the plasma catecholamine assay in this laboratory is 6.5% in the >300 pg/ml range, and 12% in the 100 pg/ml range. The intraassay coefficient of variation is less than 5%. Statistical evaluations were performed using the Kruskal-Wallis one-way analysis of variance.

RESULTS

As shown in Table 8–1, PTSD patients with and without current full-syndrome major depression did not differ significantly from each other or from control subjects in measures of SNS function. Although the number of subjects was small, the expected increases in basal heart rate, blood pressure, and plasma catecholamine levels in patients with PTSD, particularly those with comorbid major depressive disorder, were clearly not found in this study.

DISCUSSION

The results of this study do not provide obvious support for the hypothesis that combat veterans with PTSD have higher basal levels of sympathoadrenal activity than do normal control subjects. Our finding that resting heart rate and blood pressure were equivalent for the three groups is in apparent conflict with the findings of five studies to date that did report higher heart rates and blood pressure in PTSD patients than in other groups. How-

Table 8–1. Means/standard deviations and probability values for physiological variables

Measure	PTSD alone ($n = 9$) mean	PTSD + MDD ($n = 9$) mean	Control ($n = 16$) mean	P^a
Heart rate (beats per minute)	63.3 ± 8.2	63.2 ± 8.0	61.4 ± 8.7	NS
Systolic BP (mmHg)	121.2 ± 5.8	124.4 ± 11.6	118.5 ± 8.1	NS
Diastolic BP (mmHg)	77.9 ± 7.8	79.9 ± 6.1	73.8 ± 7.0	NS
Norepinephrine (pg/ml)	231.6 ± 44.4	196.8 ± 67.8	249.2 ± 86.1	NS
Epinephrine (pg/ml)	66.5 ± 37.2	54.2 ± 29.0	76.4 ± 33.8	NS

Note. MDD = major depressive disorder; BP = blood pressure.
[a]Two-tailed *P*; NS = not significant.

ever, our finding is consistent with the findings of two other studies that reported no significant group differences (see McFall et al. 1989 for review). It is possible that an explanation for the differences in findings among these studies may be found in the different waiting periods used to allow subjects to achieve a true baseline.

Studies reporting predicted differences in vital signs between PTSD patients and normal control subjects typically allowed subjects to rest for between 3 and 12 minutes before heart rate and blood pressure were measured. Such a brief rest period may not have been long enough to allow patients to reach their true basal levels. Indeed, our previous study indicated that Vietnam combat veterans with PTSD continued to display elevations in heart rate, blood pressure, and plasma epinephrine levels 30 minutes after they finished viewing a film of scenes of the Vietnam War (McFall et al. 1990; see also Murburg et al., Chapter 9, this volume). In the present study, patients were allowed to rest for 30 minutes prior to baseline measurements being taken. This longer waiting period may have allowed our PTSD patients to arrive at a level of SNS functioning that more accurately reflected their true basal state.

The lack of significant differences between basal epinephrine and norepinephrine plasma levels in PTSD patients and normal control subjects in the present study may be consistent with Pitman and Orr's (1990) negative findings for urinary epinephrine and norepinephrine, although their group used asymptomatic combat veterans as control subjects, whereas our control group consisted of combat-naive normal subjects. Our findings are in apparent conflict with those of Kosten et al. (1987), who found higher urinary output of norepinephrine and epinephrine in PTSD patients than in other groups of psychiatric patients. However, plasma and urinary measurements of catecholamines obviously represent different physiological processes. A measurement of norepinephrine and epinephrine in a 24-hour urine collection provides an index of the amount of unmetabolized catecholamines cleared by the kidney following both tonic and phasic release by the sympathoadrenal system over a full day. Many variables, including current and recent administration of a variety of drugs, posture, physical activity level, dietary status, smoking, and affective state throughout the sampling period, can influence the net measurement. In contrast, measurement of catecholamines in arterialized plasma taken from calm, resting subjects whose diet, physical activity, and pharmacological status have been controlled represents a net balance, at a particular point in time, between the rate of release of catecholamines into plasma by sympathetic nerves and the adrenal, and the rate of removal of catecholamines from plasma by neuronal reuptake and metabolism and by the kidneys. It has previously been shown that resting plasma norepinephrine levels correlate closely with direct measurements of peripheral sympathetic nerve activity in humans and that these measures are reproducible within individuals over periods of months to years (Wallin 1981).

Research to date consistently shows that PTSD patients experience phasic increases in sympathoadrenal activity that distinguish them from asymptomatic control subjects and from other psychiatric patient groups. These phasic increases may be provoked by exposure of the patients to trauma-related stimuli. In contrast, the present study, together with some of the research cited earlier in this chapter, suggests that levels of tonic or basal SNS activity in PTSD patients may not differ from levels found in control subjects. Even in the presence of a syndrome meeting criteria for the diagnosis of comorbid major depression, PTSD patients in this study showed no evidence of basal SNS hyperactivity. Our data further suggest that the syndrome of major depression seen as a comorbid complication of PTSD may differ in important biological aspects from primary major depression. Further clarification of the biological differences between the syndromal depression complicating PTSD and primary major depression is critical to increasing our understanding of the pathophysiology and treatment of both disorders.

REFERENCES

American Psychiatric Association: Diagnostic and Statistical Manual of Mental Disorders, 3rd Edition, Revised. Washington, DC, American Psychiatric Association, 1987

Anisman H: Neurochemical changes elicited by stress: behavioral correlates, in Psychopharmacology of Aversively Motivated Behavior. Edited by Anisman H, Bignami G. New York, Plenum, 1978, pp 119–171

Aston-Jones G, Ennis M: Sensory-evoked activation of locus coeruleus may be mediated by a glutamate pathway from the rostral ventrolateral medulla, in Frontiers in Excitatory Amino Acid Research. Edited by Cavalheiro A, Lehman J, Turski L. New York, AR Liss, 1988, pp 471–478

Aston-Jones G, Shipley MT, Ennis M, et al: Restricted afferent control of locus coeruleus neurons revealed by anatomic, physiologic and pharmacologic studies, in The Pharmacology of Noradrenaline in the Central Nervous System. Edited by Marsden CA, Heal DJ. Oxford, UK, Oxford University Press, 1990, pp 187–247

Axelrod J, Mueller RA, Henry JP, et al: Changes in enzymes involved in the biosynthesis and metabolism of noradrenaline and adrenaline after psychosocial stimulation. Nature 225:1059–1060, 1970

Barnes RF, Veith RC, Borson S, et al: High levels of plasma catecholamines in dexamethasone-resistant depressed patients. Am J Psychiatry 140:1623–1625, 1983

Best JD, Halter JB: Release and clearance rates of epinephrine in man: importance of arterial measurements. J Clin Endocrinol Metab 55:263–268, 1982

Best JD, Halter JB: Blood pressure and norepinephrine spillover during propranolol infusion in man. Am J Physiol 248:R400-R406, 1985

Blanchard EB, Kolb LC, Pallmeyer TP, et al: A psychophysiological study of posttraumatic stress disorder in Vietnam veterans. Psychiatr Q 54:220–229, 1982

Blanchard EB, Kolb LC, Gerardi RJ, et al: Cardiac response to relevant stimuli as an adjunctive tool for diagnosing post-traumatic stress disorder in Vietnam veterans. Behavior Therapy 17:592–606, 1986

Brown MR. Fishcr LA, Webb V, et al: Corticotropin-releasing factor: a physiologic regulator of adrenal epinephrine secretion. Brain Res 328:355–357, 1985

Chiang C, Aston-Jones G: Microinjection of lidocaine, GABA or synaptic decouplers into the ventrolateral medulla blocks sciatic-evoked activation of locus coeruleus. Society for Neuroscience Abstracts 15:1012, 1989

DaCosta JM: On irritable heart: a clinical study of a form of functional cardiac disorder and its consequences. Am J Med Sci 61:17–52, 1871

Davidson LM, Baum A: Chronic stress and post traumatic stress disorders. J Consult Clin Psychol 54:303–308, 1986

Dobbs D, Wilson WP: Observations on the persistence of war neurosis. Diseases of the Nervous System 21:686–691, 1960

Elam M, Svensson TH, Thorén P: Differentiated cardiovascular afferent regulation of locus coeruleus neurons and sympathetic nerves. Brain Res 358:77–84, 1985

Elam M, Svensson TH, Thorén P: Locus coeruleus neurons and sympathetic nerves: activation by cutaneous sensory afferents. Brain Res 366:254–261, 1986

Evans MI, Halter JB, Porte D Jr: Comparisons of double- and single-isotope enzymatic derivative methods for measuring catecholamines in human plasma. Clin Chem 24:567, 1978

Gallops M, Laufer RS, Yager T: Revised combat scale, in Legacies of Vietnam: Comparative Adjustments of Veterans and Their Peers, Vol 3. Edited by Laufer RS, Yager T, Frey-Wouters E., et al. Washington, DC, U.S. Government Printing Office, 1981, p 125

Gerardi RJ, Blanchard DB, Kolb LC: Ability of Vietnam veterans to dissimulate a psychophysiological assessment for post-traumatic stress disorder. Behavior Therapy 20:229–243, 1989

Hartshorne H: On heart disease in the Army. Am J Med Sci 47:89–92, 1863

Keane TM, Caddell JM, Taylor KL: Mississippi Scale for Combat-Related Post-traumatic Stress Disorder. J Consult Clin Psychol 56:85–90, 1988

Kosten TR, Mason JW, Giller EL, et al: Sustained urinary norepinephrine and epinephrine elevation in post-traumatic stress disorder. Psychoneuroendocrinology 12:13–20, 1987

Kvetnansky R, Mikulaj L: Adrenal and urinary catecholamines in rats during adaptation to repeated immobilization stress. Endocrinology 87:738–743, 1970

Kvetnansky R, Palkovits M, Mitro A, et al: Catecholamines in individual hypothalamic nuclei of acutely and repeatedly stressed rats. Neuroendocrinology 23:257–267, 1977

Kvetnansky R, Kopin IJ, Saavedra JM: Changes in epinephrine in individual hypothalamic nuclei after immobilization stress. Brain Res 155:387–390, 1978

Kvetnansky R, Nemeth S, Vigas M, et al: Plasma catecholamines in rats during adaptation to intermittent exposure to different stressors, in Stress: The Role of Catecholamines and Other Neurotransmitters, Vol 1. Edited by Usdin E, Kvetnansky R, Axelrod J. New York, Gordon & Breach Science Publishers, 1984, pp 537–562

Lehnert H, Reinstein DK, Wurtman RJ: Tyrosine reverses the depletion of brain norepinephrine and the behavioral deficits caused by tail-shock stress in rats, in Stress: The Role of Catecholamines and Other Neurotransmitters, Vol 1. Edited by Usdin E, Kvetnansky R, Axelrod J. New York, Gordon & Breach Science Publishers, 1984, pp 81–91

Louis WJ, Doyle AE, Anavekar SN: Plasma noradrenaline concentration and blood pressure in essential hypertension, phaeochromocytoma and depression. Clinical Science and Molecular Medicine 48:239s–242s, 1975

Malloy PF, Fairbank JA, Keane TM: Validation of a multimethod assessment of post-traumatic stress disorders in Vietnam veterans. J Consult Clin Psychol 51:488–494, 1983

McFall ME, Murburg MM, Roszell DK, et al: Psychophysiologic and neuroendocrine findings in posttraumatic stress disorder: a review of theory and research. Journal of Anxiety Disorders 3:243–257, 1989

McFall ME, Murburg MM, Ko GN, et al: Autonomic responses to stress in Vietnam combat veterans with posttraumatic stress disorder. Biol Psychiatry 27:1165–1175, 1990

Murburg MM, McFall ME, Veith RC: Catecholamines, stress, and post-traumatic stress disorder, in Biological Assessment and Treatment of Posttraumatic Stress Disorder. Edited by Giller EL Jr. Washington, DC, American Psychiatric Press, 1990, pp 27–64

Musacchio JM, Julou L, Kety SS, et al: Increase in rat brain tyrosine hydroxylase activity produced by electroconvulsive shock. Proc Natl Acad Sci U S A 63:1117–1119, 1969

Nakagawa R, Tanaka M, Kohnoy, et al: Regional responses of rat brain noradrenergic neurones to acute intense stress. Pharmacol Biochem Behav 14:729–732, 1981

Palkovits M, Kobayashi RM, Kizer JS, et al: Effects of stress on catecholamines and tyrosine hydroxylase activity of individual hypothalamic nuclei. Neuroendocrinology 18:144–153, 1975

Pallmeyer TP, Blanchard EB, Kolb LC: The psychophysiology of combat-induced post-traumatic stress disorder in Vietnam veterans. Behav Res Ther 24:645–652, 1986

Perry BD, Southwick SM, Giller EL Jr: Altered platelet alpha2-adrenergic receptor affinity states in posttraumatic stress disorder. Am J Psychiatry 144:1511–1512, 1987

Pitman RK, Orr SP: Twenty-four hour urinary cortisol and catecholamine excretion in combat-related post-traumatic stress disorder. Biol Psychiatry 27:245–247, 1990

Pitman RK, Orr SP, Forgue DF, et al: Psychophysiologic assessment of posttraumatic stress disorder imagery in Vietnam combat veterans Arch Gen Psychiatry 44:970–975, 1987

Pitman RK, Orr SP, Forgue DF, et al: Psychophysiologic responses to combat imagery of Vietnam veterans with post-traumatic stress disorder versus other anxiety disorders. J Abnorm Psychol 99:49–54, 1990

Reiner PB: Correlational analysis of central noradrenergic neuronal activity and sympathetic tone in behaving cats. Brain Res 378:86–96, 1986

Rudorfer MV, Ross RJ, Linnoila M, et al: Exaggerated orthostatic responsivity of plasma norepinephrine in depression. Arch Gen Psychiatry 42:1186–1192, 1985

Saavedra JM, Fernandez-Pardal J, Torda T, et al: Dissociation between rat hypothalamic and brainstem PNMT after stress and between hypothalamic catecholamines and PNMT after midbrain hemitransection, in Stress: The Role of Catecholamines and Other Neurotransmitters, Vol 1. Edited by Usdin E, Kvetnansky R, Axelrod J. New York, Gordon & Breach Science Publishers, 1984, pp 137–146

Spitzer RL, Williams JBW, Gibbon M: Structured Clinical Interview for DSM-III-R—Patient Version (SCID-P, 4-1-87 revision). New York, New York State Psychiatric Institute, 1987

Stone EA: Stress and catecholamines, in Catecholamines and Behavior, II: Neuropsycho-pharmacology. Edited by Friedhoff AJ. New York, Plenum, 1975, pp 31–72

Swanson LW, Sawchenko PE, Rivier J, et al: Organization of ovine corticotropin-releasing factor immunoreactive cells and fibers in the rat brain: an immunohistochemical study. Neuroendocrinology 36:165–186, 1983

Valentino R: Corticotropin-releasing factor: putative neurotransmitter in the noradrenergic nucleus locus ceruleus. Psychopharmacol Bull 25:306–311, 1989

Veith RC, Best JD, Halter B: Dose-dependent suppression of norepinephrine appearance rate in plasma by clonidine in man. J Clin Endocrinol Metab 59:151–155, 1984

Veith RC, Barnes RF, Villacres EC, et al: Plasma catecholamines and norepinephrine kinetics in depression and panic disorder, in Catecholamines: Clinical Aspects. Edited by Belmaker R. New York, AR Liss, 1988, pp 197–202

Veith RC, Lewis N, Linares OA, et al: Sympathetic nervous system activity in major depression: basal and desipramine-induced alterations in plasma norepinephrine kinetics. Arch Gen Psychiatry (in press)

Wallin BG: Sympathetic activity in human extremity nerves and its relationship to plasma norepinephrine, in Norepinephrine. Edited by Ziegler MG, Lake CR. Baltimore, MD, Williams & Wilkins, 1984, pp 431–449

Weiss JM, Stone EA, Harrell NW: Coping behavior and brain norepinephrine level in rats. Journal of Comparative and Physiological Psychology 72:153–160, 1970

Weiss JM, Bailey WH, Pohorecky LA, et al: Stress-induced depression of motor activity correlates with regional changes in brain norepinephrine but not in dopamine. Neurochem Res 5:9–23, 1980

Wenger MA: Studies of autonomic balance in Army Air Force personnel. Comparative Psychology Monographs 19 (ser no 101):1–111, 1948

Zilberg JJ, Weiss DS, Horowitz MJ: Impact of event scale: a cross-validation study and some empirical evidence supporting a conceptual model of stress response syndromes. J Consult Clin Psychol 50:407–414, 1982

Chapter 9

Stress-Induced Alterations in Plasma Catecholamines and Sympathetic Nervous System Function in PTSD

M. Michele Murburg, M.D.
Miles E. McFall, Ph.D.
Grant N. Ko, M.D.
Richard C. Veith, M.D.

Some investigators (Keane et al. 1985; Kolb 1987; see also McFall and Murburg, Chapter 7, this volume, for review) have hypothesized that the increased physiological reactivity to trauma-relevant stimuli seen in posttraumatic stress disorder (PTSD) is due to conditioned activation of the sympathetic nervous system (SNS). According to this model, unconditioned emotional, behavioral, and physiological responses to life-threatening situations become conditioned to otherwise neutral internal and external stimuli so that these conditioned stimuli come to elicit elements of the original "fight-flight" response, including increased SNS activation. To date, a number of studies have

This research was supported by National Institutes of Health Biomedical Support Grant No. 507RR0543-26 administered through the University of Washington School of Medicine. Additional support was provided by a Career Development Award (MMM) from the Veterans Administration (VA), by the Veterans Administration Medical Center Geriatric Research Education and Clinical Center, and by the Research Service of the VA. An earlier version of this paper, with much of the same data, appeared in *Biological Psychiatry* 27:1165–1175, 1990, and is used with permission. The skillful technical assistance of David Flatness, David Federighi, and Nancy Lewis is appreciated.

tested this hypothesis in combat veterans with PTSD using paradigms in which autonomic responses to combat-related stimuli were measured (see McFall and Murburg, Chapter 7, for review). These studies have generally found that PTSD patients displayed greater increases in heart rate and blood pressure than did normal or psychiatric control groups in response to trauma-relevant stimuli (Blanchard et al. 1982, 1986; Malloy et al. 1983; Pitman et al. 1987). Time-dependent sensitization has been proposed as an alternative explanation for this autonomic hyperresponsiveness. According to this model, stress exposure causes biological changes that result in sensitization of autonomic and behavioral responses to subsequent exposure to related stimuli (see Antelman and Yehuda, Chapter 4; Charney et al., Chapter 6; Rausch et al., Chapter 14, this volume).

Neuroendocrine studies investigating peripheral catecholamine function in traumatized populations and PTSD patients have reported increased heart rate, blood pressure, and urinary norepinephrine and epinephrine levels, and reduced number of platelet alpha$_2$ (α_2)–adrenergic binding sites in these subjects compared with control subjects (Davidson and Baum 1986; Kosten et al. 1987; Perry et al. 1988). Although suggesting that net SNS activity may be increased following trauma, these studies have not been designed to discriminate tonic changes in SNS activity from phasic changes that might occur in response to trauma-related stimuli. In the current study we measured changes in emotional state, heart rate, blood pressure, and plasma catecholamine levels in response to combat-related and combat-unrelated stressors in combat veterans with PTSD and in control subjects. We hypothesized that combat veterans with PTSD would show greater physiological and emotional responses to the combat-related stressor, but not to the combat-unrelated stressor, than would control subjects.

METHODS

Subjects

Ten Vietnam veterans with PTSD and 14 control subjects participated. All subjects were males who were free from diagnosable medical illness. The subjects had abstained from alcohol and all drugs for at least 2 weeks prior to participation and for at least 4 weeks prior to study had not taken psychotropic drugs or medications that are known to alter plasma catecholamine levels. All subjects abstained from caffeine, nicotine, and nourishment (except for ad libitum water) for 12 hours before the procedure began.

The PTSD patients were combat veterans who met DSM-III-R criteria (American Psychiatric Association 1987) for PTSD by the Structured Clinical Interview for DSM-III-R (SCID; Spitzer et al. 1987). These patients exceeded published cutoff scores on tests (see Table 9–1) that had previously been found to identify high levels of combat exposure and PTSD in a large percentage of veterans (Keane et al. 1988; Laufer et al. 1981; Zilberg et al. 1982). Other Axis I disorders in this group were diagnosed based on the patient version of the SCID (SCID-P; Spitzer et al. 1987). Comorbid diagnoses included major depression (40%); major depression in partial remission (30%); dysthymia (30%); bipolar disorder, depressed (10%); generalized anxiety disorder (20%);

Table 9–1. Characteristics of subjects

	PTSD	Control
n	10	14
Mean age	40.5	39.6
Mean % of ideal body weight	117	111
Length of combat (months)	11.4	4.7[a]
Mean CES	12	7.7[a]
Mean SCID PTSD score	11	3.6[a]
Mean MSCR PTSD score	121.3	69[a]
Mean IES score		
Intrusion subscale	25	10[a]
Avoidance subscale	23.8	12[a]
Current comorbidity (mean number of diagnoses/person)	1.8	0.2

Note. CES = Combat Exposure Scale; SCID = Structured Clinical Interview for DSM-III-R; IES = Impact of Event Scale; MSCR = Mississippi Scale for Combat, Revised.
[a]Values given are for the three Vietnam combat veterans in this sample.

obsessive-compulsive disorder (10%); social phobia (20%); and adjustment disorder (10%). Nine subjects had a history of substance use disorder that had been in remission for at least 2 weeks prior to the study. The literature to date indicates that presence of psychiatric conditions other than PTSD does not influence psychophysiological response to combat-related laboratory stressors (McFall et al. 1989; see also McFall and Murburg, Chapter 7, this volume).

Control subjects were two Vietnam combat veterans with psychiatric disorders other than PTSD, one asymptomatic Vietnam combat veteran without PTSD, four military veterans without combat exposure (three of whom were free from psychiatric disorder and one of whom had a mild simple phobia), and seven nonveterans without mental disorder.

Stimulus Materials

The experimental stressors consisted of two 10-minute narrated videotapes depicting combat-unrelated and combat-related situations, respectively. The combat-unrelated stressor film showed the aftermath of serious automobile accidents, while the combat stressor film consisted of combat footage taken during the Vietnam War. In a previous study using similar techniques (Malloy et al. 1983), the majority of subjects with PTSD became so upset when viewing war-related films that they were unable to complete the experiment. Therefore, to ensure that subjects would view both films, and to prevent possible carry-over effects from the combat film to the automobile film, the latter was administered before the combat film in every case in the present study.

Procedure

Subjects were admitted individually to the Special Studies Unit at the Seattle VA Medical Center at noon. Participants remained in a supine position throughout the study. An intravenous (iv) catheter was inserted in the dorsum of the hand or wrist to permit repeated nontraumatic blood sampling. The catheterized hand was then placed in a warming box at 60°C to arterialize the venous blood. Subjects rested for 30 minutes after the iv catheter was properly operating, and then baseline blood samples, mood state assessments (affect ratings), and vital sign measurements were performed every 10 minutes for 30 minutes.

The automobile accident film was then shown to subjects. Vital signs were measured five times, at 2-minute intervals, during viewing, and blood samples were drawn 5 and 10 minutes after the film began. Affect ratings were completed immediately after the film ended. The film was followed by a 30-minute recovery period, during which five measurements of vital signs were made at 2-minute intervals followed by two more measurements at 10-minute intervals. Blood samples were drawn 5, 10, 20, and 30 minutes after the film ended. Affect ratings were obtained again at the end of the recovery period. Subjects rested for another 30 minutes and then had vital signs and affect ratings measured and blood drawn to determine whether the variables had returned to baseline levels. The sequence of assessments for each variable during the combat film and subsequent recovery phase was identical to that described for the automobile film and recovery period. Thirty minutes after the combat film recovery phase had elapsed, final measurements of vital signs and affect ratings were made, and blood samples were obtained.

Dependent Measures

Affect ratings consisted of assessments of subjects' mood state that were made using self-ratings of 17 descriptive adjectives on a 5-point scale indicating the extent to which subjects experienced each affect "now." A total score (possible range 0–68) was calculated for the 17 adjectives at each time point. Blood pressure and heart rate were measured using an automated ultrasonic detector (Dinamap, Critikon, Tampa, Florida).

Circulating levels of norepinephrine and epinephrine were measured in arterialized forearm venous plasma, as described in Murburg et al., Chapter 8, this volume.

RESULTS

Data were consolidated to establish a single score for each variable during each of the following assessment intervals: baseline, automobile stress film, automobile film recovery, precombat film rest, combat film, combat film recovery, and end. Subjects' consolidated scores for a particular period represented an average of the individual measurements made during that period, with the exception of the precombat film rest and end periods, during which only one measurement was made. The means (± SEM) for dependent measures during each assessment period are presented in Table 9–2.

Comparisons Between PTSD and Control Subjects

Mann-Whitney tests were performed to evaluate the statistical significance of comparisons between PTSD and control subjects. One-tailed probability values were used to test hypothesized directional contrasts, and two-tailed values were applied to comparisons for which no directional hypotheses were formulated. Difference from baseline score was calculated for all dependent variables, and between-group comparisons were made for each experimental period.

During the automobile film, PTSD subjects reported significantly greater subjective emotional arousal than did control subjects ($Z = -2.26$, $P < 0.03$). However, this greater affective arousal in PTSD subjects compared with control subjects was not accompanied by significant elevations in vital signs or in plasma catecholamines. During the recovery period following the automobile film, PTSD patients did not differ significantly from control subjects.

During the pre–combat film rest interval, PTSD subjects had higher heart rates than did control subjects ($Z = -2.17$; $P < 0.03$) but did not differ significantly from control subjects on any other measure. The combat film evoked significantly greater heart rate ($Z = -2.87$, $P < 0.002$), diastolic blood pressure ($Z = -2.58$, $P < 0.005$), affect raftings ($Z = -3.25$, $P < 0.006$), and plasma epinephrine ($Z = -1.76$, $P < 0.04$), but not systolic blood pressure or plasma norepinephrine responses, in PTSD subjects than in control subjects.

During the post–combat film recovery period, PTSD patients continued to show elevated affect ratings ($Z = -2.73$, $P < 0.003$), heart rate ($Z = -1.70$, $P < 0.04$), systolic blood pressure ($Z = -2.14$,

Table 9–2. Results: affect ratings, vital signs, and plasma catecholamines

Experimental period	AR	HR	SBP	DBP	NE	EPI
PTSD subjects						
Baseline	12.1 ± 3.1	63.2 ± 2.2	124.0 ± 3.6	78.5 ± 2.6	244.0 ± 15.5	70.4 ± 10.2
Automobile film (Δ)[a]	10.2 ± 2.1	1.6 ± 1.0	2.7 ± 1.4	1.4 ± 0.6	−11.0 ± 14.6	3.1 ± 5.2
Automobile recovery (Δ)	−2.5 ± 2.3	1.4 ± 0.9	1.3 ± 2.4	0.9 ± 0.9	−12.2 ± 14.3	8.2 ± 6.7
Rest (Δ)	−1.7 ± 1.6	3.0 ± 1.8	0.8 ± 2.4	−0.8 ± 1.5	3.0 ± 14.1	5.6 ± 7.3
Combat film (Δ)	23.7 ± 3.7	6.8 ± 1.8	5.9 ± 2.6	4.1 ± 1.1	11.5 ± 17.4	15.1 ± 7.1
Combat recovery (Δ)	11.4 ± 3.7	4.5 ± 1.2	6.7 ± 2.2	4.5 ± 1.5	0.3 ± 14.6	24.6 ± 4.2
End/Rest (Δ)	8.5 ± 5.1	5.9 ± 2.2	2.9 ± 2.6	2.6 ± 1.9	−0.9 ± 2.1	35.1 ± 13.8
Control subjects						
Baseline	4.8 ± 1.0	63.0 ± 3.0	121.5 ± 2.8	7.5 ± 1.9	229.7 ± 21.4	76.5 ± 9.7
Automobile film (Δ)	4.4 ± 1.5	1.2 ± 1.1	2.2 ± 2.1	0.3 ± 1.4	14.6 ± 118	4.5 ± 5.5
Automobile recovery (Δ)	−1.2 ± 0.5	0.7 ± 0.7	0.8 ± 1.7	−0.4 ± 1.4	−6.7 ± 9.0	0.6 ± 6.6
Rest (Δ)	−1.1 ± 0.4	−1.4 ± 1.0	4.2 ± 2.3	1.0 ± 1.8	1.0 ± 10.1	−2.2 ± 8.5
Combat film (Δ)	6.2 ± 1.4	0.6 ± 1.1	2.6 ± 2.2	0.6 ± 1.3	−10.4 ± 9.0	−8.3 ± 7.8
Combat recovery (Δ)	0.3 ± 0.6	2.3 ± 1.2	0.9 ± 2.1	0.6 ± 1.5	−3.8 ± 10.8	−6.1 ± 7.4
End/Rest (Δ)	0.6 ± 1.0	1.1 ± 1.1	5.3 ± 2.6	1.9 ± 1.6	−6.5 ± 17.8	5.5 ± 9.7

Note. AR = affect ratings; DBP = diastolic blood pressure (mmHg); EPI = plasma epinephrine (pg/ml); HR = heart rate (beats per minute); NE = plasma norepinephrine (pg/ml); SBP = systolic blood pressure (mmHg).
[a] Δ indicates change from baseline level.

$P < .016$), diastolic blood pressure ($Z = -2.58$, $P < .005$), and plasma epinephrine ($Z = -3.02$, $P < 0.0125$), but not plasma norepinephrine. One hour after the combat film had ended, PTSD subjects continued to show significantly greater increases in heart rate than did control subjects ($Z = -2.17$, $P < 0.03$), but were comparable to control subjects on all other measures.

Comparisons Within Subject Groups

Wilcoxon signed rank tests were performed to evaluate statistical significance of comparisons between experimental conditions for each subject group. These comparisons determined whether subjects within each group responded differentially to the two experimental stressors.

PTSD subjects. For PTSD subjects, viewing the automobile film was accompanied by an increase only in systolic blood pressure ($Z = 1.78$, $P < 0.05$), diastolic blood pressure ($Z = -1.78$, $P < 0.05$), and affect ratings ($Z = -2.80$, $P < 0.01$) compared with baseline. The recovery phase following the automobile film was not associated with significant changes in any measurement relative to baseline.

The combat film evoked significant increases in heart rate ($Z = 2.80$, $P < 0.01$), systolic blood pressure ($Z = 1.89$, $P < 0.05$), diastolic blood pressure ($Z = 2.45$, $P < 0.01$), epinephrine ($Z = 2.19$, $P < 0.05$), and affect ratings ($Z = -2.80$, $P < 0.01$). During the recovery phase following the combat film, PTSD subjects continued to exhibit increased affect ratings ($Z = -2.42$, $P < 0.01$), heart rate ($Z = -2.50$, $P < 0.01$), systolic blood pressure ($Z = 2.19$, $P < 0.05$), diastolic blood pressure ($Z = 2.34$, $P < 0.01$), and plasma epinephrine ($Z = 2.70$, $P < 0.01$). At the final assessment, PTSD subjects continued to have increased heart rate ($Z = -2.31$, $P < 0.01$) and plasma epinephrine ($Z = -2.37$, $P < 0.01$) compared with baseline. PTSD subjects reacted more strongly to the combat film than to the auto film, with significantly higher affect ratings ($Z = 2.67$, $P < 0.01$), heart rate ($Z = 2.80$, $P < 0.01$), and diastolic blood pressure ($Z = -1.84$, $P < 0.05$). Plasma epinephrine was also higher in PTSD subjects during the combat film than during the automobile film, but this difference did not quite achieve significance (Z = 1.60, $P < .05$). Similarly, the group showed significantly greater elevations in affect ratings (Z = 2.80, $P < 0.01$), heart rate (Z = 2.24, $P < 0.05$), systolic blood pressure (Z = -1.99, $P < 0.05$), diastolic blood pressure (Z = 1.88, $P < 0.05$), and plasma epinephrine (Z = 1.89, $P < 0.05$) during the combat film recovery interval than during the automobile film recovery interval.

Control subjects. Control subjects exhibited increased affect ratings relative to baseline (Z = -2.27, $P < .01$), but exhibited no increases in measures of physiological arousal in response to the automobile accident film. During the recovery period following the automobile film, control subjects actually had lower affect rating scores than at baseline (Z = -2.09, $P < 0.04$). The combat film evoked a significant increase only in affect ratings (Z = -3.18, $P < 0.002$) in control subjects. No significant differences between baseline and either the post–combat film recovery period or the end of study assessment were found for any variable. Comparisons between control subjects' responses to the automobile film versus the combat film and to the automobile recovery period versus the combat recovery period showed only a significantly greater epinephrine response to the automobile film (Z = -2.04, $P < 0.02$).

DISCUSSION

The results of this study indicate that exposure to combat-related laboratory stimuli is associated with increased emotional distress and autonomic activation in Vietnam combat veterans with PTSD. This autonomic activation is manifested by increased arterialized plasma levels of epinephrine, as well as by elevated heart rate, systolic blood pressure, and diastolic blood pressure. The pattern of emotional and autonomic responses exhibited by veterans with PTSD differed from that of control subjects, who showed minimal changes in autonomic functioning during exposure to combat-related stimuli. Moreover, the increases in plasma epinephrine and other indices of SNS activity in PTSD subjects were more pronounced in response to the combat-related stressor than to the combat-unrelated stressor, whereas control subjects showed a greater epinephrine response to the automobile film. These findings are consistent with previous psycho-physiological studies in which PTSD subjects have been found to exhibit relatively greater autonomic responsiveness to trauma-specific cues (McFall et al. 1989; see also McFall and Murburg, Chapter 7, this volume), and lend support to the hypothesis that conditioning and sensitization may play roles in the pathophysiology of PTSD.

These findings are also quite interesting in light of the discussion by Aston-Jones et al. (Chapter 2, this volume) of locus coeruleus (LC) responses to meaningful cues in nonhuman primates. The combat film would of course be expected to be more "meaningful" than the auto accident film to combat veterans with PTSD, whereas for control subjects the automobile film would have represented a more directly meaningful stressful situation. Because greater increases in plasma epinephrine occurred in response to the combat film in PTSD patients and in response to the automobile film in control subjects, it is possible that sympathoadrenal as well as LC activation occurs selectively in response to psychologically or physiologically meaningful stressors in humans. The lack of an increase in control subjects' plasma epinephrine levels in response to the combat film (which caused a level of emotional distress simliar to that caused by the automobile film) suggests that the increase in plasma epinephrine in response to stressor exposure is not due solely to affective arousal.

In this study, measurements of autonomic activity in PTSD subjects remained elevated and in fact reached their highest levels during the recovery period following the combat film. Several subjects spontaneously reported that viewing the combat film activated distressing war-related memories that persisted into the recovery period. These memories may have served as repeated stressors, which in turn would have continued to activate the sympathoadrenal system. Consistent with this possibility, other investigators (Horowitz et al. 1973) have documented increased emotional distress and preoccupation with intrusive thoughts subsequent to exposure to films with stressful content. It is also possible, however, that mechanisms which normally terminate sympathoadrenal response to stressors may be impaired in PTSD patients.

In this study, plasma epinephrine, but not norepinephrine, levels increased in response to meaningful stressor stimuli. Plasma epinephrine derives primarily from the adrenal medulla, whereas norepinephrine is released from postganglionic sympathetic nerves. It has been suggested by a number of investigators that the sympathetic neural and adrenomedullary components of the SNS may be differentially activated, depending on the causal stimulus (Folkow 1984; Goldstein et al. 1987; Halter et al. 1984; Hjemdahl et al. 1984; Robertson et al. 1979; Ward et al. 1983). Thus, the combat-related stressors may have provoked a greater adrenomedullary than sympathoneural response in our PTSD group. This possibility is consistent with a growing body of evidence indicating that the SNS is capable of differential, rather than all-or-none, activation (Villacres et al. 1987).

It is important to emphasize that the interpretation of stress-induced plasma catecholamine responses requires careful attention to several physiological determinants. In a number of studies, certain psychological stressors such as the Stroop test have been found to cause greater increases in venous plasma levels of epinephrine than of norepinephrine (Robertson et al. 1979; Ward et al. 1983). However, norepinephrine levels in venous plasma are largely influenced by regional tissue factors (Goldstein et al. 1987; Hjemdahl et al. 1984). Because the outflow of sympathetic muscle nerves may decrease during some kinds of mental stress (Delius et al. 1972), with consequent decreased vascular resistance and increased blood flow and norepinephrine clearance through the muscle (Goldstein et al. 1987; Hjemdahl et al. 1984), the muscles become a site of net norepinephrine removal under such conditions. Thus, venous plasma levels of norepinephrine would be lower than those found in arterial or mixed venous samples (Hjemdahl et al. 1984).

In comparing the accuracy of arterial and venous plasma norepinephrine levels with norepinephrine release rates obtained by a radioisotope dilution technique, Goldstein et al. (1987) determined that the radioisotope dilution technique was the most sensitive in detecting SNS activation. Because SNS activation is accompanied by increased cardiac output and therefore increased total body norepinephrine clearance, arterial plasma norepinephrine levels in Goldstein et al.'s study were a less sensitive indicator of SNS activation than was the norepinephrine release rate. Again, because of the regional tissue effects on plasma norepinephrine values, venous plasma norepinephrine was not a good indicator of SNS activity.

Norepinephrine measured (as in this present study) in arterialized plasma reflects sympathetic activity more accurately than norepinephrine measured in venous plasma, but less accurately than in the kinetic studies described by Goldstein et al. (1987) and others (Best and Halter 1982; Esler 1982; Veith et al. 1986). Thus, we cannot rule out the possibility that the lack of change in arterialized plasma levels of norepinephrine in this study resulted from our failure to detect a small increase in norepinephrine release that may have been obscured by a simultaneous increase in total body norepinephrine clearance. Similarly, we cannot exclude the possibility that decreased clearance of epinephrine from plasma accounts for some or all of the elevation of epinephrine levels observed here. Moreover, regional increases in sympathetic outflow to specific organs such as the heart may have occurred in response to trauma-related stimuli, but may have been obscured by factors such as the relatively small contribution by the cardiac branch of the SNS to circulating plasma norepinephrine, and possibly by simultaneous decreases in sympathetic outflow to other organs. More sophisticated (and invasive) sampling methods would be needed to investigate regional differences in SNS responses to trauma-related stimuli.

REFERENCES

American Psychiatric Association: Diagnostic and Statistical Manual of Mental Disorders, 3rd Edition, Revised. Washington, DC, American Psychiatric Association, 1987

Best JD, Halter JB: Release and clearanced rates of epinephrine in man: importance of arterial measurements. J Clin Endocrinol Metab 55:263–268, 1982

Blanchard EB, Kolb LC, Pallmeyer TP, et al: A psychophysiological study of post-traumatic stress disorder in Vietnam veterans. Psychiatr Q 54:220–229, 1982

Blanchard EB, Kolb LC, Gerardi RJ, et al: Cardiac response to relevant stimuli as an adjunctive tool for diagnosing post-traumatic stress disorder in Vietnam veterans. Behavior Therapy 17:592–606, 1986

Davidson LM, Baum A: Chronic stress and posttraumatic stress disorders. J Consult Clin Psychol 54:303–308, 1986

Delius W, Hagbarth KE, Hongell A, et al: Maneuvers affecting sympathetic outflow in human muscle nerves. Acta Physiol Scand 84:82–94, 1972

Esler M: Assessment of sympathetic nervous function in humans from noradrenaline plasma kinetics. Clin Sci 62:247–254, 1982

Folkow B: Introductory remarks: plasma catecholamines as markers for sympathoadrenal activity in man. Acta Physiol Scand Suppl 527:7–9, 1984

Goldstein DS, Eisenhofer G, Sax FL, et al: Plasma norepinephrine pharmacokinetics during mental challenge. Psychosom Med 49:591–605, 1987

Halter JB, Stratton JR, Pfeifer MA: Plasma catecholamines and hemodynamic responses to stress states in man. Acta Physiol Scand Suppl 527:31–38, 1984

Hjemdahl P, Freyschuss U, Juhlin-Dannfelt A, et al: Differentiated sympathetic activation during mental stress evoked by the Stroop test. Acta Physiol Scand Suppl 527:25–29, 1984

Horowitz MJ, Becker SS, Malone P: Stress: different effects on patients and nonpatients. J Abnorm Psychol 82:547–551, 1973

Keane TM, Zimmering RT, Caddell JM: A behavioral formulation of post traumatic stress disorder in Vietnam veterans. Behavior Therapist 8:9–12, 1985

Keane TM, Caddell JM, Taylor KL: Mississippi Scale for Combat-Related Posttraumatic Stress Disorder: three studies in reliability and validity. J Consult Clin Psychol 56:85–90, 1988

Kolb LC: A neuropsychological hypothesis explaining posttraumatic stress disorders. Am J Psychiatry 144:989–995, 1987

Kosten TR, Mason JW, Giller EL, et al: Sustained urinary norepinephrine and epinephrine elevation in post-traumatic stress disorder. Psychoneuroendocrinology 12:13–20, 1987

Laufer RS, Frey-Wouters E, Donnellan J, et al: Legacies of Vietnam, Vol III: Post-War Trauma: Social and Psychological Problems of Vietnam Veterans and Their Peers. Washington, DC, U.S. Government Printing Office, 1981, pp 125–129

Malloy PF, Fairbank JA, Keane TM: Validation of a multimethod assessment of posttraumatic stress disorder in Vietnam veterans. J Consult Clin Psychol 51:488–494, 1983

McFall ME, Murburg MM, Roszell DK, et al: Psychophysiologic and neuroendocrine findings in post-traumatic stress disorder: a review of theory and research. Journal of Anxiety Disorders 3:243–257, 1989

Perry BD, Southwick SM, Giller EL: Adrenergic receptor regulation in PTSD. Paper presented at the 141st annual meeting of the American Psychiatric Association. Montreal, Quebec, May 1988

Pitman RK, Orr SP, Forgue DF, et al: Psychophysiologic assessment of posttraumatic stress disorder imagery in Vietnam combat veterans. Arch Gen Psychiatry 44:970–975, 1987

Robertson D, Johnson GA, Robertson RM, et al: Comparative assessment of stimuli that release neuronal and adrenomedullary catecholamines in man. Circulation 59:637–643, 1979

Spitzer RL, Williams JBW, Gibbon M: Structured Clinical Interview for DSM-III-R—Patient Version (SCID-P, 4-1-87 revision). New York, New York State Psychiatric Institute, 1987

Veith RC, Featherstone JA, Linares OA, et al: Age differences in plasma norepinephrine kinetics in humans. J Gerontol 41:319–324, 1986

Villacres EC, Hollifield M, Katon WJ, et al: Sympathetic nervous system activity in panic disorder. Psychiatry Res 21:313–321, 1987

Ward MM, Meford IN, Parker SD, et al: Epinephrine and norepinephrine responses in continuously collected human plasma to a series of stressors. Psychosom Med 45:471–486, 1983

Zilberg NJ, Weiss DS, Horowitz MJ: Impact of Event Scale: a cross-validation study and some empirical evidence supporting a conceptual model of stress response syndromes. J Consult Clin Psychol 50:407–414, 1982

Chapter 10

Relationship Between Catecholamine Excretion and PTSD Symptoms in Vietnam Combat Veterans and Holocaust Survivors

Rachel Yehuda, Ph.D.
Earl L. Giller, Jr., M.D., Ph.D.
Steven M. Southwick, M.D.
Boaz Kahana, Ph.D.
David Boisoneau
Xiaowan Ma
John W. Mason, M.D.

A number of studies have assessed autonomic function using measurement of vital signs in patients with combat-related PTSD (Blanchard et al. 1982; Butler et al. 1990; Malloy et al. 1983; Paige et al. 1990; Pitman et al. 1987; see also McFall and Murburg, Chapter 7, this volume). However, our laboratory has been the first to utilize psychoneuroendocrine approaches to characterize and better understand catecholamine regulation in this disorder (for review, see Mason et al. 1990; Yehuda et al. 1990b). We have reported sustained elevations of mean 24-hour urinary norepinephrine and epinephrine concentrations in PTSD patients compared with patients in other diagnostic groups (Kosten et al. 1987), as well as a decreased number of platelet alpha2 (α_2)–adrenergic receptors in PTSD patients compared with normal subjects (Perry et al. 1987, 1990; see also Perry,

Chapter 12, this volume). These findings, which are consistent with reports of phasically increased plasma epinephrine levels in PTSD patients (McFall et al. 1990), have led to the emerging hypothesis that alterations in central and peripheral catecholamine systems contribute to symptoms of PTSD (for review, see Giller 1990).

In assessing the potential importance of the observed changes in catecholamine for the diagnosis, and possibly the pathogenesis, of chronic PTSD, we have recently conducted two follow-up studies. The first study was designed to determine the relationship between urinary catecholamine levels and the *severity* of PTSD symptoms. Most biological studies in PTSD, including our own, have tended to focus primarily on inpatients who were quite symptomatic when they were studied and accordingly represent a relatively homogeneous group with respect to severity of symptoms. In consistently utilizing such a group it has been difficult to determine the extent to which catecholamine alterations in PTSD represent "trait" or "state" abnormalities. Given the fact that several investigators, including our own group, have suggested that measures of catecholamine dysfunction may be useful in supplying diagnostic information about PTSD (Mason et al. 1990; Yehuda et al. 1990b), it was of interest to determine the relative stability of these changes by assessing catecholamine excretion in patients over a wide range of symptom severity and/or at various phases of illness.

The second study was performed to assess whether neuroendocrine parameters such as urinary catecholamine excretion, which was found to be abnormal in Vietnam combat veterans with PTSD, were also abnormal in civilians with chronic PTSD, especially civilians who may not have sought hospitalization for their symptoms. To address both these issues we extended our psychoneuroendocrine studies to a group of Holocaust survivors. Like combat veterans, Holocaust survivors constitute a relatively homogeneous group in regard to severity of stressor and length of time that has transpired since the trauma. Furthermore, Holocaust survivors have undergone a chronic, rather than an acute, exposure to stress and have experienced the long-standing symptoms of reexperiencing traumatic memories, depression, anxiety, low morale, and the effects on emotional well-being as a result of the trauma (Kahana et al. 1988).

It was also of interest to determine whether differences in urinary catecholamines between PTSD patients and normal subjects are more likely related to chronic exposure to trauma (i.e., having undergone the experience of the concentration camp), or rather to having a current posttraumatic stress disorder (PTSD). To address this issue in the second study, we subdivided Holocaust survivors into those meeting and those not meeting the diagnostic criteria for PTSD. Both survivor subgroups were similar in having undergone chronic, traumatic stress, but differed in their current level of symptomatology. By subdividing the Holocaust survivor group in this way, it was possible to evaluate whether the psychoneuroendocrine profile has diagnostic sensitivity for chronic PTSD—a possibility suggested by our previous work (Mason et al. 1990; Yehuda et al. 1991)—or whether it is a marker for long-term biological changes associated with chronic exposure to trauma, a possibility that was not addressed in our prior studies.

In this chapter we summarize our findings of the relationship between urinary catecholamine excretion and PTSD symptoms in Vietnam veterans, as well as the results of a pilot study exploring catecholamine excretion in Holocaust survivors. In both studies, our research strategy has been to measure 24-hour urinary excretion of norepinephrine, epinephrine, and, more recently, dopamine, concurrently with symptom severity along a wide range of symptoms, in traumatized individuals and to examine the relationship between urinary catecholamines and symptom severity.

BIOLOGICAL SAMPLING AND STATISTICAL METHODS

The procedures utilized in both studies were similar regarding data collection and biochemical methodology. Subjects were asked to collect 24-hour urine samples, which were stored in freezers during the collection period to preserve catecholamines. We avoided sampling during the week of admission to the hospital (inpatients), on days of unusual physical activity or stress, and also during periods when unusual procedures, including endocrine challenge tests, were being performed. Completeness of collections was monitored by nursing staff for the inpatients and by determinations of urinary creatinine excretion for nonhospitalized subjects. Mean creatinine excretions in the present studies ranged from 0.8 to 2.0 g/day in these studies, which is within the normal range (Yehuda et al. 1990a).

The frozen urine samples were thawed in a standardized fashion and 2.5-ml aliquots adjusted to pH 2.0 with concentrated HCl following the addition of 20 μl EDTA/reduced glutathione solution per ml urine. The aliquots were then refrozen at −70°C until analyzed for catecholamines by high-pressure liquid chromatography (HPLC). Urinary norepinephrine, epinephrine, and dopamine excretion rates were measured by HPLC (Yehuda et al. 1992).

In the present studies, differences between groups were determined using one-way analysis of variance (ANOVA) (one-tailed), and posthoc comparisons were made using the Fisher's least significant difference test. Comparisons between inpatients and outpatients on clinical symptoms were made using the Student's t test (one-tailed). Correlational analyses were performed on biological and clinical measures from PTSD patients using Pearson's coefficient r. Bonferroni corrections were applied for all multiple comparisons.

SUBJECTS AND METHODS

Study 1: Catecholamine Excretion in Inpatients and Outpatient Combat Veterans with PTSD

Twenty-two nonmedicated male Vietnam combat veterans (14 inpatients and 8 outpatients) with a primary diagnosis of PTSD, and 16 age-comparable nonpsychiatric males participated in this study (age range 30–50). The subjects were interviewed with several structured scales to determine the degree of combat exposure, comorbidity of psychiatric disorders, and severity of current PTSD. Combat exposure was rated on a scale of 1 to 14 using the Combat Exposure Scale (CES; U.S. Government Printing Office 1981), with scores ranging from 7 to 14 (moderate to heavy exposure) in our sample. PTSD was diagnosed using the Structured Clinical Interview for DSM-III-R (Spitzer et al. 1987). Other diagnoses were made according to Research Diagnostic Criteria (RDC; Spitzer et al. 1978) using the Schedule for Affective Disorders and Schizophrenia (SADS; Endicott and Spitzer 1978). Severity of PTSD symptoms was assessed using the Impact of Event Scale (IES; Horowitz et al. 1979) and the Figley PTSD Interview (Figley and Stretch 1980). Depressive symptoms were measured with the Hamilton Depression Rating Scale (Ham-D; Hamilton 1959). Symptom ratings were made at the termination of the 24-hour urine collection.

Study 2: Catecholamine Excretion in Holocaust Survivors With and Without PTSD

Twenty-three Holocaust survivors (10 males and 13 females) and 13 demographically matched individuals who had not been through the Holocaust (8 males and 5 females) participated in the study (age range 62–75). These individuals were not seeking treatment and were recruited following an announcement that volunteers were needed to participate in a study examining the biological aspects of stress in Holocaust survivors. Eleven of the Holocaust survivors and 6 of the control subjects were taking some form of medication at the time of biological testing. Subjects were interviewed with several structured scales to determine medical health, past and current stress history, and current psychiatric disorder. Medical health information was obtained using the OARS checklist (Blazer 1978), and past and current stress history was determined using the Antonovsky Life Crises Scale (Antonovsky 1979) and the Recent Life Events Scale (Kahana et al. 1982). Diagnostic assessments were performed using the SCID for current and lifetime psychiatric disorders (Spitzer and Williams 1987), and the Clinician Administered PTSD Scale (CAPS; Blake et al. 1990) for assessment of current and lifetime PTSD. To study severity of PTSD symptoms and the effect of these symptoms on individuals' lives as continuous variables, the Civilian Mississippi PTSD Scale (Keane et al. 1990) was also administered to all subjects ($N = 36$).

RESULTS

Study 1

Mean 24-hour urinary excretion of dopamine, norepinephrine, and epinephrine in inpatients and outpatients with PTSD and in the normal comparison group is summarized in Figure 10–1. Although the mean urinary excretion of dopamine, norepinephrine, and epinephrine was higher in both PTSD groups compared with normal subjects, posthoc testing showed that only inpatients had significantly higher catecholamine excretion compared with normal subjects. The tendency for outpatients to show higher mean dopamine and norepinephrine excretion compared with normal subjects was not statistically significant.

The clinical symptom data for the inpatient and outpatient PTSD groups are summarized in Table 10–1. As can be clearly seen from the ranges of the scores on the clinical instruments, there was a wide range of PTSD and depressive symptoms in the patient group. Inpatients were found to be significantly more symptomatic than outpatients, as measured by the IES, because of both "intrusive" and "avoidant" symptoms. Inpatients also showed a nonsignificant 30% greater mean Figley score compared with outpatients. Depressive symptoms were comparable in both groups.

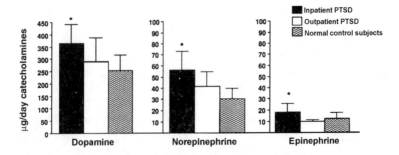

Figure 10–1. Urinary catecholamine excretion in combat veterans. PTSD inpatients showed a significantly higher mean catecholamine excretion compared with outpatients with PTSD and normal control subjects.

Correlational analysis revealed significant relationships between 24-hour urinary dopamine and norepinephrine excretion and PTSD symptoms. Both dopamine and norepinephrine were significantly correlated with the total IES scores (Table 10–2). After applying Bonferroni corrections, significant correlations were observed between catecholamines and "intrusive" symp-

Table 10–1. Severity of PTSD and depressive symptoms in combat veterans with PTSD

Rating scale	Reference	Range of scores	Inpatients	Outpatients
Figley PTSD	Figley and Stretch 1988	4–48	30.9 ± 10.4	22.4 ± 10.7
Impact of Event Scale	Horowitz et al. 1979			
Total		7–61	40.4 ± 13.1[*]	22.1 ± 17.7
Intrusive		3–33	22.8 ± 8.0[**]	11.6 ± 8.7
Avoidance		1–38	18.08 ± 7.4[***]	10.5 ± 12.1
Ham-D	Hamilton 1959	7–44	21.1 ± 11.8	18.0 ± 8.0

Note. Results are expressed as mean score ± SD. Ham-D = Hamilton Depression Rating Scale.
[*]$t = 2.6$, df = 18, $P < 0.0125$; [**]$t = 2.9$, df = 18, $P < 0.008$; [***]$t = 1.8$, df = 18, $P < 0.090$.

Table 10–2. Correlations between catecholamines and PTSD and depressive symptoms in Vietnam veterans

	Impact of Event Scale[a]				
	Figley[b]	Total	Intrusive	Avoidant	Ham-D[c]
Dopamine	.59[*]	.63[*]	.68[*]	.49[**]	.12
Norepinephrine	.37	.58[*]	.59[*]	.46[**]	.01
Epinephrine	.49[**]	.38	.27	.40	.15

Note. Ham-D = Hamilton Depression Rating Scale.
[a]Horowitz et al. 1979.
[b]Figley and Stretch 1988.
[c]Hamilton 1959.
*$P < 0.0125$, Bonferroni P value; **$P < 0.05$, nonsignificant trend.

toms (Figure 10–2). The tendency for catecholamines to be correlated with severity of avoidance symptoms was not statistically significant. Urinary excretion of dopamine, however, was positively correlated with scores on the Figley scale (which assesses intrusive, avoidant, and hyperarousal symptoms). Urinary epinephrine excretion was not significantly correlated with any of the PTSD measures, and none of the three catecholamines were correlated with Ham-D scores.

Study 2

None of the 13 age-matched volunteers met DSM-III-R criteria for lifetime or current psychiatric disorder, including PTSD. Of the 23 Holocaust survivors, 11 met criteria for current PTSD (7 men and 4 women). Among the 12 survivors not meeting the full criteria for PTSD, about half had at least two PTSD symptoms, most commonly sleep disturbance and nightmares; 5 of these 12 individuals met the diagnostic criteria for past PTSD, usually beginning within 6 months following liberation, and had not met diagnostic criteria for this disorder for at least a decade. None of the individuals were currently seeking psychiatric treatment for their symptoms, and only 3 had sought treatment for PTSD symptoms in the past.

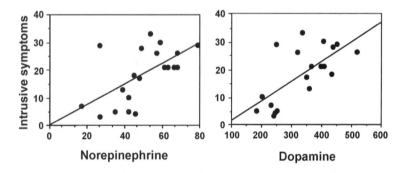

Figure 10–2. Correlation between urinary norepinephrine and dopamine excretion and severity of intrusive symptoms in combat veterans with PTSD.

The clinical symptom data in the Holocaust survivors with and without PTSD are summarized in Table 10–3. As expected, Holocaust survivors with PTSD scored significantly higher than Holocaust survivors without PTSD on the Civilian Mississippi PTSD scale and on all subscales of the CAPS. Mean 24-hour urinary excretion of dopamine, norepinephrine, and epinephrine in Holocaust survivors with and without PTSD and in normal subjects is quantified in Figure 10–3. One-way ANOVA revealed significant differences in both dopamine and norepinephrine excretion, which were shown by posthoc testing to reflect that Holocaust survivors with PTSD had higher urinary dopamine and norepinephrine excretion compared with Holocaust survivors without PTSD. In this small pilot sample, normal control subjects were not significantly different from either of the two traumatized groups. Urinary epinephrine excretion was not significantly different among the three groups. Urinary norepinephrine and dopamine levels in the Holocaust survivor group were significantly correlated with symptom severity as assessed by the CAPS (Table 10–4). Figure 10–4 presents some of these correlations more clearly for the purpose of comparison with the Vietnam veterans sample.

Table 10–3.   Severity of PTSD symptoms in the Holocaust survivor group

Rating scale	Reference	Range of scores	PTSD	Non-PTSD
Civilian Mississippi	Keane et al. 1990	57–120	$99.10 \pm 14.3^{*}$	73.6 ± 10.8
CAPS Total	Blake et al. 1990	0–103	$71.00 \pm 19.2^{**}$	20.4 ± 17.0
Intrusive		0–39	$20.54 \pm 7.6^{***}$	8.10 ± 8.8
Avoidance		0–39	$22.09 \pm 12^{****}$	6.45 ± 6.5
Hyperarousal		0–56	$28.36 \pm 14.6^{*****}$	5.82 ± 6.0

Note.   Results are expressed as mean score ± SD.
CAPS = Clinician Administered PTSD Scale.
$^{*}t = 4.3$, df = 20, $P < 0.0001$; $^{**}t = 6.6$, df = 20, $P < 0.0001$; $^{***}t = 3.5$, df = 20, $P < 0.0001$; $^{****}t = 4.5$; df = 20; $P < 0.0001$.

DISCUSSION

The results of the present studies, while replicating the previous finding of increased 24-hour urinary catecholamine excretion in combat veterans with PTSD compared with those in other diagnostic groups (Kosten et al. 1987), specifically emphasize the role of current symptomatology as contributing to the increased catecholamine excretion observed. Furthermore, preliminary data

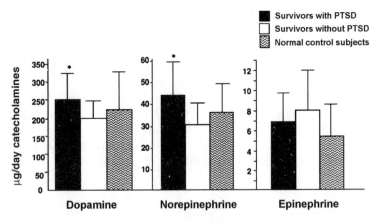

Figure 10–3. Urinary catecholamine excretion in Holocaust survivors with and without PTSD compared with age-comparable control subjects. Mean dopamine and norepinephrine excretion was significantly higher only in the survivor group with PTSD.

Table 10–4. Correlations between catecholamines and severity of PTSD symptoms in Holocaust survivors

	CAPS[a] total	Intrusive	Avoidant	Hyperarousal
Dopamine	.40*	.34**	.17	.44*
Norepinephrine	.34**	.29	.44*	.14
Epinephrine	.13	.14	.18	.21

[a]Blake et al. 1990
*$P < 0.05$; **$P < 0.015$ (trend).

from Holocaust survivors with and without PTSD suggest that the catecholamine alterations we have observed in combat veterans can be generalized to nonveterans with chronic PTSD.

In Kosten et al.'s study, urine samples and clinical ratings (using the Brief Psychiatric Rating Scale [BPRS; Overall and Gorham 1962]) were obtained from patients at four different phases of hospitalization. PTSD patients showed consistently higher norepinephrine and epinephrine excretion at every time point sampled compared with patients with major depressive disorder, paranoid schizophrenia, or undifferentiated schizophrenia. The relationship between symptom severity and catecholamine excretion could not be addressed in that study largely because of the lack of longitudinal symptom improvement during the course of hospitalization in the PTSD group. Rather, the findings from that study showed that the sustained urinary norepinephrine and epinephrine elevations in PTSD patients at each time point during the course of hospitalization were paralleled by sustained elevations in sum BPRS scores. The refractory nature of chronic PTSD symptoms in patients who are hospitalized in a general psychiatric ward is, unfortunately, not unusual. Thus, in order to investigate the relationship between catecholamine excretion and PTSD symptoms, it was necessary to include subjects across a wide range of symptom severity, and to focus subject recruitment on outpatients (who, we assumed, would be less symptomatic) as well as inpatients. This was the case in the study

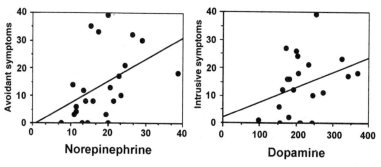

Figure 10–4. Correlation between urinary norepinephrine and dopamine, and intrusive and avoidance symptoms in Holocaust survivors with and without PTSD.

of both combat veterans and Holocaust survivors.

In the first of the present studies, inpatient combat veterans with PTSD were found to be more symptomatic than outpatient combat veterans with PTSD. The greater degree of symptomatology in the inpatient group was paralleled by increased 24-hour urinary excretion of dopamine, norepinephrine, and epinephrine. In contrast, no significant differences were observed between outpatients with PTSD and normal control subjects. However, the lack of statistical significance may merely reflect the fact that the sample size was very small. It may be that a larger sample would allow for the detection of significant differences in catecholamine excretion between outpatients and normal subjects.

In the study of Holocaust survivors, the increased symptomatology in the group with PTSD was also paralleled by increased urinary excretion of dopamine and norepinephrine. In comparing the level of hormone excretion in these two samples, it is of interest to note that the actual mean excretion of dopamine and norepinephrine in the outpatient combat veterans group with PTSD is quite similar to that of the Holocaust survivor group with PTSD. To more clearly depict this relationship, the mean norepinephrine execretion of all six groups is summarized in Figure 10–5.

From a methodological perspective, it is problematic to compare the present data from Vietnam veterans with PTSD and Holocaust survivors in one statistical design for several reasons. First, the method of recruitment differed substantially: the combat veterans were recruited after seeking treatment for PTSD, whereas the Holocaust survivors were normal volunteers from the community. Second, there is a substantial age difference between the two groups, with Holocaust survivors being an average of 25 years older than Vietnam veterans. Related to this, the chronicity of illness has been longer in the Holocaust group. Moreover, the Holocaust group is composed of both males and females, whereas only males are represented in the Vietnam veterans. Having mentioned these caveats, however, an informal examination of the means does show a similarity between Holocaust survivors with PTSD and outpatient combat veterans with PTSD.

In both studies, we added the assessment of urinary dopamine excretion to the psychoendocrine profile. Measures of urinary dopamine have not typically been included in psychoendocrine studies, and therefore little is known about the possible psychological and physiological correlates of this amine. Nonetheless, an elevated urinary dopamine excretion was observed in inpatients with PTSD, and, to a lesser extent, in the two other PTSD groups (i.e., the veteran outpatient group and the Holocaust survivor group with PTSD). The observation of increased dopamine in these two samples is consistent with results of a pilot study that found significant elevations in plasma dopamine in 12 Vietnam combat veterans with PTSD who were compared with 8 males with major depressive disorder and 8 healthy subjects (Hamner et al. 1990). In both samples, dopamine excretion was significantly related to severity of PTSD, particularly intrusive and hyperarousal symptoms, although severity of symptoms in

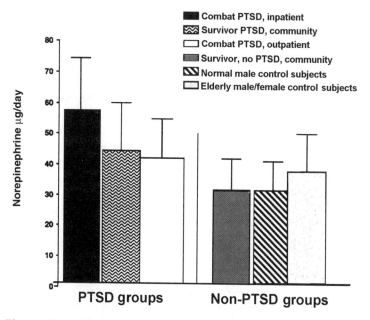

Figure 10–5. Comparison of norepinephrine excretion in combat veterans, Holocaust survivors, and normal control subjects.

the two studies was determined using different PTSD scales.

Correlational analysis also indicated a strong relationship between urinary norepinephrine excretion and overall severity of PTSD symptoms. In the case of Vietnam combat veterans, norepinephrine excretion appeared to be more associated with intrusive symptoms, whereas in the Holocaust survivor group norepinephrine excretion appeared to be related to severity of avoidant symptoms. This particular difference, however, may reflect the different comparison groups in the two studies. In the study of combat veterans, correlational analysis was based on data from inpatients and outpatients, all of whom were diagnosed as having PTSD. In the Holocaust survivor group, correlational analysis was performed on subjects who were less symptomatic overall, with half the subjects not meeting the criteria for the diagnosis of PTSD.

In contrast to the above findings, 24-hour mean urinary epinephrine excretion was not found to correlate with scores on any of the symptom scales utilized in either combat veterans or Holocaust survivors. The only observable difference in mean excretion of epinephrine was between combat PTSD inpatients on the one hand, and outpatients and control subjects on the other. Increased epinephrine was not observed in the Holocaust sample. Interestingly, in the previously published study (Kosten et al. 1987), inpatients with PTSD showed significantly higher urinary epinephrine excretion compared with patients who had been diagnosed with other psychiatric disorders. It may be that urinary epinephrine excretion reflects acute adrenomedullary activity in response to stress. This stress may be of a more general nature, reflecting a general functional impairment or associated with extreme severity of illness that requires hospitalization, or reflecting adjunctive symptoms that are more directly relevant to inpatient hospitalization, such as increased anger, suicidality, and impulsivity. These traits have been associated with increased urinary epinephrine excretion in individuals without PTSD (Funkenstein 1956; Nesse et al. 1984). Alternatively, increased epinephrine excretion could be related to exposure to trauma-related stimuli, including patients' war stories, conflicts with authority figures, or simply each patient's own painful memories. Indeed, other studies have shown an increase in plasma epinephrine levels in PTSD patients exposed to trauma-related, but not trauma-unrelated, stimuli (McFall et al. 1990; see also Murburg et al., Chapter 9, this volume). Because most of the PTSD subjects in both of our studies were free of other Axis I diagnoses, it is unlikely that the increased urinary excretion in PTSD inpatients was specifically related to other major Axis I conditions.

CONCLUSIONS

Mason et al. (1990) have suggested that the magnitude and persistence of changes in catecholamines might be potentially useful as diagnostic indicators. We now also provide evidence that urinary dopamine levels may be useful in this regard. The pilot results from Holocaust survivors support the idea that catecholamine levels are related to persistence of PTSD, rather than to the fact of having been traumatized. The present data also suggest that in addition to diagnostic "trait-like" measures in symptomatic individuals, catecholamine levels may reflect severity within the diagnostic grouping. These results provide encouragement for further exploration of the relationship between catecholamines and specific symptom clusters in PTSD.

REFERENCES

Antonovsky A: Health, Stress and Coping. San Francisco, CA, Jossey-Bass, 1979

Blake D, Weathers F, Nagy L, et al: Clinican-Administered PTSD Scale (CAPS-1). Boston, MA, National Center for Posttraumatic Stress Disorder, Behavioral Science Division, February 1990

Blanchard EB, Kolb LC, Pallmeyer TP, et al: A psychophysiological study of posttraumatic stress disorder in Vietnam veterans. Psychiatr Q 54:220–229, 1982

Blazer D: Durham Survey: Description and Application in Multidimensional Functional Assessment OARS Methodology: A Manual, 2nd Edition. Durham, NC, Duke University Center Study Aging and Human Development, 1978, pp 75–88

Butler RW, Braff D, Rausch JL, et al: Physiological evidence of exaggerated startle response in a subgroup of Vietnam veterans with combat-related PTSD. Am J Psychiatry 147:1308–1312, 1990

Endicott J, Spitzer RL: A diagnostic interview: the Schedule for Affective Disorders and Schizophrenia. Arch Gen Psychiatry 35:837–844, 1978

Figley CR, Stretch RH: Vietnam Veterans Questionnaire, 1980. (Available from CR Figley, Family Research Institute, Purdue University, West Lafayette, IN)

Funkenstein DH: Norepinephrine-like and epinephrine-like substances in relation to human behavior. J Nerv Ment Dis 124:58–68, 1956

Giller EL: Biological Assessment and Treatment of Posttraumatic Stress Disorder. Washington, DC, American Psychiatric Press, 1990

Hamilton M: The assessment of anxiety states by rating. Br J Med Psychol 32:50–55, 1959

Hamner MB, Diamond BI, Hitri A: Plasma dopamine and prolactin levels in PTSD. Biol Psychiatry 27:72A, 1990

Horowitz M, Wilner N, Alvarez W: Impact of Event Scale: a measure of subjective distress. Psychosom Med 41:209–218, 1979

Kahana E, Fairchild T, Kahana B: The Elderly Care Research Center Life Events Scale, Adaptation, in Research Instruments in Social Gerontology, Clinical and Social Psychology. Edited by Mangen DJ, Peterson WA. Minneapolis, MN, University of Minnesota Press, 1982

Kahana E, Kahaha B, Harel Z, et al: Coping with extreme trauma, in Human Adaptation to Extreme Stress: From the Holocaust to Vietnam. Edited by Wilson, Harel Z, Kahana B. New York, Plenum, 1988

Keane T, Weathers F, Blake D: The Civilian Mississippi Scale. Boston, MA, National Center for Posttraumatic Stress Disorder, Behavioral Science Division, 1990

Kosten TR, Mason JW, Giller EL, et al: Sustained urinary norepinephrine and epinephrine elevation in post-traumatic stress disorder. Psychoneuroendocrinology 12:13–20, 1987

Malloy PF, Fairbank JA, Keane TML: Validation of multimethod assessment of posttraumatic stress disorders in Vietnam veterans. J Consult Clin Psychol 51:488–494, 1983

Mason JW, Giller EL Jr, Kosten TR, et al: Psychoendocrine approaches to the diagnosis and pathogenesis of posttraumatic stress disorder, in Biological Assessment and Treatment of Posttraumatic Stress Disorder. Edited by Giller EL Jr. Washington, DC, American Psychiatric Press, 1990, pp 65–86

McFall ME, Murburg MM, Ko GN, et al: Autonomic responses to stress in Vietnam combat veterans with posttraumatic stress disorder. Biol Psychiatry 27:1165–1175, 1990

Nesse RM, Cameron OG, Curtis GC, et al: Adrenergic function in patients with panic anxiety. Arch Gen Psychiatry 41:771–776, 1984

Overall J, Gorham D: The Brief Psychiatric Rating Scale. Psychol Rep 10:799–812, 1962

Paige SR, Teid GM, Allen MG, et al: Psychophysiological correlates of posttraumatic stress disorder in Vietnam veterans. Biol Psychiatry 27:419–430, 1990

Perry BD, Giller EL, Southwick SM: Altered platelet alpha₂ adrenergic binding sites in post-traumatic stress disorder. Am J Psychiatry 144:1511–1512, 1987

Perry BD, Southwick SM, Yehuda R, et al: Adrenergic receptor regulation in posttraumatic stress disorder, in Biological Assessment and Treatment of Posttraumatic Stress Disorder. Edited by EL Giller. Washington, DC, American Psychiatric Press, 1990, pp 87–114

Pitman RK, Orr SP, Forgue DF, et al: Psychophysiologic assessment of posttraumatic stress disorder imagery in Vietnam combat veterans. Arch Gen Psychiatry 44:970–975, 1987

Spitzer RL, Endicott J, Robins E: Research Diagnostic Criteria: rationale and reliability. Arch Gen Psychiatry 35:773–782, 1978

Spitzer RL, Williams JBW, Gibbon M: Structured Clinical Interview for DSM-III-R—Patient Version (SCID-P, 4-1-87 revision). New York, New York State Psychiatric Institute, 1987

U.S. Government Printing Office: Long-term stress reactions: some causes, consequences and naturally occurring support systems, in Legacies of Vietnam, Vol IV: Comparative Adjustment of Veterans and Their Peers. Washington, DC, U.S. Government Printing Office, 1981

Yehuda R, Southwick SM, Nussbaum G, et al: Low urinary cortisol excretion in PTSD. J Nerv Ment Dis 178:366–369, 1990a

Yehuda R, Southwick SM, Perry BD, et al: Interactions of the hypothalamic-pituitary-adrenal axis and the catecholaminergic system in posttraumatic stress disorder, in Biological Assessment and Treatment of Posttraumatic Stress Disorder. Edited by Giller EL. Washington DC, American Psychiatric Press, 1990b, pp 115–134

Yehuda R, Giller EL, Southwick SM, et al: Hypothalamic-pituitary-adrenal dysfunction in posttraumatic stress disorder. Biol Psychiatry 30:1031–1048, 1991

Yehuda R, Southwick S, Giller EL, et al: Urinary catecholamine excretion and severity of PTSD symptoms in Vietnam combat veterans. J Nerv Ment Dis 180:321–325, 1992

Chapter 11

Plasma Norepinephrine and MHPG Responses to Exercise Stress in PTSD

Mark B. Hamner, M.D.
Bruce I. Diamond, Ph.D.
Ana Hitri, Ph.D.

N oradrenergic systems have been implicated in the patho-physiology of anxiety disorders (Heninger and Charney 1988; Lader 1974). However, the role of noradrenergic and other catecholaminergic systems in posttraumatic stress disorder (PTSD) has not been well defined. PTSD has a considerable phenomenological overlap with other anxiety syndromes (e.g., panic disorders; see Mellman and Davis 1985) in which abnormalities of norepinephrine function have been postulated (Heninger and Charney 1988).

Van der Kolk et al. (1985) hypothesized that hyperactivity of locus coeruleus (LC) norepinephrine neurons and eventual central nervous system (CNS) catecholamine depletion, analogous to animal models of learned helplessness secondary to inescapable shock, are involved in PTSD. Norepinephrine depletion has been described in animals restrained from escaping significant physi-

Presented in part at the 44th annual meeting of the Society of Biological Psychiatry in San Francisco, CA, May 4–8, 1989, and at the annual meeting of the American Psychiatric Association in New York, NY, May 13–17, 1990. Supported by the Veterans Administration and by a Medical College of Georgia Biomedical Research Grant (10-16-04-3802-02). The authors thank Emelia O'Neal, M.Ed., Richard Borison, M.D., Ph.D., Timothy Sprecker, B.S., Robert Chumbley, B.S., and Patrick Boudewyns, Ph.D., for their assistance with this project.

cal stressors such as electric footshock (Anisman and Sklar 1979; Anisman et al. 1981; Maier and Seligman 1976; Weiss et al. 1975). These animals often have difficulty escaping novel stressors and decreased motivation to learn new contingencies, and demonstrate evidence of chronic distress. As van der Kolk et al. (1985) described, these findings are similar to many PTSD symptoms and associated complications—for example, chronic anxiety, decreased motivation, social and occupational dysfunction, and global constriction). Conversely, animals exposed to repeated stress may have increased CNS norepinephrine function depending on the type of stressor (for review, see Murburg et al. 1990). Although these studies, together with other animal studies described in this volume (see Aston-Jones et al., Chapter 2; Simson and Weiss, Chapter 3; Antelman and Yehuda, Chapter 4; Zacharko, Chapter 5; Charney et al., Chapter 6; Rausch et al., Chapter 14), document that central catecholamine function is complexly altered by stress in animals, there have been few studies to date to support the hypothesis that abnormalities of CNS or peripheral norepinephrine function are present in PTSD patients.

Psychophysiological studies have demonstrated that enchanced physiological responses occur in PTSD following trauma-related psychological stimuli (Blanchard et al. 1982; Kolb 1987; Pitman et al. 1987). Kosten et al. (1987) demonstrated higher urinary norepinephrine and epinephrine excretion in PTSD subjects compared with other psychiatric patients. McFall et al. (1990; see also Murburg et al., Chapter 9, this volume) recently reported exaggerated plasma epinephrine responses to viewing combat films in Vietnam veterans with PTSD. These studies suggest that increased sympathetic nervous system (SNS) activity is present in PTSD. It has recently been reported that the α_2 (α_2)–adrenergic antagonist yohimbine induces panic anxiety and flashback phenomena in Vietnam combat veterans, implicating a role for central norepinephrine dysfunction in PTSD (see Charney et al., Chapter 6, this volume).

These basic and clinical data together support the hypothesis that noradrenergic function is altered in PTSD. The purpose of our study was to investigate the effects of a significant physical stressor on plasma catecholamines in combat veterans with PTSD using an exercise treadmill stress-test paradigm. Plasma levels of norepinephrine and 3-methoxy-4-hydroxyphenylglycol (MHPG), the primary CNS metabolite of norepinephrine, were measured at rest and following maximal exercise intensity. Plasma MHPG may reflect, in part, central norepinephrine turnover (Elsworth et al. 1982), although MHPG is also produced by metabolism of norepinephrine in peripheral sympathetic neurons (see Veith and Murburg, Chapter 16, this volume). We hypothesized that strenuous exercise, a known stimulus for catecholamine elevations, would result in altered norepinephrine and MHPG responses in PTSD subjects consistent with norepinephrine dysregulation.

METHODS

Twelve male Vietnam war combat veterans meeting DSM-III-R criteria for PTSD (American Psychiatric Association 1987) were recruited from an inpatient PTSD treatment program as previously described (Boudewyns et al. 1990). The subjects were free of organic mental disorder, schizophrenia, major mood disorder, or recent substance use disorder. All patients had undergone weekly urine drug screens (which were negative) during hospitalization. These patients were compared with eight age-matched healthy veterans of Vietnam war-era military service. Control subjects had no history of psychiatric illness or other significant medical illness. Two controls had been in Vietnam combat, and six had no combat experience. All subjects gave informed consent for participation in the study as approved by the Medical College of Georgia Human Assurance Committee and by the Department of Veterans Affairs Medical Center Research and Development Committee. They had a baseline psychiatric evaluation and physical examination and were free of psychoactive medication or substance use or abuse for at least 1 month prior to the study. No participant was involved in a regular exercise program, and none had undergone significant athletic training.

Following an overnight fast, participants had an indwelling 22-gauge catheter placed in a forearm vein between 8:00 and 9:30 A.M. The catheter was kept patent using a heparin lock with saline flush. Baseline blood samples were then collected after 30 minutes with subjects in a sitting position. After a brief warm-up, a standard grade-incremented exercise treadmill stress test was performed. Subjects walked at 3 miles per hour starting at 0% grade, with the grade increased by 2.5% every 2 minutes. The subjects were encouraged to exercise as long as possible in order to achieve maximal exercise intensity. Electrocardiographic and respiratory levels were monitored continuously, and blood pressure was measured every 2 minutes. Expired air volume was measured using a Parkinson-Hower GS-4 dry gas meter. Oxygen uptake was measured and calculated using a Beckman metabolic cart. Maximal exercise intensity was estimated by participants achieving an oxygen uptake increase of less than 2.1 ml/kg^{-1} min^{-1} between final workloads and by achieving greater than 95% of age-predicted maximum heart rate. Within 1 minute following exercise, blood was again collected via the indwelling catheter from subjects who were in the sitting position.

The Spielberger State Anxiety Scale (Spielberger 1971) was completed before and after exercise, and participants were asked after exercising whether they had experienced an exacerbation of PTSD-reexperiencing phenomena or other anxiety symptoms. Blood samples were refrigerated and centrifuged, and the plasma was frozen at −80°C until norepinephrine and MHPG were measured by high-pressure liquid chromatography using electrochemical detection as described elsewhere (Minegishi and Ishizaki 1984). The Student's t test, the Mann-Whitney U test, and the Wilcoxon test for two related samples were used to analyze our data. Results from this study are reported as the mean ± standard deviation.

RESULTS

Ten of the 12 PTSD patients and all 8 control subjects achieved maximal exercise intensity. The two PTSD subjects who did not achieve maximal exercise intensity stopped because of fatigue. Data are reported for the 10 PTSD patients who achieved maximal exercise intensity as well as for all control subjects. There were no complications resulting from the tests, and the electrocardiogram interpretation revealed no evidence of cardiac ischemia or other cardiac abnormalities in any of the individuals.

Oxygen uptake (Vo_2), pulse, systolic and diastolic blood pressure at rest and following maximal exercise, and the length of time on treadmill are quantified in Table 11–1. Resting diastolic blood pressure was higher in control subjects (85 ± 9 mmHg in PTSD subjects vs. 75 ± 8 mmHg in control subjects) but was clinically within normal limits. Resting pulse and systolic blood pressure were comparable between groups. Maximum blood pressure and heart rate responses to exercise were similar as was length of time on the treadmill needed to attain maximal exercise intensity. Importantly, there was no difference in the maximal level of exercise intensity reached by both groups as demon-

Table 11–1. Oxygen uptake, heart rate, and blood pressure response to exercise in PTSD patients and control subjects

	PTSD ($n = 10$)	Control ($n = 8$)	P^a
Heart Rate (beats per minute)			
Resting	77 ± 10	79 ± 9	0.738
Maximum	178 ± 12	186 ± 9	0.142
Significance[b]	$t = -23.5$, df = 9, $P < 0.001$	($t = -32.5$, df = 7, $P < 0.001$	
Diastolic blood pressure (mmHg)			
Resting	75 ± 8	85 ± 9	0.041
Maximum	80 ± 7	80 ± 7	0.841
Significance	$t = -0.98$, df = 9 P not significant	$t = -0.83$, df = 7 P not significant	
Systolic blood pressure (mmHg)			
Resting	112 ± 7	118 ± 9	0.174
Maximum	183 ± 16	184 ± 11	0.852
Significance	$t = -10.8$, df = 9, $P < 0.001$	$t = -17.0$, df = 7, $P < 0.001$	
Maximum Vo_2^c uptake (ml/kg^{-1}min^{-1})	30.7 ± 5.7	31.8 ± 5.6	0.656
Time of treadmill (min)	16 ± 2	17 ± 3	0.528

[a]Between group comparisons were made using two-tailed t tests and were comparable except for resting diastolic blood pressure, which was higher in control subjects ($t = 2.2$, df = 16, $P = 0.041$).
[b]Within group comparisons all made using two-tailed t tests.
[c]Oxygen uptake, a measure of exercise intensity, was comparable between groups ($t = -0.43$, df = 16, $P = 0.656$).

strated by the almost identical Vo2 values in each group (30.7 ± 5.7 ml/kg^{-1} in PTSD and 31.8 ± 5.6 ml/kg^{-1}min^{-1} in controls).

The average age of PTSD subjects and control subjects was 38 ± 3 years and 39 ± 4 years, respectively ($t = -0.08$, df = 16, $P = 0.935$). Weight was also comparable in the two groups (162 ± 21 vs. 174 ± 20 lbs, respectively; $t = -1.22$, df = 16, $P = 0.242$).

The catecholamine data are as follows. Preexercise (resting) norepinephrine was essentially the same in PTSD patients (1.44 ± 0.42 ng/ml) and control subjects (1.31 ± 0.79 ng/ml) (Figure 11–1). Norepinephrine increased significantly in both groups after exercise (PTSD subjects: 2.84 ± 1.6 ng/ml, $t_{[calc]} = 2.739$, df = 18, $P < 0.05$, two-tailed postexercise vs. preexercise; control subjects: 3.33 ± 1.5 ng/ml, $t_{[calc]} = 3.39$, df = 14, $P < 0.01$, two-tailed postexercise vs. preexercise).

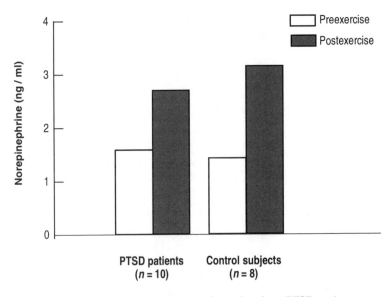

Figure 11–1. Mean plasma norepinephrine levels in PTSD patients and control subjects before and after maximal exercise stress. Norepinephrine levels were comparable between groups in both the pre- and postexercise conditions. Levels of norepinephrine increased significantly with exercise stress in both groups ($P < 0.05$; see results section).

The percent increase in mean plasma norepinephrine was 97% in PTSD subjects and 150% in control subjects. There was a trend for lower preexercise MHPG levels in PTSD subjects (5.58 ± 2.3 ng/ml) versus control subjects (14.8 ± 19 ng/ml) ($t_{[calc]} = 1.53$, df $= 16$, $P = 0.14$, two-tailed) (Figure 11–2). However, plasma MHPG levels increased significantly in PTSD patients only postexercise (17.38 ± 19 ng/ml, $Z = -2.8031$, $P = 0.0051$ by two-tailed Wilcoxon signed rank test). In control subjects, postexercise plasma MHPG levels remained unchanged from preexercise levels (9.63 ± 11 ng/ml, $Z = 0.0$, $P = 1.0$ by two-tailed Wilcoxon test). When the two PTSD patients who did not obtain maximal exercise intensity were included in the sample ($n = 12$), the MHPG response remained significant ($Z = -3.0594$, $P = 0.0022$).

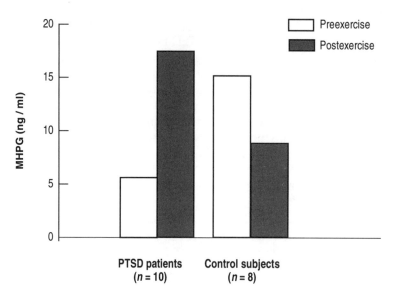

Figure 11–2. Mean plasma MHPG levels in PTSD patients and control subjects before and after maximal exercise stress. MHPG levels were comparable between groups both pre- and postexercise. However, there was a trend toward lower preexercise (i.e., resting) MHPG levels in PTSD patients. MHPG levels increased significantly with exercise stress in PTSD patients only ($Z = -2.803$, $P = 0.0051$, Wilcoxon test, two-tailed).

Thus, MHPG levels in PTSD subjects with exercise stress demonstrated a differential response and became comparable with the MHPG levels in control subjects in the pre- and postexercise states.

Although peripheral norepinephrine levels increased in PTSD patients with exercise, Spielberger anxiety scores remained unchanged from baseline ratings in both PTSD patients and control subjects (Table 11–2). As expected, PTSD subjects had significantly higher anxiety ratings pre- and postexercise ($P < 0.05$). No PTSD subject reported a clear exacerbation of anxiety symptoms or of reexperiencing phenomena (e.g., flashbacks) with exercise stress.

DISCUSSION

This pilot study suggests that PTSD patients may have an exaggerated MHPG response to exercise stress. The results must be interpreted with caution because of the small sample size and because catecholamine measurements were cross-sectional (pre- or postexercise) rather than serial in time. The similar norepinephrine levels contrast with findings from psychophysiological studies suggesting increased SNS arousal (Blanchard et al. 1982; Kolb 1987; Pitman et al. 1987), and with a previous report of increased urinary norepinephrine excretion in PTSD (Kosten et al. 1987). This finding may, however, be comparable to a report of

Table 11–2. State anxiety scores in PTSD patients and control subjects: response to exercise stress

	Baseline	Postexercise
PTSD ($n = 10$)	25 ± 6[a]	24 ± 4[b]
Control ($n = 8$)	12 ± 3	12 ± 2[c]

[a]PTSD scores significantly higher than control scores at baseline ($t = 5.69$, df = 16, $P < 0.001$) and postexercise ($t = 7.16$, df = 16, $P < 0.001$).
[b]No significant change in PTSD scores postexercise ($t = 0.34$, df = 9, $P = 0.744$, two-tailed).
[c]No significant change in control scores postexercise ($t = 0$, df = 7, $P = 1.00$, two-tailed).

normal norepinephrine levels in panic disorder patients (Villa-cres et al. 1987). Also, the cross-sectional measurement of plasma norepinephrine may not as accurately reflect total SNS activity as do the urinary excretion studies (Kosten et al. 1987). The increased norepinephrine levels secondary to maximal exercise in both PTSD patients and control subjects are consistent with previous studies demonstrating similar responses in normal subjects (Galbo et al. 1975; Kotchen et al. 1971; McMurray et al. 1987; Ziegler et al. 1985). The exaggerated MHPG response to exercise stress suggests an increased sensitivity to noradrenergic activation in these PTSD patients. In healthy subjects, a combination of exercise and mental stress (memory and calculation tests) has been reported to significantly increase urinary MHPG excretion (Peyrin et al. 1987), whereas neither mental stress nor exercise alone produced significant changes in MHPG. Peyrin et al. (1987) suggested that "physical work under mental loading" was required to facilitate this noradrenergic activity. Conceivably, in our PTSD patients, chronic psychological stress may predispose to similar noradrenergic changes with exercise stress. Conversely, because our healthy control subjects had minimal psychological stress prior to exercise (i.e., low state anxiety scores), their MHPG levels did not change significantly with exercise.

Whether these peripheral MHPG changes reflect central abnormalities of norepinephrine function as discussed for other patient populations (Elsworth et al. 1982; Kopin et al. 1983) is unclear. In panic disorder patients, Charney et al. (1984) demonstrated increased plasma MHPG responses to yohimbine, an α_2-adrenergic receptor antagonist that increases central norepinephrine function. These investigators also demonstrated decreased plasma MHPG in panic disorder patients with clonidine challenge (Charney and Heninger 1986). More recently, this group has found increased MHPG responses to yohimbine in PTSD patients as well (see Charney et al., Chapter 6, this volume). It is possible that in our study, changes in MHPG values secondary to the acute physical stress reflect changes primarily in peripheral norepinephrine metabolism. The trend toward lower resting MHPG levels in PTSD patients may suggest decreased and/or central or peripheral norepinephrine neuron activity and needs further study in a larger number of patients. This finding is interesting in light of a previous report of low MHPG levels in untreated panic disorder patients (Edlund et al. 1987). Other reports, however, have found resting MHPG levels in panic disorder patients to be similar to control values (Charney and Heninger 1985; Nesse et al. 1984). The comparable norepinephrine levels following maximal exercise in PTSD and control groups may suggest that SNS norepinephrine depletion, per se, is not present. Together, these data may be consistent with preclinical studies suggesting that animals exposed to certain repeated stressors may have increased central and peripheral norepinephrine synthesis, as recently reviewed (Murburg et al. 1990).

The PTSD patients did not experience an exacerbation of their anxiety symptoms with exercise in this study. Because exercise is a relatively nonspecific stressor, this might suggest that certain psychological stimuli are more relevant in producing acute exacerbations of anxiety (Kolb 1987). The minimal changes in anxiety symptoms in PTSD subjects after exercise contrasted with the significant increases in peripheral norepinephrine and MHPG levels. The data suggest that these increased peripheral catecholamine levels may not always be associated with increased anxiety in these patients. This possibility contrasts with reports that certain groups of other anxiety disorder patients may be sensitive to exercise (Roy-Byrne and Unde 1988). To our knowledge, however, effects of exercise on plasma catecholamines or anxiety have not been investigated previously in PTSD.

In summary, the findings of this study suggest that changes in noradrenergic function are present in PTSD as reflected by an exaggerated MHPG responsiveness to exercise stress. Further study of the noradrenergic system in PTSD is warranted.

REFERENCES

American Psychiatric Association: Diagnostic and Statistical Manual of Mental Disorders, 3rd Edition, Revised. Washington, DC, American Psychiatric Association, 1987

Anisman HL, Sklar LS: Catecholamine depletion in mice upon reexposure to stress: mediation of the escape deficits reduced by inescapable shock. Journal of Comparative and Physiological Psychology 93:610–625, 1979

Anisman HL, Ritch M, Sklar LS: Noradrenergic and dopaminergic interactions in escape behavior. Psychopharmacology (Berlin) 74:263–268, 1981

Blanchard EB, Kolb LC, Pallmeyer TP: A psychophysiological study of post-traumatic stress disorder in Vietnam veterans. Psychiatr Q 54:220–228, 1982

Boudewyns PA, Hyer L, Woods MG, et al: PTSD among Vietnam veterans: an early look at treatment outcome using direct therapeutic exposure. Journal of Traumatic Stress 3(suppl 3):359–368, 1990

Charney DS, Heninger GR: Noradrenergic function and the mechanism of action of antianxiety treatment and the effect of long-term alprazolam treatment. Arch Gen Psychiatry 42:458–467, 1985

Charney DS, Heninger GR: Abnormal regulation of noradrenergic function in panic disorders: effects of clonidine in healthy subjects and patients with agoraphobia and panic disorder. Arch Gen Psychiatry 43:1042–1054, 1986

Charney DS, Heninger GR, Breier A: Noradrenergic function in panic anxiety: effects of yohimbine in healthy subjects and patients with agoraphobia and panic disorder. Arch Gen Psychiatry 41:751–763, 1984

Edlund MJ, Swann AC, Davis CM: Plasma MHPG in untreated panic disorder. Biol Psychiatry 22:1488–1491, 1987

Elsworth JD, Redmond DE, Roth RH: Plasma and CSF 2-methoxy-4-hydroxyphenylethylglycol (MHPG) as indices of brain norepinephrine metabolism in primates. Brain Res 235:115–124, 1982

Galbo H, Holst JJ, Christensen NJ: Glucagon and plasma catecholamine responses to graded and prolonged exercise. J Appl Physiol 38:70–76, 1975

Heninger GR, Charney DS: Monoamine receptor systems and anxiety disorders. Psychiatr Clin North Am 11:309–326, 1988

Kolb LC: A neuropsychological hypothesis explaining post-traumatic stress disorders. Am J Psychiatry 144:989–995, 1987

Kopin IJ, Gordon EK, Jimerson DC, et al: Relation between plasma and cerebrospinal fluid level of 3-methoxy-5-hydroxyphenylethylglycol. Science 219:73–75, 1983

Kosten TR, Mason JW, Giller EL, et al: Sustained urinary norepinephrine and epinephrine elevation in post-traumatic stress disorder. Psychoneuroendocrinology 12:13–20, 1987

Kotchen TA, Hartley LH, Rice TW, et al: Renin, norepinephrine, and epinephrine responses to graded exercise. J Appl Physiol 31:178–184, 1971

Lader M: The peripheral and central role of the catecholamines in the mechanisms of anxiety. International Pharmacopsychiatry 9:125–137, 1974

Maier SF, Seligman MEP: Learned helplessness: theory and evidence. J Exp Psychol 105:3–46, 1976

McFall ME, Murburg MM, Ko GN, et al: Autonomic responses to stress in Vietnam combat veterans with post-traumatic stress disorder. Biol Psychiatry 27:1165–1175, 1990

McMurray RG, Forsythe WA, Mar MH, et al: Exercise intensity-related responses of beta-endorphin and catecholamines. Med Sci Sports Exerc 19:570–574, 1987

Mellman TA, Davis GC: Combat-related flashbacks in PTSD: phenomenology and similarity to panic attacks. J Clin Psychiatry 49:379–382, 1985

Minegishi A, Ishizaki T: Determination of free 3-methoxy-4-hydroxyphenylglycol with several other monoamine metabolites in plasma by high performance liquid chromatography with anlperometric detection. J Chromatogr 311:51–57, 1984

Murburg MM, McFall ME, Veith RC: Catecholamines, stress, and posttraumatic stress disorder, in Biological Assessment and Treatment of Posttraumatic Stress Disorder. Edited by Giller EL Jr. Washington, DC, American Psychiatric Press, 1990, pp 27–64

Nesse RM, Cameron OG, Curtis GC, et al: Adrenergic function in patients with panic anxiety. Arch Gen Psychiatry 41:771–776, 1984

Peyrin L, Pequignot JM, Lacour JR, et al: Relationships between catecholamine or 3-methoxy-4-hydroxyphenylglycol changes and the mental performance under submaximal exercise in man. Psychopharmacology (Berlin) 93:188–192, 1987

Pitman RK, Orr SP, Forgue DF, et al: Psychophysiologic assessment of post-traumatic stress disorder imagery in Vietnam combat veterans. Arch Gen Psychiatry 44:970–975, 1987

Roy-Byrne PR, Unde TW: Exogenous factors in panic disorder: clinical and research implications. J Clin Psychiatry 49:56–61, 1988

Spielberger CD: Trait-state anxiety and motor behavior. J Mot Behav 3:265–279, 1971

Van der Kolk BA, Greenberg MS, Boyd H, et al: Inescapable shock, neurotransmitters, and addiction to trauma: toward a psychobiology of post-traumatic stress. Biol Psychiatry 20:314–325, 1985

Villacres EC, Hollifield M, Katon WJ, et al: Sympathetic nervous system activity in panic disorder. Psychiatry Res 21:313, 1987

Weiss JM, Glazer HI, Phorecky LA, et al: Effects of chronic exposure to stressors on subsequent avoidancescape behavior and or brain norepinephrine. Psychosom Med 37:522–524, 1975

Ziegler MG, Milano AJ, Hull E: The catecholaminergic response to stress and exercise, in The Catecholamines in Psychiatric and Neurologic Disorders. Edited by Lake CR, Ziegler MG. Boston, MA, Butterworth Publishers, 1985, pp 37–53

Chapter 12

Neurobiological Sequelae of Childhood Trauma: PTSD in Children

Bruce D. Perry, M.D., Ph.D.

T raumatic events can have a profound and lasting impact on the emotional, cognitive, behavioral, and physiological functioning of an individual. These adverse effects have been described in combat veterans since the Civil War (Birkhimer et al. 1985; Bleich et al. 1986; Bury 1918; Da Costa 1871; Dobbs and Wilson 1960; Fraser and Wilson 1918). Only recently, however, has the distinct trauma-associated syndrome characterized by prominent affective symptoms (e.g., dysphoria, irritability, anxiety) and a "hyperactive" sympathetic nervous system (SNS; Brende 1982; Horowitz et al. 1980) been called posttraumatic stress disorder (PTSD; American Psychiatric Association 1987).

The symptoms of PTSD fall into three clusters: 1) recurring intrusive recollection of the traumatic event such as dreams and "flashbacks," 2) persistent avoidance of stimuli associated with the trauma or numbing of general responsiveness, and 3) persistent symptoms of increased arousal characterized by hypervigilance, increased startle response, sleep difficulties, irritability, anxiety, and physiological hyperreactivity. While the disorder

The author would like to thank the staff, residents, and students of St. Joseph's Carondelet Child Center and the members of the Laboratory of Developmental Neurosciences. These studies were supported in part by the Carondelet Center for the Study of Childhood Trauma, the Brain Research Foundation of Chicago, and the Harris Center for Developmental Studies.

was described originally in combat veterans, a high percentage of rape victims, sexual abuse victims, survivors of natural or man-made disasters, and witnesses to violence also experience symptoms of PTSD (e.g., Blanchard et al. 1983; Boehnlein et al. 1985; McLeer et al. 1988; Terr 1983). Many victims of these traumatic events are children.

The present chapter reviews childhood PTSD with a specific focus on neurobiological sequelae of childhood trauma and presents some preliminary evidence of altered functioning of brainstem catecholaminergic systems in childhood PTSD. In specific, it is hypothesized that the abnormal patterns of catecholamine activity associated with prolonged "alarm reactions" induced by traumatic events during infancy and childhood can result in altered development of the central nervous system (CNS). Furthermore, it is hypothesized that this altered development includes a "dysregulated" brain stem that in turn results in a host of signs and symptoms related to abnormal brain-stem functioning, including altered cardiovascular regulation, affective lability, behavioral impulsivity, increased anxiety, increased startle response, and sleep abnormalities. Finally, early life experience is discussed, in the context of childhood trauma, as an "expresser" of genetic predispositions.

THE SCOPE OF CHILDHOOD TRAUMA

Posttraumatic stress disorder has been described in survivors of sexual abuse (Browne and Finkelhor 1986; Conte 1985), victims of violence (Boehnlein et al. 1985), witnesses to violent acts (Eth and Pynoos 1985), survivors of natural disasters (McFarlane 1987), survivors of catastrophic accidents (Martini et al. 1990), and burn victims (Perry et al. 1987), among others. Although no epidemiological data regarding childhood PTSD are available, conservative estimates can be made based upon the incidence of traumatic events in the childhood population. Conservative estimates of childhood sexual abuse suggest an incidence of 200,000 new cases each year (Finkelhor 1984). Maltreatment of children (i.e., physical, emotional, or sexual abuse) is estimated to exceed 1.5 million children per year (U.S. Department of Health and Human Services 1988). Prevalence values for sexual (roughly 10% to 35%)

and physical abuse (5% to 15%) vary (see Conte 1985; Greenwood et al. 1990), but even with conservative estimates (there are approximately 65 million children in the United States below the age of 16), the number of children exposed to one of these severe traumas is 9.5 million. Children are often witnesses to, in addition to being victims of, violence. Eth and Pynoos (1985) have estimated that approximately 3 million children each year witness violence in their homes. Each year thousands of children survive natural or man-made disasters and traumatizing medical problems such as burns.

Taken together, a conservative estimate of children currently at risk for PTSD exceeds 15 million, and this number grows, as traumatized children carry their scars to adulthood and new children are traumatized each year. It is estimated that 15% of Vietnam veterans (1.5 million people) experience PTSD (Helzer et al. 1987); yet if one assumes that only 10% of the children traumatized since 1964 develop symptoms (a very conservative estimate), there would be 4.5 million "veterans" of childhood with PTSD. Despite the scope of this serious public health problem, relatively little research has been dedicated to this area. Some critical initial steps toward understanding the effects of childhood trauma—descriptive and clinical studies—have been carried out.

THE CLINICAL PICTURE: CHILDHOOD PTSD

Clinical descriptive studies of PTSD in children have been pioneered by Dr. Lenore Terr (Terr 1983). Although fitting roughly into the three main clusters described above, the symptoms of PTSD in children present a more confusing diagnostic picture for the clinician, often appearing as attention-deficit hyperactivity disorder, conduct disorder, anxiety disorders, and mood disorders (Terr 1991).

Over the last several years, childhood PTSD has been the focus of study at the Center for the Study of Childhood Trauma in Chicago. A number of interesting observations have been made regarding the clinical picture of childhood PTSD. In the population at the center, comorbid DSM-III-R diagnoses were seen in 85% of the children with PTSD. In many cases the only clear distinguishing features of PTSD were 1) documented history of a severe traumatic event(s), 2) exacerbation of symptoms with reexposure to trauma-specific stimuli, and 3) autonomic nervous system (ANS) hyperarousal. These three features were noted in children who exhibited psychotic, anxiety, and affective symptoms as well as symptoms of disordered conduct (often aggressive or sexualized, dependent upon the original trauma). One of the more interesting groups we have identified is a set of children severely traumatized during the first 3 years of life, resulting in an apparent posttraumatic pervasive developmental delay. In almost all cases the children do not understand their symptoms as being related to their history of trauma, and often, especially in the children abused before age 4, cognitive recall of the trauma is not present. In this regard, it is easy to see how the diagnosis of PTSD is underreported in children—a child presents with any array of psychiatric symptoms with no understanding or recall of traumatic events in his or her early life, often with an adult caretaker who is unaware of (e.g., sexual abuse), or unwilling to give (e.g., physical abuse) history regarding the trauma. A very consistent physical finding in these children, however, is ANS hyperarousal.

Many factors appear to be important in the development of PTSD following trauma: the nature of the trauma, the degree to which body integrity is threatened, and the family support system following a trauma, among others (see Eth and Pynoos 1985). We observed two important factors that appeared to play a role in the specific set of symptoms a given child will exhibit following trauma: 1) family history of psychiatric disorder and 2) age at which trauma occurred. Consistent with diathesis-stress models of mental illness, we observed that, in general, if an individual had a family history of schizophrenia, the symptoms expressed following childhood trauma included some prepsychotic- and psychotic-range symptoms; if affective or anxiety disorders were in the family history, the expressed symptoms pertained to disorders of mood and anxiety; and if there was a strong history of alcoholism and sociopathy, symptoms pertained more to conduct disorder. All of this was superimposed on a developmental matrix so that severe trauma occurring before age 4 resulted in a much higher probability of prepsychotic and psychotic symptomatology. On the other hand, children with a stable first 3 years of life but traumatized later in childhood tended to have more affective and anxiety symptoms similar to those observed in adult PTSD (Perry 1993a, 1993b). These observations may shed light on recent studies suggesting a relationship between childhood sexual and physical abuse and borderline personality disorder (Ogata et al. 1990). In this regard we have found the same ANS hyperarousal and downregulated platelet alpha$_2$ (α_2)–adrenergic receptors in borderline personality disorder (Southwick et al. 1990a, 1990b) as we observed in adult PTSD (Perry 1988; Perry et al. 1987, 1990).

This complex clinical picture complicates neurophysiological research in childhood PTSD. Indeed, most of the useful clinical research that informs the future directions of this field has not been performed within the conceptual framework of the DSM-III-R diagnostic entity of PTSD. Much of the important descriptive work comes from studies of the effects of sexual or physical abuse (e.g., Browne and Finkelhor 1986; Dodge et al. 1991) and of early-life loss as a predisposing feature for mood disorders (e.g., Breier et al. 1987, 1988). Despite a relative abundance of clinical descriptive studies from these areas, we know very little about the pathophysiology underlying the many physical signs and symptoms of childhood PTSD (Ornitz and Pynoos 1989). Studies of the neurobiology of PTSD in adults that suggest altered functioning of catecholamines, as discussed throughout this volume, provide direction for studies in children. Involvement of CNS catecholamines in the pathophysiology of childhood PTSD is not surprising considering the key role they play in the stress response (Murburg et al. 1990; see also Aston-Jones et al., Chapter 2; Simson and Weiss, Chapter 3, this volume).

CATECHOLAMINES AND STRESS

In 1914, Walter B. Cannon first coined the phrase "fight or flight" to describe the body's appropriate response to a stressful stimulus. When an individual is exposed to real or perceived danger, a series of complex, interactive neurophysiological reactions occur in the brain, the ANS, the hypothalamic-pituitary-adrenocortical (HPA) axis, and the immune system. These responses evolved to provide the critical total body mobilization required for the individual to survive a life-threatening danger. In the initial phases, first labeled the "alarm reaction" and the "stage of resistance" by Hans Selye in 1936, portions of the brain involved in arousal, attention, and concentration become activated, resulting in hypervigilance to the danger accompanied by a decrease in attention to less pressing environmental stimuli—a soldier in the midst of a fire fight, for example, may not know he has been wounded until the end of the fight.

The neurophysiology of the "alarm reaction" has been studied extensively in human and in animal models (Murburg et al. 1990; Selye 1936; Stone 1975, 1988). Acute "stress" is associated with a variety of physiological responses including the activation of the HPA axis with concomitant peripheral release of ACTH, epinephrine, and cortisol; a significant increase in centrally controlled peripheral SNS tone; and the "activation" of a variety of neurochemical systems in the CNS.

One of the most critical of these systems is the noradrenergic nucleus in the locus coeruleus (LC) (Korf 1976). This region controls noradrenergic tone and activity throughout the midbrain and in important forebrain areas including the cortex (Foote et al. 1983). The LC has been shown to be critical in many regulatory functions including the regulation of affect, "irritability," locomotion, arousal, attention, and startle (Andrade and Aghajanian 1984; Bhaskaran and Freed 1988; Foote et al. 1983; Korf 1976).

Another key neural system in the brain, also an adrenergic/noradrenergic system, is the ventral tegmental nucleus (VTN), which is involved in regulation of the sympathetic nuclei in the pons/medulla (Moore and Bloom 1979). Both the LC and the VTN have adrenergic receptors that are involved in modulation of the adrenergic or noradrenergic afferentation and efferent outflow (Perry et al. 1983; Vantini et al. 1984; see also Aston-Jones et al., Chapter 2; Simson and Weiss, Chapter 3, this volume). The critical role of CNS catecholamines and their receptors is discussed in detail elsewhere (Giller et al. 1990; Murburg et al. 1990; Perry 1988; Perry et al. 1990; see also Aston-Jones et al., Chapter 2; Simson and Weiss, Chapter 3, this volume). For the present discussion it is sufficient to know that acute stress results in an increase in LC and VTN activity.

The neurophysiological activation seen during acute stress is usually rapid and reversible. When the stressful event is of sufficient duration, intensity, or frequency, however, these changes are not reversible. Stress-induced "sensitization" occurs, with the neurochemical systems that mediate the stress response (e.g., LC noradrenergic systems) changing, becoming more "sensitive" to future stressful events. The molecular mechanisms underlying this phenomenon are not well understood but likely are related to changes in receptor sensitivity following transiently increased neurotransmitter activity, similar to that which is seen in cocaine sensitization (Kalivas and Duffy 1989; Kleven et al. 1990; see also Charney et al., Chapter 6, this volume). The major increases in catecholamine activity evident during the stress response result in increased receptor stimulation and intracellular receptor–mediated signals. In turn, these changes in intracellular second and third messengers result in altered gene expression of a variety of important structural and regulatory proteins including receptor/effector systems (Goelet and Kandel 1986; Kandel and Schwartz 1982). Finally, the altered expression of these proteins alters the responsiveness of the catecholaminergic systems mediating stress. It is this altered responsiveness that can be related to the hypervigilance, increased startle, affective lability, anxiety, dysphoria, increased SNS activity, and reactivity seen in PTSD (Krystal et al. 1989; Perry et al. 1990).

CATECHOLAMINES AND DEVELOPMENT

In the adult, with a mature brain, the increases in catecholamine activity associated with the stress response may result in sensitization. In the developing brain, however, neurotransmitters and hormones play key roles in neuronal migration, differentiation, synaptic proliferation, and overall brain development (Lauder 1988). Therefore, the tremendous increases in neurotransmitter activity seen with severe or prolonged stress would be expected to have a significant impact on brain development.

While each neuron, indeed each cell, in an individual's brain contains the same genetic material, each expresses a slightly different portion. As the brain develops, neurons divide, migrate, and differentiate in response to "microenvironmental" cues that confer information to, and direct specific differentiation of, the cell. Each neuron's unique structural, biochemical, and functional character, then, is a function of its unique environmental history—that is, the specific pattern, timing, and quantity of these microenvironmental cues. Some of the most important of these cues are receptor-mediated signals from neurotransmitters and hormones. Indeed, catecholaminergic cues during development are important in determining critical functional properties of mature neurons, including the density of neurotransmitter receptors (e.g., Miller and Friedhoff 1988; Perry et al. 1990). Alterations in the pattern, timing, and quantity of catecholamine (or any critical neurotransmitter system) activity during development might be expected to result in altered development of catecholamine receptor/effector systems and the functions mediated in part by these systems. A trauma-induced prolonged stress response is likely to result in an abnormal pattern, timing, and intensity of catecholamine activity in the developing brain. The development of the human brain continues beyond birth and remains vulnerable to the abnormal patterns of neurotransmitter and hormone activity seen following trauma. Young children victimized by trauma are at risk for developing permanent vulnerabilities—that is, permanent changes in neuronal differentiation and organization. In this regard, childhood PTSD is a developmental disorder.

It appears that there are developmental phases during which an individual is most vulnerable to traumatic stressors. These most vulnerable periods occur during the development of the complex stress-mediating CNS systems, including the catecholamines. It is likely that the functional capabilities of the CNS systems mediating stress in the adult are determined by the nature of the "stress" experiences during the development of these systems (i.e., in utero, during infancy and childhood) (Perry 1988; Perry et al. 1990). A number of fascinating studies in animals demonstrate the exquisite sensitivity of the developing CNS to stress (see Suoumi 1986). In rats exposed to perinatal handling stress, major alterations in the ability of the rat to "learn" and to respond appropriately to stressors are seen later in life (Weinstock et al. 1988). The most interesting aspect of these studies is that exposure to unpredictable stress resulted in deficits, whereas exposure to consistent, daily stress resulted in "improved" or superior behavior, that is, "resilience."

One can speculate on equivalent "controlled" or daily stress and uncontrollable, nonscheduled stressors in the development of a human. An infant who is allowed to have an "optimal" degree of frustration—one who can control, during rapprochement, his or her own optimal degree of "tension" and "anxiety" (i.e., stress) and return to mother for comfort—is one whose developing CNS is establishing an appropriate neurochemical milieu for the development of a flexible, maximally adaptive physiological apparatus for responding to future stressors. A child who is reared in an unpredictable, abusive, or neglectful environment (see Spitz and Wolf 1946) will likely have evoked in his developing CNS a milieu that will result in a poorly organized, "dysregulated" CNS catecholaminergic system. One would hypothesize that such an individual would be susceptible to the development of more severe signs and symptoms when exposed to psychosocial stressors through the course of his or her life.

Some studies in humans suggest that this is indeed the case. Increased psychiatric symptoms and disorders are observed in adults who have severe, unpredictable early-life stressors (Brown et al. 1977; Lloyd 1980; Rutter 1984). A provocative study by Breier and co-workers (1988) focused on the effects of parental loss during childhood on the development of psychopathology in adulthood. The authors examined a number of adults who had suffered a parental loss during childhood and found that the subjects with psychiatric disorders and symptoms had significant biological and immunological changes related to early parental loss relative to control groups. The authors concluded that early parental loss (i.e., a traumatic event) accompanied by the lack of a supportive relationship subsequent to the loss (i.e., an external stress-reducing factor) is related to the development of adult psychopathology.

If an early life trauma results in an abnormal pattern of stress-mediating neurotransmitter and hormone, and if this abnormal set of cues alters development of CNS catecholaminergic systems in an adverse fashion, this should be manifest when examining functions putatively mediated by these CNS catecholamines (see Moore and Bloom 1979). One would predict a host of abnormalities related to catecholaminergic regulation of affect, anxiety, arousal/concentration, impulse control, sleep, startle, and ANS regulation, among others. Clearly the clinical symptoms of PTSD support altered functioning in many of these domains. In the next sections of this chapter we review some of our preliminary investigations of the pathophysiology of severe chronic childhood PTSD.

STUDIES IN CHILDHOOD PTSD

Over the past several years, a variety of studies have been in progress at the Center for the Study of Childhood Trauma. Although multiple groups of children with PTSD have been studied, in the present chapter we will discuss our studies with the severe chronic PTSD group. All of the children in this group have been victims of severe, repeated trauma (usually physical or violent sexual abuse, or both) typically occurring during the first 5 years of life. Diagnosis was made using a modification of the Structured Interview for PTSD (Davidson et al. 1990). It was hypothesized that because this group experienced trauma early in development, major disruptions of brain-stem organization/development would be more easily observed.

Platelet Alpha2-Adrenergic Receptors in Childhood PTSD

Alpha2-adrenergic receptors, both pre- and postsynaptic, play important roles in mediating the effects of the catecholaminergic systems of the LC and VTN (Perry et al. 1983; Vantini et al. 1984; see also Simson and Weiss, Chapter 3, this volume) and thereby in mediating both acute and chronic stress (Stone 1975, 1988; U'Prichard and Kvetnansky 1980). Over the last few years, we have demonstrated downregulated and desensitized platelet α_2-adrenergic receptors in combat veterans with PTSD (Perry 1988; Perry et al. 1987, 1990). We have been able to demonstrate that, using this marker, we can track the overall "tone" of the SNS (Perry 1988; Perry et al. 1990; Southwick et al. 1990a, 1990b). This indirect method has been useful in examining regulation and dysregulation of the brain-stem catecholaminergic systems involved in the regulation of the SNS.

We performed an initial pilot study using these peripheral receptor measures in childhood PTSD (Perry et al., manuscript submitted for publication). Platelet α_2-adrenergic binding sites were measured in a small group ($n = 8$) of children (mean age = 11.1 years, range = 9–13) with PTSD using standard methodologies (Perry 1988). When compared with an age-comparable control group, the PTSD group had fewer total binding sites (Figure 12–1), a finding that is similar to our observations in adult PTSD. Downregulation of peripheral adrenergic receptors is not unexpected. This quite likely reflects downregulation in the presence of "higher than control" levels of circulating catecholamines as-

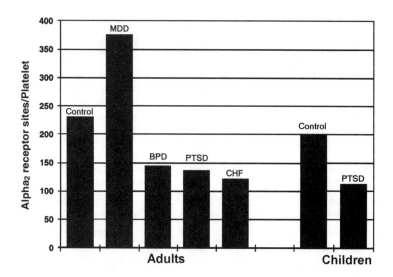

Figure 12–1.   Platelet alpha$_2$ (α_2)–adrenergic receptor binding sites in childhood PTSD. Alpha$_2$ receptor sites were measured using standard methods (Perry 1988), and comparison of these values was made across a variety of disorders. These values all derive from our laboratory, and the adult values summarize findings reported previously (Perry 1988; Perry et al. 1987, 1990; Southwick et al. 1990a, 1990b). Groups include adult control ($n = 24$), major depression (MDD, $n = 8$), borderline personality disorder (BPD, $n = 14$), adult PTSD ($n = 25$), congestive heart failure (CHF, $n = 23$), children control ($n = 14$), and childhood PTSD ($n = 8$).

sociated with the hyperreactive SNS seen in PTSD (Kosten et al. 1987; see also Murburg et al., Chapter 1, this volume).

These receptor measures are relatively invasive and difficult to employ for longitudinal studies in already traumatized children. We elected to seek other measures for our larger studies. Because the goal was to examine potential dysregulation of brain-stem catecholamines, we elected to utilize simple measures, such as autonomic regulation of heart rate, that are regulated, in part, by brain-stem catecholamines (Murphy et al. 1988). We first demonstrated a relationship between a baseline heart rate measure and platelet α_2 receptor density. Using the children with PTSD and control subjects from the preliminary receptor studies (Figure 12–1), an estimate of resting heart rate (obtained by the mean of two baseline periods on either side of an orthostatic challenge [see below]) was found to be correlated with the density of platelet α_2-adrenergic receptors ($r = -0.839; P < 0.001$). This correlation is not surprising considering that overall sympathetic tone is a major determinant of both heart rate and platelet α_2 receptor density.

Cardiovascular Lability in Childhood PTSD

A prominent feature of the children we have studied with PTSD is significant cardiovascular lability, which is manifested in a variety of ways. First of all, the majority of our PTSD population has a resting tachycardia. Of the 34 children meeting DSM PTSD diagnostic criteria, 85% had a resting heart rate greater than 94 beats per minute (bpm). (The value for an age-comparable group of normal children is 84 [Matthews et al. 1987].) Forty percent had resting rates above 100 bpm.

This lability was even more evident following a simple orthostatic challenge (Figure 12–2). In this simple procedure, a child was supine for 9 minutes, during which time a baseline heart rate was established. At 9.5 minutes, the child stood up and remained standing for another 10 minutes. Heart rate was monitored throughout this procedure. Two general patterns of heart rate change following orthostatic challenge were seen (see legend to Figure 12–2 for details). In general, the two PTSD patterns are generally described by higher-than-control basal rate and either a

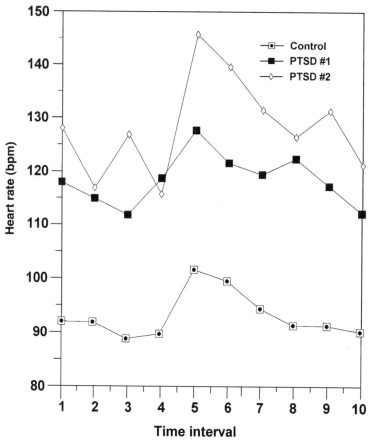

Figure 12–2. Heart rate changes following orthostatic challenge in children with PTSD. Examples of the two major patterns of change in heart rate observed in children with severe chronic PTSD are given. Heart rate was monitored every 2 minutes for 20 minutes. During the first 4 time intervals, children were resting quietly in a supine position; after 9 minutes (4.5 time intervals), children stood up and remained standing for the duration of the challenge period. A control pattern is illustrated by the open squares (child, age 11.4 years, with psychiatric disorder other than PTSD). The two PTSD patterns are generally described by a higher-than-control basal rate and either a dramatic overshoot of heart rate with a slow return to a baseline (open diamonds) or a more normal increase in heart rate but a sluggish return to a baseline rate (closed squares).

dramatic overshoot of heart rate with a slow return to a baseline (open diamonds in Figure 12–2) or a more normal increase in heart rate but a sluggish return to a baseline rate (closed squares in Figure 12–2).

Clearly these simple studies reflect abnormal regulation of simple reflexes mediated in part by brain-stem catecholamines. Central regulation of autonomic function, including cardiovascular reflexes, is very complex (see Loewy and Spyer 1990), but the power of these findings suggests poorly integrated brain-stem functioning. Cardiovascular afferentation influences the activity of the LC (Elam et al. 1984; Svensson 1987). This finding would suggest that in addition to any primary dysfunction of the LC related to altered developmental afferentation, these children with overactive and poorly regulated cardiovascular systems may have overactive and poorly regulated afferentation to the LC. This in turn may be related to some of the symptoms observed in PTSD.

The cardiovascular findings above are from one end of the spectrum of abused and traumatized children. Although caution should be used in generalizing the findings to other populations with childhood PTSD, it is likely that similar pathophysiological mechanisms may also be important in other traumatized children. Our preliminary studies in other children with PTSD suggest that this is the case.

Clonidine Treatment of Childhood PTSD

The receptor and cardiovascular evidence above suggested that one of the key features of our PTSD population was overactive (increased) sympathetic tone and overreactive, poorly regulated (exaggerated orthostatic responses) brain-stem catecholaminergic systems. For this reason, an open trial of clonidine was carried out. Clonidine is an α_2-adrenergic receptor partial agonist that acts via a combination of presynaptic inhibition and postsynaptic α_2 receptors, some on important sympathetic nuclei, which may be the mechanism by which it is an effective antihypertensive medication. In limited open trials, clonidine has been found to be effective in treatment of adult PTSD (Kolb et al. 1984).

Seventeen children with PTSD (13 male, 4 female; mean age

10.4 years, range = 6.0–14.2) were drug free for at least 4 weeks, during which time baseline symptoms were assessed by using the Psychiatric Symptom Assessment Scale (PSAS; Bigelow and Berthot 1989), a 23-item modification of the Brief Psychiatric Rating Scale. As part of the clinical program, a weekly PSAS was performed, independently, by each child's teacher, individual therapist, and primary child care worker. For the 4-week drug-free period prior to starting clonidine, these PSAS scores were meaned. Clonidine was started after appropriate physical examination, laboratory work, and consents had been obtained. Initial dosage was 0.05 mg bid, which was rapidly titrated up to 0.1 mg bid as tolerated. The only side effect of any significance was sedation, which was typically transient. Altering the dosage schedule to 0.05 qid significantly decreased sedation.

The effects of clonidine on psychiatric symptoms were profound (Figure 12–3). This group of children had a wide range of presentations (see descriptions above). The largest degree of improvement was in the areas of behavioral impulsivity, anxiety, arousal, concentration, and mood. Interestingly, in the few children that had prepsychotic or psychotic symptoms, improvement was seen in these symptoms as well as in the more "traditional" PTSD symptoms. In addition to improvement in psychiatric symptoms, there appeared to be a decrease in physiological "lability," likely underlying the improvement in the other symptoms. Basal heart rate of this group prior to clonidine treatment was 110 ± 12 bpm (as compared with 88 ± 10 bpm in an age comparable non-PTSD psychiatric population). Following 4 weeks of clonidine, the group mean dropped to 96 ± 8 bpm. In addition, the D-scale (autonomic arousal) score of the Structured Interview for PTSD (Davidson et al. 1990) prior to medication, 15.3 ± 4, dropped to 6 ± 3. Overall, clonidine treatment, in this population, significantly improved the signs and symptoms of childhood PTSD.

This observed pharmacologically induced decrease in arousal symptoms suggests that α_2-adrenergic receptors play a pivotal role in mediating the signs and symptoms of PTSD in this group of severely traumatized children. The role of the α_2 receptor in regulating the LC and VTN is well known (Perry et al. 1983; Vantini et al. 1984; see also Aston-Jones et al., Chapter 2; Simson and Weiss, Chapter 3, this volume). The capacity of clonidine to modulate and "buffer" LC and VTN activity is related to its special qualities as a partial agonist. In physiological systems, a partial agonist can act as both an agonist and an antagonist depending on the system's tonic activity. If the tonic activity falls below a certain level, the partial agonist will act by stimulating unoccupied receptors, thereby increasing agonism; when the tonic activity becomes too high, the partial agonist will compete with the endogenous agonist for the receptor sites and *decrease* activity of the system by virtue of lower intrinsic activity than the full-agonist neurotransmitter. In this way, clonidine activates

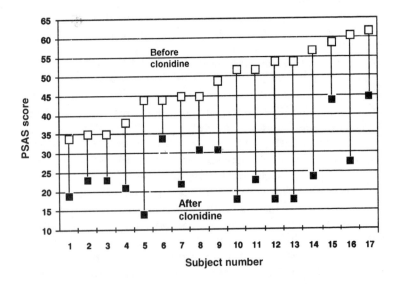

Figure 12–3. The effects of clonidine on psychiatric symptoms in childhood PTSD. Seventeen children with severe chronic PTSD received clonidine (dose range: 0.05 mg bid to 0.1 mg tid) for a 4-week period. Prior to and during this time, weekly assessments of symptoms were made independently by teacher, individual therapist, and primary child care worker using the Psychiatric Symptom Assessment Scale (PSAS). Values represent means of these three independent assessments from the 2 weeks prior to (open squares) and after the fourth week (closed squares) of clonidine treatment.

some parts of the noradrenergic terminal areas and prevents overreactivity in others. The summed effect is to help poorly regulated brain-stem catecholaminergic systems work in a more organized, efficient fashion, thereby decreasing symptoms related to dysregulation of the brain stem.

IMPLICATIONS AND FUTURE DIRECTIONS

Severe trauma during childhood can have a devastating effect on the development of the brain and on all functions mediated by this complex organ—emotional, cognitive, behavioral, and physiological. In many cases the sequelae of childhood trauma present with signs and symptoms similar to those of adult PTSD, but often they present with very different symptoms. The concept of childhood PTSD must be considered within the broader concept of the diathesis-stress model of mental illness. The diathesis-stress model suggests that a predisposition (genetic or developmental) for a specific psychiatric disorder exists that can be differentially expressed in an individual depending on the degree of biopsychosocial stressors. The concept of PTSD loses meaning if we consider all of the effects of childhood trauma as part of this "disorder." Indeed, it is clear that early life trauma/stress plays an important role as an expresser of genetically determined vulnerabilities to a variety of neuropsychiatric disorders, including schizophrenia (e.g., Garmezy 1978), major depression (Lloyd 1980), and Tourette's syndrome (Leckman et al. 1990). It is important to study childhood trauma/stress as expressers of genetic vulnerabilities to medical conditions as well (Coddington 1972a, 1972b), including cardiovascular diseases such as essential hypertension, sudden cardiac death, or cardiac dysrhythmias. Associations between stress during childhood and adolescence and the development of cardiovascular disease have been made for many years (see Boyce and Chesterman 1990). It is interesting to note that associations have also been made between vulnerability to affective disorders and cardiovascular disease. Early life stress/trauma is a common link between many associated medical and psychiatric conditions, including those that are neuroimmunological, cardiovascular, and neuroendocrinological. This is not surprising considering the critical role of development in determining the final phenotype (and therefore function) of all physiological functioning in the adult.

For a number of reasons, the long-term effects of childhood trauma remain relatively unexplored. In part this has been due to a variety of complex clinical and social issues, some of which are being addressed at present by multidisciplinary research teams working closely with the state and local social agencies involved in providing services for these traumatized children. With the high incidence of sexual abuse, physical abuse, and violence in our society, the need to understand these complex issues is ever pressing. The study of traumatized children and the long-term effects of trauma provides an important conceptual starting point from which to explore the developmental nature of all psychiatric illness and, hopefully, to develop new and effective therapeutic and preventive interventions.

REFERENCES

American Psychiatric Association: Diagnostic and Statistical Manual of Mental Disorders, 3rd Edition, Revised. Washington, DC, American Psychiatric Association, 1987

Andrade R, Aghajanian GK: Locus coeruleus activity in vitro: intrinsic regulation by a calcium-dependent potassium conductance but not alpha-2 adrenoceptors. J Neurosci 4:161–170, 1984

Bhaskaran D, Freed CR: Changes in neurotransmitter turnover in locus coeruleus produced by changes in arterial blood pressure. Brain Res Bull 21:191–199, 1988

Bigelow LB, Berthot BD: The Psychiatric Symptom Assessment Scale. Psychopharmacol Bull 25:168–179, 1989

Birkhimer LJ, DeVane CL, Muniz CE: Post-traumatic stress disorder: characteristics and pharmacological response in the veteran population. Compr Psychiatry 26:304–310, 1985

Blanchard EB, Kolb LC, Pallmeyer TP, et al: A psycho-physiologic study of posttraumatic stress disorder in Vietnam veterans. Psychiatr Q 54:220–228, 1983

Bleich A, Siegel B, Garb R, et al: Post-traumatic stress disorder following combat exposure: clinical features and psychopharmacological treatment. Br J Psychiatry 149:365–369, 1986

Boehnlein JK, Kinzie JD, Ben R, et al: One-year follow-up study of post-traumatic stress disorder among survivors of Cambodian concentration camps. Am J Psychiatry 142:956–959, 1985

Boyce WT, Chesterman E: Life events, social support, and cardiovascular reactivity in adolescence. J Dev Behav Pediatr 11:105–111, 1990

Breier A, Albus M, Pickar D, et al: Controllable and uncontrollable stress in humans: alterations in mood, neuroendocrine, and psychophysiological function. Am J Psychiatry 144:1419–1425, 1987

Breier A, Kelsoe JR, Kirwin PD: Early parental loss and development of adult psychopathology. Arch Gen Psychiatry 45:987–993, 1988

Brende JO: Electrodermal responses in post-traumatic syndromes. J Nerv Ment Dis 170:352–361, 1982

Brown GW, Harris T, Copeland JR: Depression and loss. Br J Psychiatry 130:1–18, 1977

Browne A, Finkelhor D: Impact of child sexual abuse: a review of the literature. Psychol Bull 99:66–77, 1986

Bury JS: Pathology of war neurosis. Lancet 1:97–99, 1918

Cannon WB: The emergency function of the adrenal medulla in pain and the major emotions. Am J Physiol 3:356–372, 1914

Coddington RD: The significance of life events as etiological factors in the diseases of children, I: a survey of professional workers. J Psychosom Res 16:7–18, 1972a

Coddington RD: The significance of life events as etiological factors in the diseases of children, II: a study of the normal population. J Psychosom Res 16:205–213, 1972b

Conte JR: The effects of sexual abuse on children: a critique and suggestions for future research. Victimology 10:110–130, 1985

Da Costa JM: On irritable heart: a clinical study of a form of functional cardiac disorder and its consequences. Am J Med Sci 61:17–52, 1871

Davidson JRT, Kudler HS, Smith RD: Assessment and pharmacotherapy of posttraumatic stress disorder, in Biological Assessment and Treatment of Posttraumatic Stress Disorder. Edited by Giller EL Jr. Washington, DC, American Psychiatric Press, 1990, pp 205–236

Dobbs D, Wilson WP: Observations on persistence of war neurosis. Diseases of the Nervous System 21:40–46, 1960

Dodge KA, Bates JE, Pettit GS: Mechanisms in the cycle of violence. Science 250:1678–1683, 1991

Elam M, Svensson TH, Thorén P: Regulation of locus coeruleus neurons and splanchinic, sympathetic nerves by cardiovascular afferents. Brain Res 290:281–287, 1984

Eth S, Pynoos RS (eds): Post-Traumatic Stress Disorder in Children. Washington, DC, American Psychiatric Press, 1985

Finkelhor D: Child Sexual Abuse. New York, Free Press, 1984

Foote SL, Bloom FE, Aston-Jones G: Nucleus locus coeruleus: new evidence of anatomical and physiological specificity. Physiol Rev 63:844–856, 1983

Fraser F, Wilson RM: The sympathetic nervous system and the "irritable heart of soldiers." BMJ 2:27–29, 1918

Garmezy N: Observations on high-risk research and premorbid development in schizophrenia, in The Nature of Schizophrenia. Edited by Wynne LC, Cromwell A, Matthysse S. New York, Wiley, 1978

Giller EL Jr, Perry BD, Southwick S, et al: Psychoendocrinology of posttraumatic stress disorder, in Posttraumatic Stress Disorder: Etiology, Phenomenology, and Treatment. Edited by Wolf ME, Mosnaim AD. Washington, DC, American Psychiatric Press, 1990, pp 158–167

Goelet P, Kandel ER: Tracking the flow of learned information from membrane receptors to genome. Trends Neurosci 9:492–499, 1986

Greenwood CL, Tangalos EG, Maruta T: Prevalence of sexual abuse, physical abuse, and concurrent traumatic life events in a general medical population. Mayo Clin Proc 65:1067–1071, 1990

Helzer J, Robins L, McEvoy L: Post traumatic stress disorder in the general population. N Engl J Med 317:1630–1634, 1987

Horowitz MJ, Wilner N, Kaltredder N, et al: Signs and symptoms of post-traumatic stress disorder. Arch Gen Psychiatry 37:85–92, 1980

Kalivas PW, Duffy P: Similar effects of daily cocaine and stress on mesocorticolimbic dopamine neurotransmission in the rat. Biol Psychiatry 25:913–928, 1989

Kandel ER, Schwartz JH: Molecular biology of an elementary form of learning: modulation of transmitter release by cyclic AMP. Science 218:433–443, 1982

Kleven MS, Perry BD, Woolveron WL, et al: Effects of repeated injections of cocaine on D-1 and D-2 dopamine receptors in rat brain. Brain Res 532:265–270, 1990

Kolb LC, Burris BC, Griffiths S: Propranolol and clonidine in the treatment of post traumatic stress disorders of war, in Post Traumatic Stress Disorders: Psychological and Biological Sequelae. Edited by van der Kolk BA. Washington, DC, American Psychiatric Press, 1984, pp 29–44

Korf J: Locus coeruleus, noradrenaline metabolism, and stress, in Catecholamines and Stress. Edited by Usdin E, Kvetnansky R, Kopin IJ. New York, Pergamon, 1976, pp 105–111

Kosten TR, Mason JW, Giller EL, et al: Sustained urinary norepinephrine and epinephrine elevation in post-traumatic stress disorder. Psychoneuroendocrinology 12:13–20, 1987

Krystal JH, Kosten T, Perry BD, et al: Neurobiological aspects of posttraumatic stress disorder: review of clinical and preclinical studies. Behavior Therapy 20:177–193, 1989

Lauder JM: Neurotransmitters as morphogens. Prog Brain Res 73:365–388, 1988

Leckman JF, Dolnansky ES, Hardin MT, et al: Perinatal factors associated with tic severity in Tourette's syndrome. J Am Acad Child Adolesc Psychiatry 29:220–226, 1990

Lloyd C: Life events and depressive disorder reviewed, I: events as predisposing factors. Arch Gen Psychiatry 37:529–535, 1980

Loewy AD, Spyer KM (eds): Central Regulation of Autonomic Functions. New York, Oxford University Press, 1990

Matthews KA, Rakaczky CJ, Stoney CM, et al: Are cardiovascular responses to behavioral stressors a stable individual difference variable in childhood? Psychophysiology 24:464–473, 1987

Martini DR, Ryan D, Nakayama D, et al: Psychiatric sequelae after traumatic injury: the Pittsburgh regatta accident. J Acad Child Adolesc Psychiatry 29:70–75, 1990

McFarlane AC: Posttraumatic phenomena in a longitudinal study of children following a natural disaster. J Am Acad Child Adolesc Psychiatry 26:764–769, 1987

McLeer SV, Deblinger E, Atkins MS, et al: Post-traumatic stress disorder in sexually abused children. J Am Acad Child Adolesc Psychiatry 27:650–654, 1988

Miller JC, Friedhoff AJ: Neurotransmitter programming of receptor density during development. Prog Brain Res 73:507–523, 1988

Moore RY, Bloom FE: Central catecholamine neuron systems: anatomy and physiology of the norepinephrine and epinephrine systems. Annu Rev Neurosci 2:113–153, 1979

Murburg MM, McFall ME, Veith RC: Catecholamines, stress, and posttraumatic stress disorder, in Biological Assessment and Treatment of Posttraumatic Stress Disorder. Edited by Giller EL Jr. Washington, DC, American Psychiatric Press, 1990, pp 27–65

Murphy JK, Alpert BS, Willey ES, et al: Cardiovascular reactivity to psychological stress in healthy children. Psychophysiology 25:144–152, 1988

Ogata SN, Silk KR, Goodrich S, et al: Childhood sexual and physical abuse in adult patients with borderline personality disorder. Am J Psychiatry 147:1008–1013, 1990

Ornitz EM, Pynoos RS: Startle modulation in children with post-traumatic stress disorder. Am J Psychiatry 147:866–870, 1989

Perry BD: Placental and blood element neurotransmitter receptor regulation in humans: potential models for studying neurochemical mechanisms underlying behavioral teratology. Prog Brain Res 73:189–207, 1988

Perry BD: Neurodevelopment and the neurophysiology of trauma, I: conceptual considerations for clinical work with maltreated children. The Advisor 6(1):1–18, 1993a

Perry BD: Neurodevelopment and the neurophysiology of trauma, II: clinical work along the alarm-fear-terror continuum. The Advisor 6(2):1–20, 1993b

Perry BD, Stolk JM, Vantini G, et al: Strain differences in rat brain epinephrine synthesis and alpha-adrenergic receptor number apparent "in vivo" regulation of brain alpha-adrenergic receptors by epinephrine. Science 221:1297–1299, 1983

Perry BD, Southwick SM, Giller EL Jr: Altered platelet alpha2-adrenergic receptor affinity states in post-traumatic stress disorder. Am J Psychiatry 144:1511–1512, 1987

Perry BD, Southwick SM, Yehuda R, et al: Adrenergic receptor regulation in posttraumatic stress disorder, in Biological Assessment and Treatment of Posttraumatic Stress Disorder. Edited by Giller EL Jr. Washington, DC, American Psychiatric Press, 1990, pp 87–114

Rutter M: Psychopathology and development, I: childhood antecedents of adult psychiatric disorder. Aust N Z J Psychiatry 18:225–234, 1984

Selye H: A syndrome produced by diverse nocuous agents. Nature 138:32, 1936

Southwick SM, Yehuda R, Giller EL Jr, et al: Altered platelet alpha-2 adrenergic binding sites in borderline personality disorders. Am J Psychiatry 147:1014–1017, 1990a

Southwick SM, Yehuda R, Giller EL Jr, et al: Altered platelet alpha-2 adrenergic binding sites in major depressive disorder and borderline personality disorder. Psychiatry Res 34:193–203, 1990b

Spitz RA, Wolf KM: Anaclitic depression: an inquiry into the genesis of psychiatric conditions in early childhood, II. Psychoanal Stud Child 2:313–342, 1946

Stone EA: Stress and catecholamines, in Catecholamines and Behavior 2: Neuropsychopharmacology. Edited by Friedhoff AJ. New York, Plenum, 1975, pp 31–72

Stone EA: Stress and brain neurotransmitter receptors, in Receptors and Ligands in Psychiatry. Edited by Sen AK, Lee T. New York, Cambridge University Press, 1988, pp 400–423

Suoumi SJ: Genetic and maternal contributions to individual differences in rhesus monkey biobehavioral development, in Psychobiological Aspects of Behavioral Development. Edited by Krasnagor N. New York, Academic, 1986, pp 397–420

Svensson TH: Peripheral, autonomic regulation of locus coeruleus noradrenergic neurons in brain: putative implications for psychiatry and psychopharmacology. Psychopharmacology (Berl) 92:1–7, 1987

Terr L: Chowchilla revisited: the effects of psychic trauma four years after a schoolbus kidnapping. Am J Psychiatry 140:1543–1550, 1983

Terr L: Childhood traumas: an outline and overview. Am J Psychiatry 148:120, 1991

U'Prichard DC, Kvetnansky R: Central and peripheral adrenergic receptors in acute and repeated immobilization stress, in Catecholamines and Stress: Recent Advances. Edited by Usdin E, Kvetnansky R, Kopin IJ. New York, Elsevier/North Holland, 1980, pp 299–308

U.S. Department of Health and Human Services: National Incidence Study. 1988

Vantini G, Perry BD, Gucchait RB, et al: Brain epinephrine systems: detailed comparison of adrenergic and noradrenergic metabolism, receptor number and in vivo regulation in two inbred rat strains. Brain Res 296:49–65, 1984

Weinstock M, Fride E, Hertzberg R: Prenatal stress effects on functional development of the offspring. Prog Brain Res 73:319–331, 1988

Chapter 13

Peripheral Adrenergic Receptors in PTSD

Bernard Lerer, M.D.
Eitan Gur, M.D.
Avraham Bleich, M.D.
Michael Newman, Ph.D.

Peripheral receptor strategies have traditionally played an important role in biological psychiatry. The primary motivation for studies of this type has been, and remains, the inaccessibility of human brain tissue to direct experimental examination. Although functional imaging with positron-emission tomography (PET) and single-photon emission computed tomography (SPECT) has already led to in vivo receptor binding studies in human brain, significant technological obstacles will need to be overcome before the promise of these techniques is fully realized. For this reason, strategies utilizing tissue derived from peripheral blood cells (and more rarely skin and other organs) are likely to remain an important research avenue for the foreseeable future.

The rationale underlying peripheral receptor studies in biological psychiatry may be summarized as follows:

1. As previously reviewed (Stahl 1977), human brain and peripheral blood cells, particularly platelets, share important similarities in terms of neurobiological processes such as uptake mechanisms, receptor regulation, and second-messenger signal transduction.
2. In certain disease states, intrinsic abnormalities (e.g., adenylate cyclase abnormalities in primary pseudohypoparathyroidism [Farfel et al. 1980]) are demonstrable in peripheral blood

cells as well as in the organs primarily manifesting the disease. According to this rationale, a trait marker (defined below) that is phenotypically relevant in brain could potentially be demonstrable in blood elements as well.

3. Pharmacological effects of psychotropic agents that have been extensively studied in the brains of laboratory animals are frequently demonstrable in human peripheral blood cells, and drug mechanisms can be studied in parallel (e.g.. monoamine oxidase inhibition and neurotransmitter reuptake blockade by antidepressant agents).

The limitations of the above approach are obvious. Extrapolation of peripheral findings to brain is based on assumptions for which empirical evidence is many times not available. Although neurochemical and other mechanisms are indeed parallel in many cases, comparisons are frequently based on brain studies in laboratory animals versus human peripheral cells. Furthermore, peripheral receptors and the transducing mechanisms to which they are linked are subject to the modulatory effect of circulating catecholamines and other hormones that are not necessarily operative in brain. This latter consideration increases the likelihood of false positive results and also of variance within the system that may be erroneously labeled as "perturbation" or "dysregulation." The potential for false negative results with regard to a particular system should also not be overlooked.

In spite of these limitations, receptors for a variety of neurotransmitters and hormones have been extensively studied in human blood elements, particularly platelets and mononuclear leukocytes, from patients with various psychiatric disorders. More recently, attention has shifted to encompass the second-messenger systems to which these receptors are linked and the molecular biology of their subcomponents.

In this chapter we focus on studies of this type pertinent to peripheral adrenergic receptor function in posttraumatic stress disorder (PTSD). The findings will be addressed in the broader context of peripheral adrenergic receptor studies in affective illness, a juxtaposition supported by the substantial clinical overlap between PTSD and major depression as well as other syndromes within the affective spectrum.

TRAIT AND STATE MARKERS

A biological marker for a psychiatric disorder may be defined as an observation of disturbed or abnormal function that is consistently associated with the illness under study. The important subdivision of biological markers into "trait" and "state" markers should be stressed.

Rigorously defined (Rieder and Gershon 1978), a *trait* marker is one that not only consistently differentiates patients affected by the disorder from unaffected individuals but is present in affected persons during the well state (in the case of an episodic remitting disorder), is under genetic control, and is demonstrable in some unaffected family members, unless the disorder is fully penetrant. Characteristics of this type may also be termed *vulnerability* or *susceptibility* markers in that they reflect an underlying biological predisposition to the illness. A trait marker should thus reflect at least some aspect of the pathogenesis of the disorder and possibly its etiology. If a clear pattern of inheritance is demonstrable, trait markers can serve as genetic linkage markers or as the basis for identifying candidate genes by "reverse genetics."

In contrast, a *state* marker is one that is demonstrable during the ill condition but not in the well state, and may reflect the severity of the affected state in a quantifiable fashion. It is not under genetic control and is absent in unaffected family members. A state marker may reflect some aspect of the pathogenesis of the disorder but could be a secondary manifestation thereof.

The phenylalanine hydroxylase deficiency of phenylketonuria is a classic example of a trait marker that fulfills the criteria noted above. Such deficiency directly reflects the phenotypic expression of an abnormal gene and is thus a genetic marker. The hypercortisolemia found in major depression is an example of a state marker that is associated with the affected state and reflects the presence of the illness rather than susceptibility to it.

Most of the findings to be discussed in this chapter are state markers or must be considered as such because the data required to classify them as trait characteristics are absent. This need not imply a "second rate" status in terms of the heuristic significance of such markers, because state markers can provide important clues to pathogenesis and may be reliable correlates of treatment response.

Important limitations at the methodological level have impeded studies of biological markers in psychiatric illness. Such limitations include problems of diagnostic heterogeneity (due to nonuniform diagnostic criteria as well as the basic heterogeneity of syndromes for which agreed-upon criteria exist and are consistently applied), the influence of pharmacological agents upon the marker (i.e.. the degree and length of time that subjects are "drug free"), variability of the marker due to conditions that are not experimentally controlled (such as circadian influences, exercise, ambient temperature), and differences in assay method and conditions. Although these considerations would seem to limit the comparability of studies to a disturbing degree, certain consistent findings have emerged in relation to some of the disorders that are the focus of this chapter.

COMORBIDITY WITH PTSD: IMPLICATIONS FOR MARKER STUDIES

The comorbid occurrence of other psychiatric conditions with PTSD has been noted by a number of investigators and is a highly consistent finding (Bleich et al. 1986; Green et al. 1989; Lerer et al. 1987a; Sierles et al. 1983). In fact, PTSD would seem to occur infrequently as a single diagnosis, raising the question of whether the syndrome is indeed justifiably classified as a separate diagnostic entity.

We have presented data on a cohort of 60 Israeli combat veterans with PTSD (consecutive referrals to the Israeli Defence Force Unit for Combat Stress Reactions who were diagnosed according to DSM-III-R criteria [American Psychiatric Association 1987]) and have shown that in all of the subjects additional diagnoses according to the Research Diagnostic Criteria (Spitzer et al. 1989) were present (Lerer et al. 1991). These data were gathered by structured interviews using the Schedule for Affective Disorders and Schizophrenia—Lifetime Version (SADS-L; Endicott and Spitzer 1978) and refer to the period following the trauma. In 27% of the subjects one additional diagnosis was documented, in 35%

two, in 23% three, and in 15% four or more. A breakdown of the concomitant diagnoses is presented in Table 13–1. In 95% of the subjects major depression was present in addition to PTSD. Although major depression was by far the most prominent comorbid diagnosis in our sample, the frequencies of phobic disorder (25%), obsessive-compulsive disorder (21.7%), and panic disorder (18.3%) were also striking.

Important differences between our observations and those of investigators in the United States studying Vietnam veterans with PTSD should be noted. Major depression is frequent in U.S. samples, although not to the extent observed in our subjects (Green et al. 1989; Southwick et al. 1991). On the other hand, a comorbid diagnosis of alcoholism and/or substance abuse tends to be considerably more frequent among Vietnam veterans with PTSD (Davidson et al. 1985; Sierles et al. 1983; Yager et al. 1984). Alcoholism has also been associated with abnormalities of peripheral adrenergic receptor function (see, e.g., Nagy et al. 1988; Tabakoff et al. 1988) and, as a comorbid diagnosis, could compli-

Table 13–1. Concomitant diagnoses in 60 Israeli combat veterans with PTSD

Diagnosis	No. of subjects	Percentage of sample[a]
Major depressive disorder	57	95
Phobic disorder	15	25
Obsessive-compulsive disorder	13	21.7
Panic disorder	11	18.3
Generalized anxiety disorder	7	11.7
Alcoholism	7	11.7
Hypomanic disorder	5	8.3
Drug abuse	4	6.7
Minor depression	4	6.7
Manic disorder	1	1.7

Note. This table reflects more than one comorbid diagnosis per subject.
[a]Refers to percentage of sample having the coexisting diagnosis. Diagnoses are according to the Research Diagnostic Criteria (Spitzer et al. 1989).

cate analysis of biochemical findings from populations manifesting both pathologies.

The observed comorbidity of PTSD with affective illness clearly demands that studies of catecholamine function in PTSD, including peripheral adrenergic receptor studies, be considered in the context of similar research in major depression and other disorders within the affective spectrum. At issue is the question of whether abnormalities associated with PTSD are truly markers for this syndrome or rather manifestations of comorbid disorders. An etiological consideration, in the case of shared characteristics, is whether they might point to a common underlying predisposition to PTSD and affective disorder, particularly major depression.

In Figure 13–1 is shown a hypothetical construct whereby predisposition to affective disorder might, because of intercur-

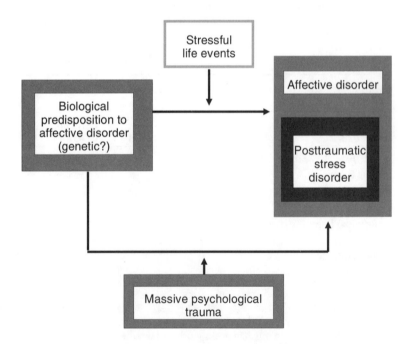

Figure 13–1. PTSD and affective disorder: hypothetical relationship

rent traumatic exposure, manifest as a clinical syndrome that has both affective characteristics and symptoms specific to PTSD that would not be encountered in nontraumatized patients with affective illness. An important step in testing this hypothesis would be to determine whether there is an increased incidence of affective illness among untraumatized relatives of patients with PTSD. A preliminary family history study suggested that this might be the case (Davidson et al. 1985) and also noted an increased incidence of alcohol abuse and anxiety syndromes.

ADRENERGIC RECEPTORS AND THEIR LINKAGE TO EFFECTOR SYSTEMS

Multiple receptors that mediate the physiological effects of the catecholamines epinephrine and norepinephrine have now been identified. The subdivision of adrenergic receptors into alpha$_1$ (α_1), alpha$_2$ (α_2), beta$_1$ (ß$_1$), and beta$_2$ (ß$_2$) types on the basis of different pharmacological potencies of agonists and antagonists, and the coupling of these receptors to different second-messenger reactions, have now been extended by the use of molecular cloning techniques to encompass ß$_3$, α_{1A}, α_{1B}, α_{2A}, α_{2B}, and α_{2C} subtypes (Harrison et al. 1991). Guanyl nucleotide binding proteins (G proteins) play a key role in coupling these receptors to the various types of intracellular effector systems. Receptors of the beta class appear to be linked to stimulation of adenylate cyclase, the stimulatory G_s protein, while α_1 receptors are linked to phosphoinositide hydrolysis via G_p (also termed G_o or G_q). Alpha$_2$ receptors inhibit adenylate cyclase via activation of an inhibitory guanyl nucleotide binding protein (G_i). "Promiscuity" in receptor coupling to second-messenger effectors has, however, been described.

At the molecular level, adenylate cyclase–linked receptors consist of seven transmembrane domains linked by a series of extracellular and cytoplasmic loops (Lefkowitz et al. 1989). G proteins consist of alpha, beta, and gamma subunits, with the alpha units conferring specificity and the beta-gamma units being similar or interchangeable for all G-protein heterotrimers. Molecular cloning studies have identified at least four forms of the alpha subunit of G_s, which may result from alternative splicing of a single precursor mRNA, and three forms of the alpha subunit of G_i, which appear to be products of three separate genes. Interaction of a ligand with a receptor results in dissociation of the alpha subunit from the complex and exchange of the guanosine diphosphate (GDP) bound to the alpha subunit for guanosine triphosphate (GTP). The dissociated alpha units then activate the relevant intracellular effectors and also hydrolyze the bound GTP to GDP via an intrinsic GTPase, thus facilitating reassociation of the inactive alpha-beta-gamma heterotrimer and terminating the signal.

Beta-adrenergic receptors are mainly located postsynaptically in the brain and are also present on human lymphocytes and leukocytes. Both cell types appear to possess ß2-adrenergic receptors exclusively. Functions of beta-adrenergic stimulation of white cells include alteration of hemolytic plaque formation, stimulation of mitogenesis by lymphocytes, and inhibition of release of hydrolytic enzymes by granulocytes. Receptors of the ß2 class have also been reported to be present on human platelets, but these appear to not be coupled to stimulation of adenylate cyclase. In rat and human brain, α2-adrenergic receptors are located pre- as well as postsynaptically. Presynaptic α2-adrenergic receptors inhibit norepinephrine release, and their downregulation results in increased levels of this neurotransmitter in the synaptic cleft. Human platelets possess an α2-adrenergic receptor, with pharmacological characteristics identical to that in brain, that is involved in the aggregation response of platelets to epinephrine and norepinephrine. The platelet receptor appears to be of the α2A subtype, while the CNS is characterized by a mixture of α2A and α2C subtypes (Harrison et al. 1991).

A variety of radiolabeled ligands have been used to label each of these receptors. Adrenergic receptors were initially labeled using [3H]-labeled dihydroalprenolol ([3H]-DHA), while ligands more recently introduced include [125I]-labeled iodocyanopindolol, [125I]-labeled hydroxybenzylpindolol, and [3H]-labeled CGP 12177. All of the above are antagonist ligands, but agonist ligands such as [3H]-labeled hydroxybenzylisoproterenol are also available. An important advantage of the use of agonist ligands is that they generally label more than one population of sites, the site with higher affinity corresponding to the state of the receptor that is capable of interacting with a G protein. Addition of GTP to the system results in elimination of this high-affinity site. Similar results are obtained when varying concentrations of an unlabeled agonist (e.g., isoproterenol) are used to displace a fixed concentration of an antagonist ligand.

Similar considerations apply to the α_2-adrenergic receptor. Antagonist ligands used to label this receptor include ^{3}H-labeled yohimbine, ^{3}H-labeled rauwolscine, and ^{3}H-labeled dihydroergocryptine, while agonist ligands include ^{3}H-labeled clonidine and ^{3}H-labeled p-aminoclonidine. Studies in human platelets indicate that although the antagonist ligands bind to one site only, use of agonist binding or agonist displacement of antagonist binding reveals the presence of a second low-affinity site, the high-affinity component of binding disappearing on addition of GTP (Limbird 1983). Further studies in a variety of tissues including human platelets have indicated that imidazoline ligands such as clonidine and idazoxan, in addition to binding to α_2 receptors, label a population of sites not coupled to G proteins, tentatively termed "imidazoline receptors" (Atlas 1991).

A variety of techniques are now available for measurement of G proteins, although, as in the case of receptors and second-messenger activity, a distinction must be made between techniques that measure G protein "amount" in terms of quantity of protein, and those that measure activity. "Amount" is most simply measured by the technique of ^{3}H-labeled GTP or ^{3}H-labeled GppNHp (guanosine-5'-[beta, gamma-imido]triphosphate) binding, analogous to the use of radiolabeled ligands for measurement of receptors. Increases in binding induced by either isoproterenol or the muscarinic agonist carbachol, for example, are presumed to reflect amounts of G_s and $G_{i/o}$, respectively. A more recently introduced technique is immunoblotting using specific antisera for individual subunits of the various G proteins. Qualitative measurements are made by electrophoresis of membrane proteins followed by transfer, or "blotting," to a medium that is then allowed to react with the specific antibody followed by an anti-IgG antibody. This method has now been quantitated and developed into an enzyme-linked immunoabsorbent assay (ELISA) (Lesch et al. 1991). G-protein activity is usually measured by the techniques of cholera toxin– or pertussis toxin–induced ADP-ribosylation. Incubation of membrane proteins with these toxins results in covalent modifications of G_s and $G_{i/o}$, respectively. The modifications, which in the in vivo situation lead to permanent activation of adenylate cyclase or prevention of cyclase inhibition or phosphatidyl inositol turnover, can be measured by incubation with ^{32}P-labeled NAD followed by electrophoresis.

The third component of the receptor–G protein–effector complex, the effector unit, is usually quantitated by measurement of enzymatic activity, either adenylate cyclase or phospholipase C in cell-free systems, or formation of cyclic AMP and inositol phosphates in systems in which intact cells are incubated. Whereas stimulation of cyclase by NaF, either alone or in the presence of $AlCl_3$, measures activity mediated via G proteins, the diterpene agent forskolin stimulates the catalytic unit directly. NaF has also been shown to stimulate phospholipase C in broken cell preparations of both brain and platelets (Kienast et al. 1987), although an agent equivalent to forskolin for this system is still lacking. An alternative to the assay of adenylate cyclase is use of ^3H-labeled forskolin in binding studies. As in the case of studies of receptor number compared with receptor-activated second-messenger formation, however, measurements of [^3H]forskolin binding have not always yielded results compatible with those of adenylate cyclase activity.

Finally, techniques using cDNA clones specific for individual protein subunits are now available for analysis of mRNA levels coding both for receptors and for G proteins. This approach has recently been extended to measurement of the mRNA coding for the adenylate cyclase catalytic unit protein (Colin et al. 1991), thus providing an alternative to the measurement of catalytic unit activity.

Studies of peripheral adrenergic receptors in patients with depression and PTSD compared with normal control subjects have thus far primarily focused on binding studies with radioligands and on studies of basal adenylate cyclase activity, responsiveness to agents acting via beta adrenoceptors, and inhibition of adenylate cyclase activity by agents acting via α_2-adrenergic receptors.

PERIPHERAL ADRENERGIC RECEPTORS IN MAJOR DEPRESSION

A comprehensive review of the large body of experimental data pertaining to peripheral blood cell adrenergic receptor number and second-messenger function in major depression is beyond the scope of this chapter. A brief overview of the findings is presented, and the reader is referred to reviews of this area for further details (Garcia-Sevilla et al. 1990; Werstiuk et al. 1990). It should be noted that methodological problems that were referred to earlier, such as diagnostic heterogeneity, drug washout, and assay differences, complicate interpretation. In this overview we focus on studies of ß-adrenergic receptor number and ß-adrenergic receptor–mediated cyclic AMP (cAMP) activity in mononuclear leukocytes, and α_2-adrenergic receptor number and α_2-adrenergic receptor–mediated inhibition of adenylate cyclase in platelets.

As shown in Table 13–2, mononuclear leukocyte ß-adrenergic receptor number has been reported to be both lower and higher in depressed patients than in control subjects. A slight prepon-

Table 13–2. Adrenergic receptor number and cyclic AMP signal transduction in major depression

Tissue	Parameter	D < C	D > C	D = C
Intact ML	Beta AR number (B_{Max})	++(+)	+	++
Intact ML	Beta AR–mediated cyclic AMP production	+++	+	+
Platelet membranes	Alpha$_2$ AR number (B_{Max})	+	++(+)	++
Platelet membranes	Alpha$_2$ AR–mediated inhibition of adenylate cyclase	+	—	++

Note. +++ = majority of studies; ++ = some studies; + = few studies; — = no studies. D = depressed patients; C = control subjects; ML = mononuclear leukocytes; AR = adrenergic receptor.

derance of studies have reported a lower level of binding in depressed subjects. Werstiuk et al. (1990) noted that when studies examining patients after a 14-day washout are considered exclusively, there are no reports of increased binding, and a majority of studies report lower levels than those found in control subjects.

Beta-adrenergic receptor–mediated cAMP studies in mononuclear leukocytes have yielded the most consistent pattern of results. No fewer than six studies have reported lower responsiveness in depressed patients than in control subjects compared with two reports of no difference and one of higher levels. When considering only studies reporting 14-day drug washout, three out of four reports found blunted responses in the depressed patients.

Studies of α_2-adrenergic receptor binding to platelet membranes are complicated by the issue of ligand choice (agonist vs. antagonist). As noted above, antagonist binding does not permit identification of more than one affinity site unless displacement with unlabeled agonist is used. Overall, a preponderance of studies report higher α_2-adrenergic receptor number in depressed patients than in control subjects, with a number of studies reporting no difference and a few noting lower binding in the depressed patients. In studies using agonist binding or agonist displacement of antagonist binding, there is a clear trend for increased binding to be reported, reflecting a larger number of high-affinity α_2-adrenergic receptor sites that are linked to adenylate cyclase.

Studies of platelet α_2-adrenergic receptor–mediated inhibition of adenylate cyclase have yielded inconsistent results, reporting either normal or diminished inhibitory activity—but not greater inhibitory activity—in depressed patients compared with control subjects.

In summary, the most consistent finding in depressed patients is of lower ß-adrenergic receptor–mediated cAMP activity in mononuclear leukocytes. There is also a trend toward lower ß-adrenergic receptor number in mononuclear leukocytes and higher α_2-adrenergic receptor number in platelet membranes, the latter particularly being evident when agonist binding or agonist displacement of antagonist binding is used.

PERIPHERAL ADRENERGIC RECEPTORS IN PTSD: NUMBER AND FUNCTION

In contrast to the extensive literature on major depression, there have been remarkably few studies of peripheral adrenergic receptor number and function in PTSD. Those studies that have been reported are summarized in Table 13–3.

Perry et al. (1987) examined 12 Vietnam veterans (11 male, 1 female) who met DSM-III criteria for PTSD (American Psychiatric Association 1980) and were medication free for 3 weeks prior to the examination. These individuals were compared with 13 age-matched control subjects. Extended saturation studies with 12 concentrations of [^{3}H]rauwolscine were carried out on the subjects' platelet membranes to determine the number (B_{Max}) of α_2-adrenergic receptor sites and their affinity (K_d) for the radioligand. Two interaction sites were revealed. For neither site was there a difference in affinity for rauwolscine between the PTSD and control groups. However, 40% fewer total rauwolscine binding sites were seen in the PTSD subjects. This difference was attributed to fewer rauwolscine 2 sites (i.e., high-affinity sites that are coupled to adenylate cyclase).

A further series of experiments conducted by Perry et al. (1990) is worthy of note. In vitro incubation of intact platelets in 100 µM of epinephrine for varying time periods was used to determine the sensitivity of α_2-adrenergic receptors to downregulation by the agonist. A progressive loss of high-affinity α_2-adrenergic receptor sites was observed in both PTSD ($n = 8$) and control ($n = 5$) subjects. However, both the extent and the rate of loss of rauwolscine binding sites were greater in the PTSD subjects than in the control subjects. This finding suggests that platelet α_2-adrenergic receptors from PTSD patients may be more sensitive to downregulation by agonist than platelet α_2-adrenergic receptors of control subjects. If the elevated urinary catecholamine excretion reported in PTSD (Kosten et al. 1987; Mason et al. 1986) reflects high ambient plasma levels, enhanced sensitivity of platelet α_2-adrenergic receptors to agonist-induced downregulation would explain the observation by Perry et al (1987) of reduced platelet α_2-adrenergic receptor high-affinity sites in PTSD patients compared with control subjects.

Table 13–3. Studies of adrenergic receptor number and function in PTSD

Authors	Tissue	Subjects (n)	Assay	Finding[a]
Perry et al. 1987	Platelet membranes	Combat PTSD (12) Civilian control subjects (13)	[^{3}H]rauwolscine Binding to α_2 AR	$\Downarrow$ Total α_2 AR sites $\Downarrow$ High-affinity site
Lerer et al. (1987b)	Intact lymphocytes	PTSD (mixed) (10)[b] Civilian control subjects (10)	Cyclic AMP production in response to: Forskolin Isoproterenol PGE$_1$	$\Downarrow$ Basal $\Downarrow$ Forskolin $\Downarrow$ Isoproterenol ND
Lerer et al. (1987b)	Platelet membranes	PTSD (mixed) (10)[b] Civilian control subjects (10)	Adenylate cyclase activation by: Forskolin AlCl$_3$/NaFl PGE$_1$	$\Downarrow$ Basal $\Downarrow$ Forskolin $\Downarrow$ AlCl$_3$/NaFl $\Downarrow$ PGE$_1$
Lerer et al. (1990)	Platelet membranes	PTSD (combat) (19) Combat control subjects (35)	Adenylate cyclase activation by: Forskolin AlCl$_3$/NaFl PGE$_1$	$\Downarrow$ Basal $\Downarrow$ Forskolin ND ND

Note.   AR = adrenergic receptor; PGE$_1$ = prostaglandin E$_1$; ND = no difference.
[a] $\Downarrow$ = indicates lower response in PTSD subjects.
[b] Same PTSD subjects in lymphocyte and platelet studies; different control groups.

The functional activity of platelet α_2-adrenergic receptors in PTSD patients, as reflected in the receptors' inhibitory coupling to adenylate cyclase, has not thus far been reported. If, as was found by Perry et al. (1987), high-affinity platelet α_2-adrenergic receptor sites are diminished in PTSD, reduced inhibitory activity would be expected, because the high-affinity α_2-adrenergic receptor site is coupled to G_i.

Lerer et al. (1987b) examined cAMP signal transduction in intact lymphocytes and in platelet membranes from patients with PTSD ($n = 10$ for each assay, all male) and compared these measurements with those from the same number of age- and sex-matched control subjects. The PTSD subjects were heterogeneous, with PTSD of both combat and noncombat origin being present. All subjects were medication free for at least 4 weeks. The control subjects had no history of traumatic exposure. The lymphocyte preparations of the PTSD subjects showed reduced basal cAMP levels and significantly lower responsiveness to stimulation with isoproterenol and forskolin (but not PGE_1 [prostaglandin E_1]). The platelet membrane preparations of the PTSD subjects showed lower responsiveness to forskolin, $AlCl_3/NaF$, and PGE. These findings suggested a significantly lower responsiveness of adenylate cyclase in PTSD patients to stimulation via the ß-adrenergic receptor (in lymphocytes), the PGE_1 receptor (in platelets), and at sites distal to adenylate cyclase–linked receptors.

Lerer et al. (1990) conducted a follow-up study in a different population: combat veterans of the 1982–1984 Lebanon War who were diagnosed as having PTSD ($n = 19$) were compared with military personnel ($n = 35$) with combat exposure but no PTSD. Only platelet membranes were examined in this study. Basal activity was lower in the PTSD subjects, and responsiveness to forskolin, but not to $AlCl_3/NaF$ and PGE_1, was lower. The less striking finding in this latter study was suggested by Lerer et al. (1990) as reflecting the less severe clinical syndrome of the patient group. Another possible explanation may be the difference in control groups. In the second study by Lerer et al., control subjects were military personnel with a history of combat exposure. Although these subjects did not suffer from PTSD, subclinical symptoms could have been present and might explain the lesser degree of biochemical difference between the control subjects and the patient group.

An important aspect of the two studies by Lerer et al. (1987b, 1990) is that they reflect abnormal responsiveness to the receptor–adenylate cyclase complex in PTSD that extends distal to the receptor. Further studies are needed to determine the relationship between the findings of Lerer et al. and those of Perry et al. (1987). They should include concurrent determination of α_2-adrenergic receptor number and function (inhibition of adenylate cyclase via G_i) and also stimulatory responses to agents acting upon adenylate cyclase at the level of G_s, and the catalytic unit, in the same subjects. These studies should encompass, in addition to PTSD patients, control groups with and without a history of traumatic exposure. Platelet membrane studies will provide information on α_2-adrenergic receptor–mediated signal transduction. To determine ß-adrenergic receptor number and function, lymphocyte studies will be needed.

CONCLUSIONS

Peripheral adrenergic receptor studies in PTSD are still in their very early stages. As a research strategy for understanding the neurobiology of PTSD, the approach is faced by the same validity issues as other peripheral marker paradigms such as urinary and plasma catecholamines and other peripheral receptors. The absence of readily available technological means for directly examining receptor number and function in the intact human brain is a strong motivating factor for studies of this type. However, positive rationales also exist, including the parallels between peripheral models and brain noted in the introduction to this chapter, as well as the theoretical possibility that peripheral abnormalities may represent trait markers that are also expressed in brain, where they have phenotypic relevance for the pathological syndrome.

In pursuing studies of this type, reliability and replicability problems that have plagued peripheral receptor studies in major affective disorder and other psychiatric syndromes should be avoided. Particular attention should be given to diagnostic homogeneity (by applying standard criteria) and to other methodological issues such as withdrawal time from medication and assay procedures. Because of the chronic nature of PTSD, longitudinal studies comparing the same subjects in the remitted and affected states are problematic. One of the most important criteria for trait marker status is therefore difficult to fulfill. Family studies are possible, however, and should be undertaken. It is also necessary to achieve some degree of control over the effects of trauma by including subjects who were exposed to the same stimuli but did not develop overt PTSD (in addition to control subjects without such exposure).

Comorbidity is another important consideration. In this chapter we have focused on comorbidity with major depression, which is of particular importance among the Israeli subjects (particularly veterans) with PTSD whom we have studied. Findings from our laboratory suggest peripheral biochemical parallels between PTSD and major depression (Lerer et al. 1987b, 1990). We did, however, find that reduced lymphocyte ß-adrenergic receptor–mediated cAMP formation was also present in subjects without concurrent major depression (Lerer et al. 1987b). In the case of platelet α_2-adrenergic receptors, the report of Perry et al. (1987) suggests that findings may be opposite in PTSD and major depression. Although platelet α_2-adrenergic receptor number was reduced in PTSD, a preponderance of studies in major depression show these receptors to be elevated compared with control subjects. Comorbidity with alcohol and substance abuse as well as with other disorders should also be taken into account. In the case of alcoholism, abnormalities of platelet cAMP signal transduction have, as previously noted, been well characterized (e.g., Nagy et al. 1988; Tabakoff et al. 1988). Studies that encompass control groups for these codiagnoses (as well as, to the extent possible, PTSD subjects without codiagnoses or, at least, without multiple codiagnoses) are the only way in which to tease apart these complex influences.

REFERENCES

American Psychiatric Association: Diagnostic and Statistical Manual of Mental Disorders, 3rd Edition. Washington, DC, American Psychiatric Association, 1980

American Psychiatric Association: Diagnostic and Statistical Manual of Mental Disorders, 3rd Edition, Revised. Washington, DC, American Psychiatric Association, 1987

Atlas D: Clonidine-displacing substance (CDS) and its putative imidazoline receptor. Biochem Pharmacol 41:1541–1549, 1991

Bleich A, Siegel B, Garb R, et al: Post-traumatic stress disorder following combat exposure: clinical features and psychopharmacological treatment. Br J Psychiatry 149:365–369, 1986

Colin SF, Chang H-C, Mollner S, et al: Chronic lithium regulated the expression of adenylate cyclase and Gi-protein a subunit in rat cerebral cortex. Proc Natl Acad Sci U S A 88:10634–10637, 1991

Davidson J, Swartz M, Storck M, et al: A diagnostic and family study of posttraumatic stress disorder. Am J Psychiatry 142:90–93, 1985

Endicott J, Spitzer RL: A diagnostic interview: the Schedule for Affective Disorders and Schizophrenia. Arch Gen Psychiatry 35:837–862, 1978

Farfel Z, Brickman AS, Kaslow HR, et al: Defect of receptor-cyclase coupling protein in pseudohypoparathyroidism. N Engl J Med 303:237–242, 1980

Garcia-Sevilla JA, Padro D, Giralt T, et al: Alpha-2 adrenoceptor-mediated inhibition of platelet adenylate cyclase and induction of aggregation in major depression. Arch Gen Psychiatry 47:125–132, 1990

Green BL, Lindy JD, Grace MC, et al: Multiple diagnosis in posttraumatic stress disorder: the role of war stressors. J Nerv Ment Dis 177:329–335, 1989

Harrison JK, Pearson WR, Lynch KR: Molecular characterization of alpha-1 and alpha-2 adrenoceptors. Trends Pharmacol Sci 12:62–67, 1991

Kienast J, Arnout J, Pfliegler G, et al: Sodium fluoride mimics effects of both agonists and antagonists on intact human platelets by simultaneous modulation of phospholipase C and adenylate cyclase activity. Blood 69:859–866, 1987

Kosten TR, Mason JW, Giller EL, et al: Sustained urinary norepinephrine and epinephrine elevation in post-traumatic stress disorder. Psychoneuroendocrinology 12:13–20, 1987

Lefkowitz RJ, Kobilka BK, Caron MG: The new biology of drug receptors. Biochem Pharmacol 38:2941–2948, 1989

Lerer B, Bleich A, Kotler M, et al: Posttraumatic stress disorder in Israeli combat veterans. Arch Gen Psychiatry 44:976–981, 1987a

Lerer B, Ebstein RP, Shestatzky M, et al: Cyclic AMP signal transduction in posttraumatic stress disorder. Am J Psychiatry 144:1324–1327, 1987b

Lerer B, Bleich A, Bennett ER, et al: Platelet adenylate cyclase and phospholipase C activity in posttraumatic stress disorder. Biol Psychiatry 3:29–45, 1990

Lerer B, Dolev A, Bleich A: Comorbidity and cross cultural variability in PTSD. Paper presented at the 144th annual meeting of the American Psychiatric Association, May 1991

Lesch KP, Aulakh CS, Tolliver TJ, et al: Differential effects of long-term lithium and carbamazepine administration on Gs-a and Gi-a protein in rat brain. Eur J Pharmacol 207:355–359, 1991

Limbird LE: Alpha-2 adrenergic systems: models for exploring hormonal inhibition of adenylate cyclase. Trends Pharmacol Sci 4:135–138, 1983

Mason JW, Giller EL, Kosten TR, et al: Urinary free cortisol levels in posttraumatic stress disorder patients. J Nerv Ment Dis 174:145–149, 1986

Nagy LE, Diamond I, Gordon A: Cultured lymphocytes from alcoholic subjects have altered AMP signal transduction. Proc Natl Acad Sci U S A 85:6973–6976, 1988

Perry BD, Southwick SM, Giller EL: Altered platelet alpha-2 adrenergic receptor affinity sites in post-traumatic stress disorder. Am J Psychiatry 144:1511–1512, 1987

Perry BD, Southwick SM, Yehuda R, et al: Adrenergic receptor regulation in posttraumatic stress disorder, in Biological Assessment and Treatment of Posttraumatic Stress Disorder. Edited by Giller EL Jr. Washington DC, American Psychiatric Press, 1990, pp 87–114

Reider R, Gershon ES: Genetic strategies in biological psychiatry. Biol Psychiatry 35:866–873, 1978

Sierles FS, Chen JJ, McFarland RE, et al: Posttraumatic stress disorder and concurrent psychiatric illness: a preliminary report. Am J Psychiatry 140:1177–1179, 1983

Southwick SM, Yehuda R, Giller EL, et al: Characterization of depression in war-related posttraumatic stress disorder. Am J Psychiatry 148:179–183, 1991

Spitzer RL, Endicott J, Robins E: Research Diagnostic Criteria for a Selected Group of Functional Disorders. New York, New York State Psychiatric Institute, 1989

Stahl SM: The human platelet: a diagnostic and research tool for the study of biogenic amines in psychiatry and neurologic disorders. Arch Gen Psychiatry 34:503–515, 1977

Tabakoff B, Hoffman PL, Lee JM, et al: Differences in platelet enzyme activity between alcoholics and nonalcoholics. N Engl J Med 318:134–139, 1988

Werstiuk ES, Steiner M, Burns T: Studies on leukocyte beta-adrenergic receptors in depression: a critical appraisal. Life Sci 47:85–105, 1990

Yager T, Laufer R, Gallops M: Some problems associated with war experience in men of the Vietnam generation. Arch Gen Psychiatry 41:327–333, 1984

Section III

Central Catecholamine Function in PTSD

Chapter 14

Neurobiology of Startle Response Abnormalities in PTSD

Jeffrey L. Rausch, M.D.
Mark A. Geyer, Ph.D.
Melissa A. Jenkins, B.A.
Curtis Breslin, M.S.
David L. Braff, M.D.

A n exaggerated startle response has been consistently described as a central feature of the heightened physiological reactivity found in patients diagnosed with DSM-III-R posttraumatic stress disorder (PTSD; American Psychiatric Association 1987). These observations date back to the descriptions of combat soldiers sensitized to stress during World War I. Campbell (1918, p. 1622) indicated that once a World War I soldier had been "un-nerved" by his experience of high explosives, he would later succumb to otherwise *trivial* stimuli. Numerous observations have since then strengthened the association of exaggerated startle responses to the syndrome of PTSD. New developments now present an opportunity to understand better whether specific aminergic influences may underlay the exaggerated startle responses in PTSD patients.

This work was supported by the Veterans Affairs and grants from the State of California Department of Mental Health (DMH 89-7000) and the National Institute of Mental Health (MH42228). M. A. Geyer was supported by a Research Scientist Development Award from the National Institute of Mental Health (MH00188).

DEFINITION

The *startle response* is defined by a constellation of *motor movements* that occur immediately after a sudden, strong sensory stimulus. This immediate reaction is distinguished from the more slowly evolving autonomic responses that may present after a sudden stimulus (Graham 1979; Wilkins et al. 1986). Indeed, a cardinal feature of the startle response is its very short latency. In the jaw muscles the response occurs in as few as 14 milliseconds (msec) after a loud noise (Davis 1984). Although the earliest detectable change in movement may occur in the jaw muscles, a rapid contraction of the eyelid may be the only evidence noted at the mildest levels of measurable startle response (Jacobson 1926). Accordingly, the human startle response can be measured reliably by the amplitude of eyeblink in response to a sudden abrupt auditory stimulus (Hoffman and Ison 1980; Landis and Hunt 1939). As such, the eyeblink movements of the orbicularis oculi muscle are considered to be a useful motor component of startle response measurement in human studies.

DESCRIPTION

Although the eyeblink has been designated as a convenient site for startle measurement, the components of the human startle response also include forward head movement; widening of the mouth; flexion of the shoulders, elbows, fingers, knees, and trunk; and pronation of the lower arms and abduction of the upper arms, as catalogued by Straus (cited in Davis 1984). These movements are largely flexor in nature. Startle responses emerge at no earlier than 6 weeks of age in humans, although the brain mechanisms that modulate the responses undergo change during early childhood and do not mature until about 8 years of age (Ornitz et al. 1986).

ANATOMY

Although the motor expression of the startle response comprises a number of reflexes, its basic neuroanatomy is relatively simple, as found from a variety of lesion studies and electrical stimulation paradigms. These studies have investigated the locus of the basic "startle circuit" in laboratory rats. The neuroanatomic foundation of the startle circuit has been well delineated in the pioneering work of Davis (1984) and others. Davis and colleagues (1984) have painstakingly delineated the brain-stem startle circuit as involving the posteroventral cochlear nucleus (VCN), the lateral lemniscus, the reticulospinal tract, and the lower motor neurons of the spinal cord. Although the fundamental brain-stem startle circuitry seems straightforward, it is the more complex physiological modulation of startle, often involving inputs from higher brain centers, that is of great interest to psychopathology researchers. For example, it has been noted that lesions of the amygdala impair fear-potentiated startle, and these observations provide preliminary evidence that the amygdala may be involved in processing information related to conditioned fear or may be part of an output pathway for the expression of conditioned fear (Hitchcock and Davis 1986). As discussed later in this chapter, evidence now exists that cortical elements may influence the tone of the startle response, insofar as cognitive or perceptual influences may affect startle in humans (Vrana et al. 1988).

PHYSIOLOGY

Startle responses have, in fact, been shown to be modulated by a variety of factors, as evidenced by various paradigmatic manipulations. This apparent plasticity of the response has proved useful to psychopathology researchers. Two examples can be considered:

1. Startle magnitude shows prepulse inhibition (PPI) or gating, as reflected by decreased startle magnitude when the startle-eliciting stimulus is preceded by a weak prestimulus or warning stimulus at an interval of 60 to 100 msec in humans (Graham 1975) and at shorter intervals in rodents (Hoffman and Ison 1980). Schizophrenic patients show a loss of this normal preattentive and theoretically "protective" gating activity (Braff et al. 1978). This same loss is seen in rats with

nucleus accumbens dopamine overactivity (Swerdlow et al. 1986).

2. Startle responses show habituation or a decrement of responding upon repeated presentation of the same, initially novel stimulus. The observed habituation is theoretically the result of the two opposite underlying processes of habituation and sensitization (Groves and Thompson 1970), and is complexly determined. Schizophrenic patients, for example, exhibit impairments of startle habituation that may be linked to abnormalities of serotonergic systems (Geyer and Tapson 1988).

BASIC STUDIES

A particularly useful model for the study of PTSD is the behavioral paradigm of *conditioned fear,* a phenomenon that can be conceptualized as a sensitization emergent from an enduring anxiety state. Anderson and Parmenter (1941), for example, described sheep and dogs that had been followed for over 12 years after the induction of "experimental neuroses." In this paradigm, an electric shock was used as an *unconditioned* stimulus, and the sound of a metronome was used as a *conditioned* stimulus. The investigators noted a chronic physiological state in these animals characterized by a startle reaction that would generalize in response to extraneous low-level stimuli, such as touch or merely scratching on the wall of the experimental chamber. The animals' responses to such stimuli included crouching, trembling, running, and even defecation. The authors characterized these behavioral states well in noting that from all appearances the animal seemed already set to react before it had cause for reacting (Anderson and Parmenter 1941).

Such exaggerated startle responses have since defined conditioned fear in the laboratory. Davis (1986) described a paradigm measuring increases in whole-body startle in laboratory rats in the presence of a light that had previously been paired with electric footshock. Davis's group demonstrated that the increased startle amplitude in the fear-conditioned rats could be pharmacologically attenuated by diazepam, morphine, or buspirone, but not imipramine (Cassella and Davis 1985).

Contributing to clinical paradigms aimed at understanding PTSD treatment, the neuropsychopharmacology and pathophysiology of human startle have been informed by observations from animal studies investigating the basis for the startle reaction. Clinical researchers have now just begun to look at startle modulation in humans to understand whether changes in gating, habituation, or sensitization occur in patients previously exposed to traumatic stimuli. Ultimately the treatment and prevention of sensitization to stress will involve not only considerations in the already stress-sensitized organism, but also knowledge pertaining to what factors may best prevent, prior to or during trauma, the acquisition of subsequent pathological responses.

CLINICAL STUDIES

It has been only recently that human startle has been measured in clinical studies of patients diagnosed with PTSD. Previously, several clinical studies (Blanchard et al. 1986; Malloy et al. 1983; Ornitz and Pynoos 1989; Pitman et al. 1987; see also McFall and Murburg, Chapter 7, this volume, for review) had demonstrated increases in heart rate, respiration, and electromyographic activity in war veterans exposed to gunfire or other abrupt auditory stimuli. A less consistent finding was a higher basal heart rate in PTSD subjects (Blanchard et al. 1982, 1986; see also McFall and Murburg, Chapter 7; Murburg et al., Chapter 8, this volume, for review). Changes in heart rate in response to traumatic stimuli had previously been shown to provide a degree of diagnostic discrimination of PTSD subjects (Blanchard et al. 1986).

More recently, startle response measures per se have been assessed in clinical PTSD populations, once the validity (Braff and Geyer 1990; Graham 1975) and the methodological advantages (Vrana et al. 1988) of eyeblink startle measures had been verified. Startle reactions of PTSD subjects have since been specifically studied by measuring the subjects' response to sudden abrupt stimuli, differentiating direct measures of startle motor reactions from other more slowly evolving autonomic responses.

In an early study of startle response physiology in human subjects, Ornitz and Pynoos (1989) recorded startle responses in six children (ages 8 to 13) meeting DSM-III (American Psychiatric Association 1980) criteria for PTSD. The children were exposed to 104-decibel bursts of white noise. During some trials, warning stimuli were administered at time intervals that normally would either facilitate (i.e., 800 and 2,000 msec) or inhibit (i.e., 120 and 250 msec) a startle response. Results of the "warned" trials indicated that children with PTSD showed a loss of startle inhibition from the prepulse warning. The PTSD children also demonstrated an exaggerated startle facilitation compared with the control children, although the startle response of the PTSD children on "unwarned" trials was significantly smaller than that of the control children.

Our own group recently studied eyeblink responses to startling acoustic or tactile stimuli in 13 Vietnam combat veterans with chronic PTSD, compared with 12 combat veterans without PTSD (Butler et al. 1990). The study was designed to examine whether the veterans with chronic PTSD would exhibit measurable startle responses at lower sound intensities than the intensities required to elicit startle in the non-PTSD patients. Subjects in either group who failed to show an eyeblink response to the startle stimulus were excluded. Thirteen of 20 identified PTSD-positive subjects (65%), and 12 of 18 control subjects (67%) were included as having measurable eyeblink reactions to the acoustic stimulus. Of these, the PTSD group had measurably greater startle responses than did the control group at the intermediate sound intensities (i.e., 95 and 100 decibels). The PTSD patients were not significantly different on measures of prepulse inhibition and were equivalent to control subjects in their responses to tactile startle stimuli. Our results suggested that there was a lower threshold for acoustic startle responses in the PTSD subjects (Figure 14–1). The identical startle responses to tactile stimuli could reflect differences between weak and strong stimuli. Alternatively, it may be that increased startle responses are specific to stimuli that resemble the traumatic event.

There is evidence that the cognitive or perceptual set may influence the startle response. Vrana et al. (1988) tested the eyeblink responses to unsignaled white noise bursts while subjects viewed photographic slides depicting either pleasant, neutral, or unpleasant scenes or objects. Independent of interest levels or arousal, eyeblink startle magnitudes evoked by the noise bursts were largest while subjects were viewing unpleasant material, and smallest while they were viewing pleasant material.

It is debatable whether white noise bursts may be cognitively associated with perceptions of gunshots (Ornitz and Pynoos 1989). It had previously been asserted that activation of conditioned responses in PTSD patients requires stimuli that resemble the traumatic event (Kolb 1984). The present data suggest that age, the cognitive/perceptual context of the stimulus, its character and modality, and the interval between preceding stimuli all may influence the startle response.

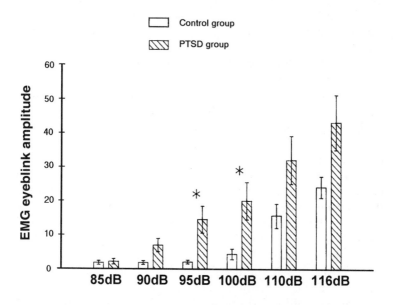

Figure 14–1. Startle response reactivity in subjects with combat-related PTSD and in control subjects. Reprinted from Butler RW, Braff DL, Rausch JL, et al: "Physiological Evidence of Exaggerated Startle Response in a Subgroup of Vietnam Veterans With Combat-Related PTSD." *American Journal of Psychiatry* 147:1308–1312, 1990. Copyright 1990, American Psychiatric Association. Used with permission.

NEUROCHEMISTRY OF STARTLE

It is not yet known whether startle response differences between PTSD patients and control subjects are correlated with specific neurochemical abnormalities. These issues are potentially important in understanding the physiological basis for PTSD and may well be important in advancing effective treatment of the condition. For example, we now know that startle responses can be increased or decreased by disparate lesions and drug manipulations, although these neurochemical influences are still being investigated in basic studies.

Generally, it appears that dopamine and possibly norepinephrine agonists increase acoustic startle (Davis 1980), whereas serotonin exerts a largely inhibitory influence (Davis et al. 1980). In the case of serotonin, for example, decreases in startle activity have been linked to increased activity in forebrain serotonergic pathways in studies using pharmacological probes (Davis 1980; Davis et al. 1984), electrolytic or neurotoxic lesions (Geyer et al. 1976, 1980), synthesis inhibitors (Conner et al. 1970), precursor manipulations, and direct intracerebral injections of serotonin (Davis et al. 1980; Geyer et al. 1975). Various serotonergic pathways (Geyer et al. 1976) and different serotonin receptors (Davis et al. 1986; Geyer and Tapson 1988) contribute differentially to these effects. Indeed, descending serotonergic pathways appear to be excitatory rather than inhibitory to startle (Davis et al. 1980).

Among the anatomically defined subdivisions of the central noradrenergic system, only the influence of the locus coeruleus (LC) itself has been studied systematically. Neurotoxic lesions of the LC or its projections decrease startle reactivity (Adams and Geyer 1981; Kehne and Davis 1985), as do several drugs that inhibit the activity of LC neurons (Davis 1980). Conversely, drugs that increase activity in the LC have the opposite effect (Davis et al. 1977). The demonstrated increases in startle induced by anxiogenic stimuli and decreases by anxiolytic drugs have been linked tentatively to noradrenergic influences (Davis et al. 1979), though the involvement of serotonin$_{1A}$ receptors has also been a recent focus of investigation (Mansbach and Geyer 1988).

Dopamine agonists such as amphetamine and apomorphine increase startle, whereas dopamine antagonists such as haloperidol have the opposite effect (Davis 1980; Davis et al. 1975). The effects of amphetamine on startle reactivity, in contrast to its effects on locomotor activity, appear to be independent of the dopaminergic projections to the nucleus accumbens (Swerdlow et al. 1990). Instead, these effects may reflect the activation of the nigrostriatal dopaminergic system and/or some complex interactions between dopaminergic and noradrenergic systems (Davis 1984). Recent results have added some complexity to what originally appeared to be a simple, direct relationship between dopamine activity and startle reactivity, because different subtypes of dopamine receptors appear to have opposite influences on startle reactivity (Melia and Davis 1988). Nevertheless, the converging evidence from a variety of studies indicates that all three monoamine neurotransmitters have important influences that combine to modulate the level of startle reactivity in mammals.

Miserendino and colleagues (1990) have demonstrated that N-methyl-D-aspartate (NMDA) receptors may be linked to the acquisition, but not the expression, of fear-potentiated startle. These receptors seem to play a critical role in synaptic plasticity, and NMDA antagonists prevent long-term facilitation as a potential mechanism underlying memory and learning. The ability of NMDA antagonists, infused into the amygdala, to block the acquisition of fear-conditioned startle suggests that NMDA-dependent processes in the amygdala may subserve associative fear conditioning (Miserendino et al. 1990).

MORPHOLOGY

Evidence also exists to suggest that fundamental morphological changes may occur in response to conditioned behavioral dishabituation and sensitization. Organisms as simple as Aplysia can be shown to overrespond to a light touch with a defensive gill withdrawal if the light touch is previously paired with an electric shock. The network of neurons responsible for the gill withdrawal has been identified by Kandel and co-workers, who found that shock-conditioning strengthens neuronal connections within this network, augmenting the signal transmission in the sensorimotor synapse (Glanzman et al. 1990). This synapse can be strengthened by applying serotonin, a transmitter known to strengthen connections between neurons associated with conditioning in the intact animal (Glanzman et al. 1989; Mackey et al. 1989). It is not known whether such an increase in transmitter release (Dale et al. 1988), or growth of new points of synaptic contact between sensory and motor neurons (Korn et al. 1981), or an activity-dependent enhancement of synaptic activity (Miserendino et al. 1990) might represent a specific aspect of the fundamental mechanisms underlying perturbations of the startle threshold in PTSD patients.

CONCLUSIONS

Animal models of fear-conditioned startle consistently suggest that enduring changes in startle response may occur with sensory cues paired to traumatic stimuli. Experimental paradigms of stress dishabituation or sensitization, and fear-conditioning are contributing important information that may allow us to make inferences about the startle response abnormalities found in PTSD patients. A vital test for future investigations will be to ascertain which neurotransmitters known to affect the startle response are implicated in both the acquisition and the retention of such heightened physiological states in patients. The identification of such specific neurotransmitter systems may support the development of receptor-specific psychopharmacological preventions of, and treatment interventions for, PTSD. The ability to quantify specific neurobiological parameters of the startle response in clinical populations can now contribute to a delineation of the appropriate subject population for studies of the pathophysiology, treatment, and prevention of acquisition of exaggerated startle reactions in persons with PTSD.

REFERENCES

Adams LM, Geyer MA: Effects of 6-hydroxydopamine lesions of locus coeruleus on startle in rats. Psychopharmacology (Berlin) 73:394–398, 1981

American Psychiatric Association: Diagnostic and Statistical Manual of Mental Disorders, 3rd Edition. Washington, DC, American Psychiatric Association, 1980

American Psychiatric Association: Diagnostic and Statistical Manual of Mental Disorders, 3rd Edition, Revised. Washington, DC, American Psychiatric Association, 1987

Anderson OD, Parmenter R: Long-term study of the experimental neurosis in the sheep and dog: with nine case histories. Psychosom Med Monograph, Vol 2, Nos 3–4, 1941

Blanchard E, Kolb L, Pallmeyer T, et al: A psychophysiological study of post traumatic stress disorder in Vietnam veterans. Psychiatr Q 54:220–229, 1982

Blanchard E, Kolb L, Gerardi R, et al: Cardiac response to relevant stimuli as an adjunctive tool for diagnosing post-traumatic stress disorder in Vietnam veterans. Behavior Therapy 17:592–606, 1986

Braff DL, Geyer MA: Sensorimotor gating and schizophrenia: human and animal model studies. Arch Gen Psychiatry 47:181–188, 1990

Braff DL, Stone C, Callaway E, et al: Prestimulus effects of human startle reflex in normals and schizophrenics. Psychophysiology 15:339–343, 1978

Butler RW, Braff DL, Rausch JL, et al: Physiological evidence of exaggerated startle response in a subgroup of Vietnam veterans with combat-related PTSD. Am J Psychiatry 147:1308–1312, 1990

Campbell CM: The role of instinct, emotion and personality in disorders of the heart. JAMA 71:1621–1626, 1918

Cassella JV, Davis M: Fear-enhanced acoustic startle is not attenuated by acute or chronic imipramine treatment in rats. Psychopharmacology (Berlin) 87:278–282, 1985

Conner RJ, Stolk JM, Barchas SD, et al: Parachlorophenylalanine and habituation to repetitive auditory startle stimuli in rats. Physiol Behav 5:1215–1219, 1970

Dale N, Schacher S, Kandel ER: Long-term facilitation in aplysia involves increase in transmitter release. Science 239:282–285, 1988

Davis M: Neurochemical modulation of sensory-motor reactivity: acoustic and tactile startle reflexes. Neurosci Biobehav Rev 4:241–263, 1980

Davis M: The mammalian startle response, in Neural Mechanisms of Startle Behavior. Edited by Eaton RC. New York, Plenum, 1984, pp 287–352

Davis M: Pharmacological and anatomical analysis of fear conditioning using the fear-potentiated startle paradigm. Behav Neurosci 100:814–824, 1986

Davis M, Svensson TH, Aghajanian GK: Effects of D- and L-amphetamine on habituation and sensitization of the acoustic startle response in rats. Psychopharmacologia 43:1–11, 1975

Davis M, Cedarbaum JM, Aghajanian GK, et al: Effects of clonidine on habituation and sensitization of acoustic startle in normal, decerebrate, and locus coeruleus lesioned rats. Psychopharmacology (Berlin) 51:243–253, 1977

Davis M, Redmond DE Jr, Baraban JM: Noradrenergic agonists and antagonists: effects on conditioned fear as measured by the potentiated startle paradigm. Psychopharmacology (Berlin) 65:111–118, 1979

Davis M, Astrachan DI, Kass E: Excitatory and inhibitory effects of serotonin on sensorimotor reactivity measured with acoustic startle. Science 209:521–523, 1980

Davis M, Kehne JH, Commissaris RL, et al: Effects of hallucinogens on unconditioned behaviors, in Hallucinogens: Neurochemical, Behavioral and Clinical Perspectives. Edited by Jacobs BL. New York, Raven, 1984, pp 35–75

Davis M, Cassella JV, Wrean WH, et al: Serotonin receptor subtype agonists: differential effects on sensorimotor reactivity measured with acoustic startle. Psychopharmacol Bull 22:837–843, 1986

Geyer MA, Tapson GS: Habituation of tactile startle is altered by drugs acting on serotonin-2 receptors. Neuropsychopharmacology 1:135–147, 1988

Geyer MA, Warbritton JD, Menkes DB, et al: Opposite effects of intraventricular serotonin and bufotenin on rat startle responses. Pharmacol Biochem Behav 3:687–691, 1975

Geyer MA, Puerto A, Menkes DB, et al: Behavioral studies following lesions of the mesolimbic and mesostriatal serotonergic pathways. Brain Res 106:256–270, 1976

Geyer MA, Petersen LR, Rose GJ: Effects of serotonergic lesions on investigatory responding by rats in a holeboard. Behav Neural Biol 30:160–177, 1980

Glanzman DL, Mackey SL, Hawkins RD, et al: Depletion of serotonin in the nervous system of aplysia reduces the behavioral enhancement of gill withdrawal as well as the heterosynaptic facilitation produced by tail shock. J Neurosci 9:4200–4213, 1989

Glanzman DL, Kandel ER, Schacher S: Target-dependent structural changes accompanying long-term synaptic facilitation in aplysia neurons. Science 249:799–802, 1990

Graham FK: The more or less startling effects of weak prestimuli. Psychophysiology 12:238–248, 1975

Graham F: Distinguishing among orienting, defense, and startle reflexes, in The Orienting Reflex in Humans: An International Conference Sponsored by the Scientific Affairs Division of the North Atlantic Treaty Organization. Edited by Kimmel H, van Olst E, Orlebeke J. Hillsdale, NJ, Lawrence Erlbaum, 1979, pp 137–167

Groves PM, Thompson RF: A dual process theory. Psychol Rev 77:419–450, 1970

Hitchcock J, Davis M: Lesions of the amygdala, but not of the cerebellum or red nucleus, block conditioned fear as measured with the potentiated startle paradigm. Behav Neurosci 100:11–22, 1986

Hoffman HS, Ison JR: Reflex modification in the domain of startle, I: some empirical findings and the implications for how the nervous system processes sensory input. Psychol Rev 87:175–189, 1980

Jacobson E: Response to a sudden unexpected stimulus. J Exp Psychol 9:19–25, 1926

Kehne JH, Davis M: Central noradrenergic involvement in yohimbine excitation of acoustic startle: effects of DSP4 and 6-OHDA. Brain Res 330:31–41, 1985

Kolb L: The post-traumatic stress disorders of combat: a subgroup with a conditioned emotional response. Milit Med 149:237–243, 1984

Korn H, Triller A, Mallet A, et al: Fluctuating responses at a central synapse: N of binomial fit predicts number of stained presynaptic boutons. Science 213:898–901, 1981

Landis C, Hunt WA (eds): The Startle Pattern. New York, Farrar and Rinehart, 1939

Mackey SL, Kandel ER, Hawkins RD: Identified serotonergic neurons LCB1 and RCB1 in the cerebral ganglia of aplysia produce presynaptic facilitation of siphon sensory neurons. J Neurosci 9:4227–4235, 1989

Malloy P, Fairbank J, Keane T: Validation of a multimethod assessment of posttraumatic stress disorders in Vietnam veterans. J Consult Clin Psychol 51:488–494, 1983

Mansbach RS, Geyer MA: Blockade of potentiated startle responding in rats by 5-hydroxytryptamine$_{1A}$ receptor ligands. Eur J Pharmacol 156:375–383, 1988

Melia KR, Davis M: Differential effects of selective dopamine agonists and antagonists on startle elicited electrically from the brainstem. Society for Neuroscience Abstracts 14:849, 1988

Miserendino MJ, Sananes CB, Melia KR, et al: Blocking of acquisition but not expression of conditioned fear-potentiated startle by NMDA antagonists in the amygdala. Nature 345:716–718, 1990

Ornitz EM, Pynoos RS: Startle modulation in children with posttraumatic stress disorder. Am J Psychiatry 146:866–871, 1989

Ornitz EM, Guthrie D, Kaplan A, et al: Maturation of startle modulation. Psychophysiology 23:624–634, 1986

Pitman R, Orr S, Forgue D, et al: Psychophysiologic assessment of posttraumatic stress disorder imagery in Vietnam combat veterans. Arch Gen Psychiatry 44:970–975, 1987

Swerdlow NR, Braff DL, Geyer MA, et al: Central dopamine hyperactivity in rats mimics abnormal sensory gating of the acoustic startle response in schizophrenics. Biol Psychiatry 21:23–33, 1986

Swerdlow NR, Mansbach RS, Geyer MA, et al: Amphetamine disruption of prepulse inhibition of acoustic startle is reversed by nucleus accumbens denervation. Psychopharmacology (Berlin) 100:413–416, 1990

Vrana SR, Spence EL, Lang PJ: The startle probe response: a new measure of emotion? J Abnorm Psychol 97:487–491, 1988

Wilkins DE, Hallett M, Wess MM: Audiogenic startle reflex of man and its relationship to startle syndromes. Brain 109:561–573, 1986

Chapter 15

Use of Tricyclics and Monoamine Oxidase Inhibitors in the Treatment of PTSD: A Quantitative Review

Steven M. Southwick, M.D.
Rachel Yehuda, Ph.D.
Earl L. Giller, Jr., M.D., Ph.D.
Dennis S. Charney, M.D.

P osttraumatic stress disorder (PTSD) has a lifetime prevalence of 1% in the general population (Helzer et al. 1987) and a 15% prevalence among Vietnam combat veterans (Kulka et al. 1990). Yet, study of the rational use of psychotropic agents for the treatment of PTSD is in its infancy. Although many different pharmacological agents have been tried, no one drug of choice or pharmacological treatment strategy has yet emerged. The most commonly used medications for the treatment of PTSD are antidepressants. However, results of treatment outcome have been varied across published reports. Clearly, antidepressants are not "curative" in PTSD, and they do not appear to treat all aspects of the disorder.

Nonetheless, by nearly all reports, antidepressants do appear to have some beneficial effects in the treatment of patients with PTSD. However, the extent to which these drugs affect com-

Support of this work was provided in part by Veterans Administration Merit Award to SMS and National Institute of Mental Health Postdoctoral-Training Grant 5-T32-MH17122 to RY.

monly occurring adjunctive symptoms of depression and anxiety versus specific PTSD symptoms is currently unclear. Furthermore, it is not known whether all three core symptom clusters (i.e., reexperiencing, avoidance, hyperarousal) in PTSD respond equally to these medications. The precise delineation of the symptoms that do respond to antidepressants in PTSD is an important next step in establishing a rational approach to pharmacotherapy of the traumatized patient. Analogously, in the schizophrenia literature, the finding that neuroleptics are useful for "positive" rather than "negative" symptoms has lead to more precise pharmacotherapy for the schizophrenic patient.

The present report is a summary of our attempt to synthesize and critically evaluate outcome findings across all published reports (Birkhimer et al. 1985; Bleich et al. 1986; Davidson et al. 1987, 1990; Falcon et al. 1985; Hogben and Cornfield 1981; Kauffman et al. 1987; Kosten et al. 1991; Lerer et al. 1987; Levenson et al. 1982; Milanes et al. 1984; Reist et al. 1989; Shen and Park 1983; Shestatzky et al. 1988; Walker 1982) on the use of tricyclic antidepressants (TCAs) and monoamine oxidase inhibitors (MAOIs) in the treatment of PTSD. The specific aim was to determine whether antidepressants differentially influence particular PTSD symptoms, or instead primarily treat comorbid major depression and anxiety disorders such as panic disorder.

Given the high clinical demand for information about the role of pharmacotherapy in the treatment of PTSD, and the relative confusion of the literature, we felt it important to provide a more rigorous analysis than is usually achieved through a standard literature review. Several meta-analytic techniques have been developed for the purpose of quantitative literature review (Landman and Dawes 1982). However these techniques, which require calculating statistical effect sizes, are more appropriately utilized in evaluating literatures with numerous controlled studies. In the PTSD literature only 4 out of 15 reports on antidepressant treatment are randomized placebo-controlled trials, while the rest are open trials and case reports.

Because we felt it important to evaluate all published studies, including case reports, standard meta-analytic techniques could not be meaningfully utilized. To perform the analysis, we first evaluated the extent to which factors such as study design, type of medication, and duration of treatment were related to reports of antidepressant efficacy in PTSD. Next, subjects from all published reports were pooled and rated with a uniform rating scale designed to assess the efficacy of antidepressant medications on particular symptom clusters. This procedure allowed all subjects reported in the literature to be evaluated as one overall sample using identical criteria for symptom improvement. Symptom improvement in all patients was rated on both the primary DSM-III-R (American Psychiatric Association 1987) symptom clusters of PTSD (i.e., reexperiencing, avoidance, and hyperarousal) and symptoms of depression and anxiety. Depression and anxiety symptoms were rated because, although not formally part of the DSM-III-R criteria for PTSD, they often are present in patients with PTSD. Furthermore, given the well-known efficacy of antidepressants in the treatment of depression and panic disorder, it is possible that antidepressants primarily affect these co-occurring symptoms rather than the core symptoms of PTSD. Statistical analysis was performed to determine the relative effectiveness of TCAs and MAOIs on the above-mentioned symptom clusters and to address methodological considerations relevant to the determination of treatment outcome.

METHODS

All published primary data papers dealing with psychopharmacological treatment of chronic (i.e., duration of more than 6 months) PTSD were included for analysis ($N = 15$ studies). Studies were evaluated for study design, drop-out rate, type of medication, comorbid psychiatric diagnoses, method of symptom assessment, range of dosage, duration of treatment, and symptom improvement. Fisher's exact probability test was used to determine whether aspects of study methodology (i.e., study design, use of structured vs. clinical ratings, duration of treatment) were related to overall symptom improvement. For these analyses each drug study was considered separately. All subjects in a particular study were considered as one group, and overall drug efficacy for that study was rated as "good to very good" if there was a greater than 50% reduction of symptoms.

Data analysis was also performed on symptom improvement data from the total pool of individual subjects. Summing across these studies, the total number of subjects was 215 (209 war-related cases, 6 civilian cases). Using the total pool of subjects, we compared the relative efficacy of MAOIs and TCAs on five symptom clusters: 1) reexperiencing (e.g., intrusive memories, nightmares, flashbacks); 2) avoidance (e.g., efforts to avoid reminders of the trauma, detachment, diminished interest, restricted affect); 3) hyperarousal (e.g., insomnia, anger, hypervigilance, physiological reactivity); 4) depression (including neurovegetative symptoms if specified); and 5) anxiety (including panic). The relative efficacy of TCAs and MAOIs on overall global improvement was also determined. Global improvement or improvement on a particular symptom cluster was judged to be good to very good if there was a 50% or greater improvement, to be moderate if there was a 20% to 50% improvement, and to be poor if there was less than 20% clinical improvement. Whenever possible, symptom improvement was rated for each individual. In larger studies that did not include anecdotal descriptions or data from individual subjects, we considered the mean improvement of all patients in that study for data analysis. This determination was made by comparing baseline scores of structured interview data with scores following antidepressant treatment. Subjects dropping out from any study prior to the end of 2 weeks of treatment were not included in data analysis. Symptom improvement was assessed by the consensus of two raters (SMS and RY). A third rater (ELG) then assessed the same studies independently. Interrater reliability using intraclass r was performed by correlating the consensus ratings of the experienced raters with the independent ratings of the third rater. Reliability was established as $r = 0.90$ for reexperiencing, $r = 0.76$ for avoidant, $r = 0.79$ for hyperarousal, $r = 0.88$ for depression, and $r = 0.68$ for anxiety. Chi-square analysis was used to compare the relative efficacy of TCAs and MAOIs.

RESULTS

The published literature to date on antidepressant trials in the treatment of chronic PTSD is summarized in Table 15–1. The literature, in total, consists of four case reports, seven open trials, and four randomized, placebo-controlled drug trials. Thirteen percent of the subjects were reported to have dropped out because of side effects. The total remaining number of subjects across studies was 128 for TCAs and 87 for MAOIs. The TCAs used included imipramine, desipramine, amitriptyline, and doxepin. Phenelzine was the only MAOI used. Ten of the 15 studies documented a relatively high incidence of comorbid psychiatric diagnoses, including major depression, dysthymia, generalized anxiety, panic, substance abuse, and character disorders. Diagnostic comorbidity was not specified in the other five studies.

When open trial and case studies were compared with ran-

Table 15–1.   Studies, subject numbers, and drop-out rates used in analyzing pharmacological treatment of chronic PTSD

Study	Design	TCA	MAOI	Dropouts
Hogben and Cornfeld (1981)	Case	—	5	NR
Levenson et al. (1982)	Case	—	1	NR
Walker (1982)	Case	—	3	2
Shen and Park (1983)	Case	—	3	NR
Milanes et al. (1984)	Open	—	10	4
Birkhimer et al. (1985)	Open[a]	15	5	NR
Falcon et al. (1985)	Open	17	—	NR
Bleich et al. (1986)	Open	25	2	NR
Davidson et al. (1987)	Open	—	10	1
Kauffman et al. (1987)	Open	8	—	0
Lerer et al. (1987)	Open	—	22	3
Shestatzky et al. (1988)	RCT	—	10	3
Reist et al. (1989)	RCT	18	—	6
Davidson et al. (1990)	RCT	22	—	3
Kosten et al. (1991)[b]	RCT	23	19	6
		128	87	28

Note. TCA = tricyclic antidepressant; MAOI = monoamine oxidase inhibitor; NR = not reported; RCT = randomized clinical trial.
[a]Retrospective study.
[b]Preliminary findings reported in Frank et al. 1988.

domized clinical trials, there were no significant differences in overall global symptom improvement (Fisher's exact test, $P = 0.28$). Seven of the 15 studies used structured symptom assessments to measure symptom changes in response to medication, while 8 of the studies used clinical ratings. Overall global symptom improvement was not significantly different in studies using structured symptom ratings (Fisher's exact test, $P = 0.18$).

Most studies used roughly equivalent doses of antidepressants. Doses ranged from 140 to 225 mg/day (mean = 181 mg) for TCAs and 30 to 75 mg/day (mean = 60 mg) for phenelzine. Duration of treatment ranged from 4 to 24 weeks (mean = 10 weeks) for TCAs and from 2 to 8 weeks (mean = 5.8) for phenelzine. To study the effect of treatment duration on global symptom improvement, the 15 studies were divided into those with treatment durations of greater than or less than 8 weeks. There was a nonsignificant trend for greater global improvement in studies with treatment duration greater than 8 weeks (Fisher's exact test, $P = 0.08$).

Monoamine oxidase inhibitors were judged to be better overall than TCAs ($\chi^2 = 33.2$; $df = 2$; $P < 0.0001$; see Table 15–2). A good to very good global response was reported in 82% of phenelzine-treated patients and 45% of patients treated with TCAs. However, the response of individual symptom clusters to TCAs and MAOIs was less robust than the overall global response (Table 15–2).

The only specific PTSD symptom cluster that showed good improvement in response to antidepressants was the "reexperiencing" cluster (Table 15–2). Overall, phenelzine was found to be significantly more effective than TCAs for this symptom cluster ($\chi^2 = 18.6$; $df = 2$; $P < 0.001$). On the other hand, symptoms of avoidance tended to respond moderately or poorly to antidepressants. In this case, TCAs were also found to be somewhat inferior to phenelzine. Similarly, symptoms of hyperarousal responded in the moderate to poor range for phenelzine. Hyperarousal was seldom rated in TCA studies.

The adjunctive symptoms of depression and anxiety also showed a poor response to antidepressants. In this case, phenelzine was significantly less efficacious than TCAs for depression ($\chi^2 = 18.6$; $df = 2$; $P < 0.001$), with only 13% of phenelzine-treated

Table 15–2. Efficacy of antidepressants on global symptom improvement and individual symptom clusters associated with PTSD

	Frequency (%)	
	TCA	**MAOI**
Global		
Good	45	82
Moderate	25	2
Poor	30	16
Not rated	0	0
Reexperiencing		
Good	22	41
Moderate	42	41
Poor	36	11
Not rated	0	6
Avoidant		
Good	0	0
Moderate	20	36
Poor	47	43
Not rated	33	22
Hyperarousal		
Good	4	9
Moderate	23	23
Poor	5	40
Not rated	69	28
Depression		
Good	13	0
Moderate	25	13
Poor	43	62
Not rated	20	25
Anxiety		
Good	11	1
Moderate	0	43
Poor	45	37
Not rated	45	20

Note. The data represent assessments of drug responses from subjects pooled across 15 antidepressant trials: 128 subjects received TCAs, and 87 subjects received phenelzine. Response to medication was judged good if symptoms improved by greater than 50%, moderate if there was between a 20% and 50% improvement, and poor if symptom improvement was less than 20%.

subjects showing a moderate response of depressive symptoms, and 38% of TCA-treated subjects showing a moderate or better response (Table 15–2). Depression was not rated in one-quarter of the studies. The response of anxiety symptoms, including panic, was in the moderate or better range in 44% of patients following phenelzine treatment, compared with 11% with TCA treatment. These symptoms were not rated in many of the studies.

DISCUSSION

The present analysis suggests that antidepressants are useful in the treatment of PTSD, but only for some symptoms. These symptoms are not necessarily the ones for which antidepressants are commonly prescribed. Although global improvement was reported as good to very good in most studies, analysis of particular symptom clusters revealed that only the "reexperiencing" cluster showed significant improvement. Approximately 75% of the subjects showed moderate or better improvement in flashbacks, nightmares, and intrusive traumatic memories, with phenelzine being more effective for these symptoms than TCAs. Symptoms of avoidance and hyperarousal responded poorly to both phenelzine and TCAs. However, within the hyperarousal cluster, symptoms of insomnia showed moderate improvement. In this regard, it should be noted that the efficacy of antidepressants for symptoms of hyperarousal and avoidance was not specified in all studies, likely because marked improvement was not observed.

Interestingly, concurrent symptoms of depression and anxiety (including panic) also failed to respond to antidepressants. This is surprising because antidepressants are very effective in treating major depression and panic disorder in non-PTSD populations. Furthermore, the hypothesis has been raised that antidepressants enhance global improvement in PTSD because of their effect on comorbid major depressive disorder (Davidson et al. 1985; Friedman 1988) and/or panic disorder (Davidson et al. 1985). However, our results suggest that global improvement in PTSD cannot be attributed to the effects of antidepressants on these concurrent disorders. Rather, in addition to their effects on reexperiencing symptoms, antidepressants may in part improve global functioning through effects on other areas of functioning such as social relationships, family, and work (Giller et al. 1988b), areas that were not systematically evaluated in these studies. It is also possible that global improvement was rated relatively high despite minimal effects on most symptom clusters, because for this chronic and often treatment-resistant population, improvements in even one symptom cluster make a substantial difference in the patient's overall presentation.

In addition to pooling subjects across all studies for the purpose of comparing the efficacy of TCAs with that of MAOIs, we also compared some relevant aspects of methodology between studies. These analyses were performed to explore the relative effect of methodological differences on overall treatment outcome and to confirm the appropriateness of pooling subjects across studies. Treatment outcome did not appear to differ depending on type of study design when the four randomized clinical trials were compared with all open trials. This is largely due to methodological differences within the randomized clinical trials. The two studies using a standard double-blind, placebo-controlled design rated global efficacy as good to very good (Davidson et al. 1990; Kosten et al. 1991). These studies also used a relatively large number of subjects in their experimental groups (i.e., Kosten et al. 1991, $n = 42$; Davidson et al. 1990, $n = 22$) and assessed symptom improvement at the end of an 8-week trial. In the other two studies (Reist et al. 1989; Shestatzky et al. 1988) that reported moderate to poor global improvement, fewer subjects were utilized, and symptom improvement was assessed following 4-week trials. In these studies, poor drug effect may have been related to the significant effect of time alone (i.e., nonspecific or placebo) on improvement.

Our analysis did show a trend toward symptom improvement with greater treatment duration. Patients treated for 8 weeks or longer tended to show greater overall symptom improvement, suggesting that antidepressant treatment trials in PTSD may need to be longer than the standard 4 to 6 weeks recommended for major depression. In Bleich et al.'s study, for example, an 85% response rate to amitriptyline occurred only after 6 months of treatment (Bleich et al. 1986). In fact, it may be that antidepressants should be taken chronically as maintenance medication to prevent relapse, as has been described for chronic depression (Giller et al. 1988a). The optimal course of antidepressant treatment for PTSD has not yet been established and awaits further assessment through follow-up and medication discontinuation studies.

When comparing global improvement in studies using standardized scales versus subjective clinical ratings, no differences were observed. However, some of the standardized scales used in these studies were designed to assess depression and anxiety, and as a result may have been too insensitive to detect changes in PTSD-specific symptoms. Furthermore, studies that did use a standardized instrument to assess PTSD symptoms typically used the Impact of Event Scale (Horowitz et al. 1972), a self-report measure, which may be less sensitive than a clinician-rated instrument.

Issues pertaining to subject heterogeneity could not be assessed in the present study. For example, we were unable to address systematically the interaction between baseline symptomatology at treatment onset and symptom improvement across studies. Nor were we able to identify a subgroup of severely symptomatic individuals for the purpose of comparing treatment efficacy. In general, inpatients tend to be more severely ill than outpatients. However, in some studies, hospitalization status was not clearly stated, or was not considered as a separate variable in data analysis. Nonetheless, an informal assessment indicated that global symptom improvement seemed to be better in studies using outpatients (Davidson et al. 1990; Kosten et al. 1991), compared with those using inpatients. Furthermore, analysis of the drop-out data in one study indicated that patients who were unable to tolerate antidepressant treatment had the highest baseline scores (Davidson et al. 1987). Thus, it may be that symptoms in the moderate, rather than the severe, range of symptom severity are best targeted by antidepressants. Moreover, the relatively poor improvement in inpatients may reflect comorbid illnesses in these groups such as affective and personality disorders (Davidson et al. 1985; Helzer et al. 1987; Kulka et al. 1990; Yehuda et al. 1990).

Another important issue is the relationship between diagnostic comorbidity and treatment outcome. The rate of diagnostic comorbidity across pharmacological studies was high, which is in agreement with nonpharmacological studies in PTSD (Davidson et al. 1985; Kulka et al. 1990). This variable was not systematically considered in our analysis because most studies did not specify comorbid diagnoses or indicate whether symptom improvement was related to the occurrence of concurrent psychopathology. The effect of a comorbid diagnosis may in fact affect global symptom improvement with antidepressants. For example, Kosten et al. (1991), in their study of PTSD patients who did not meet the criteria for major depressive disorder, reported the highest rate of symptom improvement among subjects in the randomized clinical trials. Similarly, Davidson et al. (1990), in their study, showed that recovery rates with amitriptyline were generally lower in patients who met diagnostic criteria for concurrent major depressive disorder. In this regard, it is important to note that the studies reviewed in this analysis did not typically distinguish depressive from melancholic symptoms in patients. Thus, the efficacy of antidepressants for PTSD patients with concurrent melancholia is a question that requires further exploration.

The major treatment implication from the above findings is that antidepressants are best prescribed for particular target symptoms of PTSD, especially the reexperiencing cluster, rather than for the entire syndrome as a whole. Patients who suffer from symptoms of avoidance and hyperarousal may be more effectively treated with other agents. For example, in an ongoing open trial on the efficacy of fluoxetine in PTSD, significant improvement in avoidance and hyperarousal has been observed (McDougle et al. 1991). Other drugs that have been reported to be useful in alleviating some PTSD symptoms include clonidine and propranolol for hyperarousal symptoms (Kolb et al. 1984), carbamazepine and lithium for impulsivity and aggressive behavior (Kitchner and Greenstein 1985; van der Kolk 1983), and benzodiazepines for anxiety (van der Kolk 1983). Thus, in the pharmacotherapy of PTSD, different agents may be useful for treating different symptom clusters; furthermore, a combination of pharmacological agents may prove useful in the same patient (Thomson et al. 1990).

REFERENCES

American Psychiatric Association: Diagnostic and Statistical Manual of Mental Disorders, 3rd Edition, Revised. Washington, DC, American Psychiatric Association, 1987

Birkhimer LJ, DeVane CL, Muniz CE: Posttraumatic stress disorder: characteristics and pharmacological response in the veteran population. Compr Psychiatry 26:304–310, 1985

Bleich A, Seigel B, Garb R, et al: Post-traumatic stress disorder following combat exposure: clinical features and psychopharmacological treatment. Br J Psychiatry 149:365–369, 1986

Davidson J, Swartz M, Storck MD, et al: A diagnostic and family study of PTSD. Am J Psychiatry 142:90–93, 1985

Davidson J, Walker JI, Kilts C: A pilot study of phenelzine in the treatment of post-traumatic stress disorder. Br J Psychiatry 150:252–255, 1987

Davidson J, Kudler H, Smith R, et al: Treatment of post-traumatic stress disorder with amitriptyline and placebo. Arch Gen Psychiatry 47:259–266, 1990

Falcon S, Ryan C, Chamberlain K, et al: Tricyclics: possible treatment for posttraumatic stress disorder. J Clin Psychiatry 46:385–388, 1985

Frank JB, Kosten TR, Giller EL, et al: A preliminary study of phenelzine and imipramine for post-traumatic stress disorder. Am J Psychiatry 145:1289–1291, l988

Friedman MJ: Toward rational pharmacotherapy for posttraumatic stress disorder: an interim report. Am J Psychiatry 145:281–285, 1988

Giller EL Jr, Bialos D, Harkness L, et al: Long-term amitriptyline in chronic depression. Hillside J Clin Psychiatry 7:16–33, 1988a

Giller EL Jr, Bialos D, Riddle MA, et al: MAOI treatment response: multiaxial assessment. J Affective Disord 4:171–175, 1988b

Helzer JE, Robins LN, McEvoy L: Post-traumatic stress disorder in the general population: findings of the epidemiological catchment area survey. N Engl J Med 317:1630–1634, 1987

Hogben GL, Cornfield RB: Treatment of traumatic war neurosis with phenelzine. Arch Gen Psychiatry 38:440–445, 1981

Horowitz M, Wilner N, Alvarez W: Impact of Events Scale: A measure of subjective distress. Psychosom Med 41:209–218, 1972

Kauffman CD, Reist C, Djenderedjian A, et al: Biological markers of affective disorders and posttraumatic stress disorder: a pilot study with desipramine. J Clin Psychiatry 48:366–367, 1987

Kitchner I, Greenstein R: Low dose lithium carbonate treatment of post-traumatic stress disorder: brief communication. Milit Med 50:378–381, 1985

Kolb LC, Burris BC, Griffiths S: Propranolol and clonidine in treatment of the chronic post-traumatic stress disorders of war, in Post-traumatic Stress Disorder: Psychological and Biological Sequelae. Edited by van der Kolk BA. Washington, DC, American Psychiatric Press, 1984, pp 97–105

Kosten TR, Frank JB, Dan E, et al: Pharmacotherapy for post-traumatic stress disorder using phenelzine or imipramine. J Nerv Ment Dis 179:366–370, 1991

Kulka RA, Schlenger WE, Fairbank JA, et al: Trauma and the Vietnam War Generation. New York, Brunner/Mazel, 1990

Landman JT, Dawes RM: Psychotherapy outcome: Smith and Glass's conclusions stand up under scrutiny. Am Psychol 37:504–516, 1982

Lerer B, Bleich A, Kotler M: Posttraumatic stress disorder in Israeli combat veterans. Arch Gen Psychiatry 44:976–981, 1987

Levenson H, Lanman R, Rankin M: Traumatic war neurosis and phenelzine. Arch Gen Psychiatry 39:1345, 1982

McDougle CJ, Southwick SM, St James RL, et al: An open trial of fluoxetine in the treatment of posttraumatic stress disorder (letter). J Clin Psychopharmacol 11:325–327, 1991

Milanes FJ, Mack CN, Dennison J, et al: Phenelzine treatment of post-Vietnam stress syndrome. VA Practitioner 1(6):40–47, 1984

Reist C, Kauffman CD, Haier RJ, et al: A controlled trial of desipramine in 18 men with posttraumatic stress disorder. Am J Psychiatry 46:513–516, 1989

Shen WW, Park S: The use of monoamine oxidase inhibitors in the treatment of traumatic war neurosis: a case report. Milit Med 148:430–431, 1983

Shestatzky M, Greenberg D, Lerer B: A controlled trial of phenelzine in posttraumatic stress disorder. Psychiatry Res 24:149–155, 1988

Thomson J, Dan E, Rosenheck R, et al: Medication clinic within a Vietnam Veteran Readjustment Counseling Center, in Biological Assessment and Treatment of Posttraumatic Stress Disorder. Edited by Giller EL Jr. Washington, DC, American Psychiatric Press, 1990, pp 173–183

van der Kolk BA: Psychopharmacological issues in post-traumatic stress disorder. Hosp Community Psychiatry 34:683–391, 1983

Walker JI: Chemotherapy of traumatic stress. Milit Med 147:1029–1033, 1982

Yehuda R, Southwick SM, Giller EL Jr: Axis II psychopathology in combat PTSD, in 1990 New Research Program and Abstracts, 143 annual meeting of the American Psychiatric Association, New York, May 1990, NR513, p 244

Section IV

Methodological Issues

Chapter 16

Assessment of Sympathetic Nervous System Function in PTSD: A Critique of Methodology

Richard C. Veith, M.D.
M. Michele Murburg, M.D.

I t has long been recognized that activation of the sympathetic nervous system (SNS) serves an important physiological role in the response to stress (Cannon 1929, 1939; Selye 1950). Increases in heart rate, blood pressure, and cardiac output and the fall in skeletal muscle vascular resistance associated with the classic "fight or flight," or defense reaction, are largely mediated by alterations in SNS activity. Not surprisingly, therefore, the prominence of such symptoms as anxiety, tachycardia, and an excessive startle response among individuals suffering from PTSD has stimulated efforts to determine if SNS hyperactivity is present in PTSD.

As noted by McFall and Murburg (Chapter 7, this volume), psychophysiological studies indicate that patients with PTSD exhibit elevated resting heart rate and blood pressure and demonstrate heightened cardiovascular responses to trauma-related experimental cues. Although this profile is compatible with increased SNS responsiveness, heart rate and blood pressure are only indirect indices of SNS activity, because they are subject to

This work was supported by the Medical Research Service of the Veteran's Administration.

the counterregulatory influences of the parasympathetic nervous system and several neuroendocrine systems. Reports describing increased 24-hour urinary excretion of catecholamines in PTSD patients and populations exposed to stress (Davidson and Baum 1986; Kosten et al. 1987), and both increased and more prolonged elevations of plasma epinephrine in response to combat cues in combat veterans with PTSD (McFall et al. 1990; Murburg et al., Chapter 9, this volume), constitute more compelling evidence for SNS hyperactivity in this disorder. However, as will be elaborated in this review, these measures must be interpreted cautiously.

One rationale for investigating SNS function in PTSD is the possibility that SNS disturbances might serve as diagnostic markers for the presence or severity of the disorder. Alternatively, alterations in SNS function might parallel the course of the disorder or provide an index of the effectiveness of treatment. Biological models of PTSD postulate an etiological role for brain dysfunction in the pathogenesis of this disorder (McFall et al. 1989; van der Kolk et al. 1984; see also Charney et al., Chapter 6; McFall and Murburg, Chapter 7, this volume). From this perspective, the study of SNS functioning in PTSD might constitute an indirect means of acquiring insight into those central nervous system (CNS) mechanisms that regulate the SNS or underlie the defense reaction. For example, extensive research in animals has shown that the cardiovascular and adrenomedullary components of the classic defense reaction can be elicited by stimulation of discrete brain regions (Smith and DeVito 1984; Stoddard 1991). In a series of elegant studies among freely moving baboons, Smith and co-workers (DeVito and Smith 1982; Smith et al. 1990) localized an area of the hypothalamus that is responsible for the pattern of cardiovascular changes that accompany the emotional response of the defense reaction. Thus, the presence of SNS disturbances in PTSD could allow inferences to be made regarding specific brain regions known to be important in the regulation of stress responses.

Our purpose in this chapter is to evaluate the relative merits and limitations of currently available methods for assessing SNS function in humans and to assess their implications for studies exploring possible SNS dysfunction in PTSD.

ORGANIZATION AND FUNCTION OF THE SYMPATHETIC NERVOUS SYSTEM

For the purposes of considering the assessment of SNS function in humans, the peripheral SNS can be organized into two major components: 1) the SNS nerves regulating cardiovascular function and 2) those innervating the adrenal medulla (Cryer 1980; Kopin et al. 1988). Postganglionic SNS nerves innervating the heart, major organs, skeletal muscles, and vasculature constitute the cardiovascular component of the SNS, which is principally involved in regulating blood pressure and mediating hemodynamic adaptations to stress. Accordingly, such "stressors" as hypotension, the assumption of upright posture, and exercise are potent stimuli for activating this component of the SNS, reflected by increased firing of pre- and postganglionic SNS nerves and the release of norepinephrine into the circulation (Cryer 1980; Kopin et al. 1988). The adrenomedullary component of the SNS, comprised of cholinergic preganglionic SNS nerves directly innervating the adrenal medulla, serves important homeostatic and adaptive functions primarily involving glucose regulation, thermogenesis, and metabolism (Cryer 1980; Kopin et al. 1988). This component of the SNS is preferentially activated in response to such stimuli as hypoglycemia, which produces a prompt release of epinephrine into the circulation (Cryer 1980; Kopin et al. 1988). Although the adrenal medulla is capable of synthesizing norepinephrine, it is generally accepted that less than 2% of circulating plasma norepinephrine derives from adrenal sources in humans in the absence of profound physiological stress (Esler et al. 1989).

Brain-stem cardiovascular centers serve to integrate visceral and baroreceptor afferent input and descending efferents from cortical, hypothalamic, and midbrain regions that are essential for the maintenance of blood pressure and regulation of the cardiovascular and adrenomedullary adaptations to stress. The paraventricular nucleus and the amygdala (Brown and Fisher 1984, 1985; Sawchenko and Swanson 1982; Smith and DeVito 1984; Swanson and Sawchenko 1980; see also Aston-Jones et al., Chapter 2, this volume) send direct projections to the brain-stem cardiovascular centers and intermediolateral cell columns of the spinal cord and thereby link the neocortex and hypothalamus with the brain stem and spinal cord regions that regulate SNS function. As noted by Aston-Jones and associates (Chapter 2, this volume), the nucleus paragigantocellularis (PGi) in the ventrolateral rostral medulla is a key brain region for control of the SNS. Neurons of the PGi project to the intermediolateral cell column of the spinal cord to influence SNS preganglionic nerves and also provide the major afferent input to the locus coeruleus (LC). Evidence indicating a close temporal relationship between LC activation and the simultaneous firing of peripheral SNS neurons (Elam et al. 1981, 1984; Reis et al. 1984, 1988), possibly mediated by PGi neurons, suggests that under some circumstances peripheral SNS activity might serve as an index of activation of the LC CNS noradrenergic system.

Activation of preganglionic SNS nerves results in the release of acetylcholine and an immediate increase in the rates of norepinephrine release from postganglionic nerve terminals and epinephrine release from the adrenal medulla. The rates of catecholamine release are subject to further modulation by effects of the catecholamines themselves as well as other substances—for example, angiotensin, dopamine, and prostaglandins via presynaptic receptors on SNS neurons (Charney et al. 1981; Kopin et al. 1988). Most of the norepinephrine released from SNS nerves is removed from the synaptic cleft by an energy-requiring reuptake mechanism involving an uptake transporter (Pacholczyk et al. 1991; Paton 1976). Following reuptake, norepinephrine is repackaged in storage vesicles for rerelease or is deaminated to form dihydroxyphenylglycol (DHPG), which diffuses out of the neuron and is rapidly O-methylated to form 3-methoxy-4-hydroxyphenylglycol (MHPG) (Goldstein et al. 1988). Some of the released norepinephrine activates postsynaptic adrenergic receptors on target organs or stimulates presynaptic $alpha_2$ (α_2)–adrenergic receptors, inhibiting further norepinephrine release.

Following its release from SNS nerves, norepinephrine that escapes inactivation by the norepinephrine transporter (uptake 1) may also be removed by uptake 2, a nonstereoselective process that transports norepinephrine into non-neural cells where it is metabolized by monoamine oxidase to form normetanephrine (Iversen and Salt 1970; Kopin 1985; Paton 1976; Trendelenburg 1980). Normetanephrine is partially conjugated and excreted into the urine, but is predominantly deaminated and excreted as 3-methoxy-4-hydroxymandelic acid (VMA). Approximately 10% to 20% of norepinephrine released from SNS nerves escapes reuptake and metabolism to spill over into plasma (Eisenhofer et al. 1991; Esler et al. 1988; Goldstein et al. 1983; Kopin 1985; Linares et al. 1987). Because of the efficiency of the mechanisms for terminating the actions of released catecholamines, the plasma half-lives of norepinephrine and epinephrine are approximately 2 to 4 minutes (Eisenhofer et al. 1991; Esler et al. 1988; Goldstein et al. 1983; Kopin 1985). Although it has traditionally been considered that norepinephrine and epinephrine are cleared from the plasma by similar mechanisms, recent studies have demonstrated differential effects of aging on plasma norepinephrine and epinephrine clearance (Morrow et al. 1987) and have revealed differences in the efficiency of their removal by neuronal reuptake (Eisenhofer et al. 1990). These findings have led to a reappraisal of the assumption that norepinephrine and epinephrine are cleared from the plasma by identical mechanisms.

Unlike circulating plasma norepinephrine, which has little hormonal effect at physiological concentrations and can be considered neurotransmitter overflow, epinephrine is a potent circulating hormone (Clutter et al. 1980; Cryer 1980; Kopin et al. 1988; Silverberg et al. 1978). Only modest increases in the plasma epinephrine concentration (i.e., doubling) are required to elicit metabolic or cardiovascular effects. In contrast, a five- to eightfold increase in circulating plasma norepinephrine is necessary to produce measurable increases in heart rate or blood pressure in humans (Cryer 1980; Kopin et al. 1988; Silverberg et al. 1978).

TECHNIQUES FOR ASSESSING SYMPATHETIC NERVOUS SYSTEM ACTIVITY IN HUMANS

Urinary Catecholamine Excretion

In 1948, von Euler discovered that norepinephrine is the neurotransmitter released from peripheral SNS nerves, and developed a biochemical assay for norepinephrine in urine (von Euler 1948).

By the mid-1950s, urinary measurements were being employed in large clinical studies of hypertensive subjects to estimate SNS nerve activity. Subsequent studies have demonstrated that the total urinary excretion of norepinephrine and all of its metabolites can be used as a global measure of norepinephrine synthesis rate (Hoeldtke et al. 1983). This approach has several advantages. Although somewhat cumbersome, urinary sampling is noninvasive and easily applicable to the clinical setting. Urinary norepinephrine and its metabolites are of sufficient concentrations that laboratory analysis requires less sensitive methods than those required for plasma sampling. In addition, urinary sampling potentially provides an integrated index of SNS activity over prolonged periods of time.

The reliance on urinary excretion of norepinephrine and its metabolites to assess SNS activity in humans also suffers from several limitations. Because urinary excretion is substantially downstream for the actual site of release of norepinephrine from postganglionic SNS nerves, this approach is insensitive to acute, transient alterations in SNS activity. This potential problem is amplified by the fact that only a very small fraction of norepinephrine released from SNS neurons escapes local reuptake and metabolism to be excreted in the urine (Hoeldtke et al. 1983; Kopin 1985; Linares et al. 1987). In addition, measurements of norepinephrine and its metabolites in urine are subject to the local influences of renal blood flow and sympathetic nerve activity in the kidney itself (DeVito and Smith 1982; Esler 1989). Renal SNS activity may or may not parallel SNS activity in other organs (DeVito and Smith 1982; Esler 1989; Esler et al. 1988). Such influences render urinary excretion, at best, an unpredictable correlate of systemic SNS activity, particularly if prolonged sampling is not employed.

Finally, the rates of peripheral norepinephrine synthesis and release do not necessarily coincide. For example, intraneuronal metabolism of some amount of norepinephrine probably occurs independent of release from SNS neuroeffector junctions (Eisenhofer et al. 1991; Hoeldtke et al. 1983). Leakage of norepinephrine from neuronal storage granules is estimated to account for a large proportion of DHPG production (Eisenhofer et al. 1991). The contribution of the resulting metabolites to the total urinary excretion concentration theoretically results in an overestimation of actual release. Alternatively, to the extent that released norepinephrine is recaptured, stored, and rereleased, urinary excretion products could underestimate actual norepinephrine release from SNS nerves. These factors further limit the use of total urinary excretion products as an index of total body SNS activity.

Plasma Catecholamines and Catecholamine Kinetics

The development of sensitive and specific assays for the catecholamines in the late 1960s and 1970s allowed for a more accurate assessment of SNS activity in humans than had previously been possible by the reliance on heart rate or blood pressure, or the measurement of total urinary excretion products. Plasma norepinephrine concentrations rise in response to acute stressful illness, surgery, exercise, and assumption of upright posture, and fall with blockade of SNS outflow by spinal anesthesia, thus, providing a potentially useful index of the cardiovascular component of peripheral SNS activity (Christensen and Brandsburg 1973; Cryer 1980; Halter et al. 1977; Kopin et al. 1988; Pflug and Halter 1981). Similarly, plasma epinephrine has been shown to be a sensitive index of adrenomedullary SNS activity (Cryer 1980; Kopin et al. 1988). Studies in humans indicate that the majority of circulating plasma norepinephrine derives from norepinephrine spillover from skeletal muscle and the kidney, with relatively smaller contributions from the skin and hepatomesenteric system (Esler et al. 1988). Only approximately 2% of circulating plasma norepinephrine derives from the heart (Esler et al. 1988). The brain makes no contribution to circulating norepinephrine, epinephrine, or dopamine because of the presence of a blood-brain barrier for the catecholamines (Peskind et al. 1986; Ziegler et al. 1980).

Dopamine is also present in SNS nerves and circulates in plasma in concentrations that closely approximate those of epinephrine (Van Loon 1983; Williams et al. 1986). Renal clearance studies have established that dopamine is formed in the kidney, which is probably the major source for plasma and urinary dopamine (Esler 1989; Van Loon 1983; Williams et al. 1986). Evidence that acute alterations in SNS tone are paralleled by changes in plasma dopamine has fueled speculation that dopamine may serve as a peripheral neurotransmitter (Van Loon 1983). Alternatively, as a precursor for norepinephrine synthesis, dopamine might simply be coreleased with norepinephrine during SNS activation. The urinary excretion of dopamine greatly exceeds that attributable to filtration from circulating plasma dopamine (Esler 1989). This increase derives largely from the kidney itself, where the presence of neurons rich in dopamine suggests the presence of an intrinsic dopamine neuronal system. A large fraction of the dopamine found in the kidney is extraneuronal. Dopamine is formed from the decarboxylation of circulating dihydroxyphenylalanine (DOPA). Urinary excretion of dopamine from this source is increased by high dietary sodium or protein intake (Van Loon 1983; Williams et al. 1986). Yehuda, Giller, and colleagues (Chapter 10, this volume) describe elevations of urinary dopamine in combat veterans and Holocaust survivors with PTSD. It is important to note in this context that, to date, no stimulus has been shown to differentially increase dopamine and norepinephrine spillover into plasma, renal outflow, or urine (Esler 1989).

The circulating concentrations of norepinephrine and epinephrine in plasma are determined not only by their rates of appearance into plasma but also by their rates of clearance (Best and Halter 1982; Esler et al. 1979, 1988). The rate of removal of catecholamines from plasma is a function of the cardiac output to tissues that fractionally extract norepinephrine and epinephrine and of the cellular mechanisms of catecholamine removal, particularly neuronal uptake. In the 1970s, Esler and associates (1979, 1988) developed a radioisotope dilution technique that allows for the determination of the rates of norepinephrine appearance into plasma and its clearance from plasma. This approach has proven useful in examining differences in plasma catecholamines among clinical populations at baseline and in response to physiological or pharmacological perturbations of the SNS (Esler et al. 1988; Goldstein et al. 1987; Schwartz et al. 1987; Veith et al. 1984, 1986). More recently, this approach has been extended to the assessment of organ-specific norepinephrine kinetics in humans (Esler et al. 1989, 1991b; Meredith et al. 1991). Radiotracer methods for measuring plasma epinephrine kinetics have also been described (Morrow et al. 1987; Rosen et al. 1989).

The assessment of the effects of normal human aging on SNS function is a good example of the utility of the plasma catecholamine kinetic approaches. Plasma norepinephrine concentrations are elevated in elderly persons (Schwartz et al. 1987; Veith et al. 1986). Taken at face value, it is not necessarily apparent if this finding represents an increase in SNS activity, a reduction in plasma norepinephrine clearance, or both. Plasma norepinephrine kinetic studies have demonstrated that norepinephrine clearance *is* reduced in elderly persons, but a corresponding increase in plasma norepinephrine appearance, or "spillover," is the predominant factor accounting for the age-associated elevation in plasma norepinephrine concentrations (Veith et al. 1986). Unlike the concentration of norepinephrine in plasma, the concentration of epinephrine in plasma is unaffected by aging, and there is no age-related increase in epinephrine release (Morrow et al. 1987). Interestingly, the absence of an age-related fall in plasma epinephrine clearance suggests that norepinephrine and epinephrine are cleared from plasma by different mechanisms (Morrow et al. 1987).

As illustrated in its application to the study of human aging, the plasma norepinephrine kinetic technique described by Esler et al. represents an important methodological advance over the reliance on norepinephrine concentrations in plasma alone. However, this approach, too, has several limitations. Only a small portion of the norepinephrine released at postganglionic SNS synapses (approximately 10% to 20%) escapes reuptake or local metabolism and spills over into the circulation where it can be measured (Kopin 1985). Moreover, norepinephrine released from SNS nerve terminals is not released directly into plasma, but must diffuse across the neuroeffector junction, thereby temporarily occupying a physiological space, or "compartment," that is distinct from the circulating plasma compartment (Linares et al. 1987). Thus, *estimated* norepinephrine release measured by plasma norepinephrine appearance, or "spillover," is still at least one step removed from *actual* release from SNS neuroeffector junctions. In addition, the single or noncompartmental kinetic model of Esler et al. does not accommodate the fact that the disappearance of labeled norepinephrine in plasma is biexponential, indicating that the accurate assessment of norepinephrine kinetics in plasma requires the use of at least a two-compartment model (Linares et al. 1987).

Linares and associates (1987) recognized these limitations of the Esler method and developed a compartmental model to analyze plasma norepinephrine kinetics. Compartmental analysis is now commonly used in studies of metabolic and endocrine processes to estimate physiological parameters that cannot be assayed directly (Carson et al. 1983; Linares et al. 1987, 1988; Supiano et al. 1990). A physiologically based, two-compartment mathematical model was the minimal model that accurately fit the known physiological properties of peripheral norepinephrine metabolism (Linares et al. 1987). This model includes a vascular compartment (the circulating blood pool from which norepinephrine is sampled) and an extravascular compartment (into which norepinephrine is released from SNS nerves). The extravascular compartment is lumped and includes body tissues that locally release, take up, metabolize, and "spill" norepinephrine into the circulation (e.g., SNS neurons, heart, kidney). The norepinephrine mass in the extravascular compartment most likely represents norepinephrine anywhere in the immediate vicinity of the neuroeffector junctions of SNS nerve synapses but does not include norepinephrine contained in the presynaptic nerve terminals (Linares et al. 1987). Norepinephrine in the extravascular compartment is subjected to neuronal and non-neuronal uptake and exchanges with norepinephrine in the vascular compartment. As with the noncompartmental Esler technique (Esler et al. 1979), the two-compartment model allows for estimation of the rates of appearance and clearance of norepinephrine from the vascular compartment. The unknown compartmental parameters estimated by this model that are not provided by the Esler approach include the steady-state rate of norepinephrine input into the extravascular compartment, the mass of norepinephrine in the vascular and extravascular compartments, the volume of distribution of norepinephrine in the vascular compartment, the mean residence times of norepinephrine in both compartments, the rate of irreversible norepinephrine removal from the extravascular compartment, and estimates of the rate constants governing the transfer of norepinephrine between compartments. Thus, the two-compartment model is a more powerful analytic approach that offers a closer approximation of actual norepinephrine release (i.e., norepinephrine release rate into the extravascular compartment) than can be obtained by the use of plasma norepinephrine concentrations alone or by the original Esler model.

The increased interpretive power of the two-compartment mathematical model is well illustrated in a report by Linares et al. (1988), who examined the effects of upright posture and dietary sodium manipulations on plasma norepinephrine and norepinephrine kinetics. The orthostatic challenge test has long been viewed as a useful provocative stimulus for activation of the cardiovascular component of the SNS. Indeed, Linares et al. demonstrated that standing significantly increased norepinephrine release into the extravascular compartment and norepinephrine appearance into plasma. In addition, however, the associated rise in plasma norepinephrine was shown to be partially due to a decrease in plasma norepinephrine clearance resulting from a fall in the volume of distribution of norepinephrine in the vascular (plasma) compartment. The latter was likely a reflection of a reduction in blood flow to tissues from which norepinephrine is extracted. Dietary sodium restriction also elevated plasma norepinephrine. Although this response has traditionally been viewed as an indication of increased SNS activity, Linares and associates (1988) showed that the elevation of plasma norepinephrine associated with dietary sodium restriction is attributable entirely to a reduction in norepinephrine clearance due to a fall in plasma norepinephrine volume of distribution. Thus, the two-compartment analysis revealed that the long-held belief that a low-salt diet stimulates SNS activity is invalid.

Despite their potential usefulness, plasma norepinephrine kinetic strategies to estimate overall SNS activity have several important limitations. The inherent requirement of these studies for the use of radioactive tracers, multiple indwelling catheters, frequent blood samples, and highly technical analytic methods limits the clinical applicability of this approach. These models also require that kinetic assessments be performed at steady-state plasma norepinephrine concentrations, which precludes the use of kinetic analysis to estimate SNS responses to stimuli that would be expected to provoke acute, transient activation of the

SNS. Finally, it must be recognized that despite the advantages offered by the two-compartment analysis, current mathematical models undoubtedly do not yet provide an accurate representation of the known complexity of the SNS.

The site of plasma catecholamine sampling deserves special emphasis when the use of plasma catecholamine determinations to estimate SNS activity is considered. The majority of clinical studies utilizing plasma catecholamines for this purpose have relied upon antecubital venous measurements, which have been shown to have several problems (Best and Halter 1982; Goldstein et al. 1987; Hjemdahl et al. 1984). Recent studies have demonstrated that antecubital venous blood does not provide as accurate a measure of systemic SNS activity as arterial or arterialized venous sampling (Best and Halter 1982; Esler et al. 1989; Goldstein et al. 1987; Hjemdahl et al. 1984; Veith et al. 1984). (Arterialized samples are obtained from a hand vein while heating the hand in a warming box or heating pad, which sufficiently increases local blood flow to "arterialize" the venous sample). This diminished accuracy is due, in part, to the 40% to 50% fractional extraction of circulating catecholamines that occurs as they traverse the forearm tissues and are subjected to neuronal uptake at SNS synapses. Furthermore, the forearm is a site of net norepinephrine production, resulting in higher norepinephrine levels in antecubital venous blood compared with simultaneously obtained arterial or arterialized venous measurements (Abumrad et al. 1981; Veith et al. 1984). Thus, antecubital venous norepinephrine levels are greatly influenced by the local production and release of norepinephrine from forearm tissues and largely provide an index of skeletal muscle, not total body, SNS activity.

Because circulating epinephrine is derived exclusively from the adrenal medulla, the fractional extraction of epinephrine by the forearm results in an approximate 50% fall in plasma epinephrine in venous compared with arterial blood. This reduction results in resting plasma epinephrine values that often fall below the sensitivity of many assay techniques.

These sampling issues become particularly important if SNS activity or regional blood flow, which affects clearance, differs in skeletal muscle compared with the rest of the body. In fact, precisely these factors necessitate revision of the traditional view that mental or cognitive stress preferentially activates the adrenomedullary component of the SNS, as suggested by several studies that observed greater elevations of venous plasma epinephrine than norepinephrine following such stressors (Barnes et al. 1982; Dimsdale and Moss 1980; Hjemdahl et al. 1984). Hjemdahl and associates (1984), using the Stroop Color Word Test to induce mental stress in normal subjects, demonstrated an increase in heart rate, blood pressure, and cardiac output. These effects were associated with an increase in both norepinephrine and epinephrine measured in arterial blood. Although venous epinephrine levels increased, there was no change in antecubital venous norepinephrine. These findings were confirmed and extended by Goldstein and associates (1987), who investigated SNS responses to a somewhat less noxious "stress," a video challenge task. They observed increases in heart rate, blood pressure, and cardiac output that were associated with a significant increase in forearm blood flow. Arterial norepinephrine, but not antecubital venous norepinephrine, was increased without a significant change in arterial or venous epinephrine.

Both studies are compatible with a "defense reaction"–like hemodynamic response (Folkow 1982; Hilton 1982) with marked cardiac stimulation and peripheral vasodilatation. Had these studies, like several earlier investigations, relied upon venous catecholamine measurements alone, they would have been interpreted as indicating a preferential effect of mental stress on adrenomedullary SNS activity (Hjemdahl et al.'s study) or the absence of an effect of mental stress on plasma catecholamines (Goldstein et al.'s study), thereby overlooking the important effect of these challenges on the cardiovascular component of the SNS. The conclusion that cognitive challenge tests preferentially increase cardiac SNS activity and that antecubital venous plasma norepinephrine changes are not sufficiently sensitive to detect the associated increase in SNS outflow to the heart was recently confirmed by Esler et al. (1989), who compared venous plasma norepinephrine, systemic plasma norepinephrine appearance rate, and regional cardiac norepinephrine spillover following a mental arithmetic task. Significantly, neither plasma norepinephrine nor systemic norepinephrine appearance determinations reflected the increase in cardiac SNS activity associated with mental stress. It is important to consider these sampling issues in appraising the clinical studies of SNS function in psychiatric disorders, the majority of which have utilized venous catecholamine measurements.

Microneurographic Techniques

Beginning in the late 1960s, Hagbarth and Vallbo developed clinical electrophysiological techniques for directly measuring the firing rate of SNS nerves in skeletal muscle and skin (Hagbarth and Vallbo 1968). The clinical application of this microneurographic technique has been extended by Wallin and associates (Vallbo et al. 1979; Wallin 1984), who demonstrated the stability of SNS "tone" measured within individuals over extended periods of time and investigated muscle SNS responses to a number of physiological stimuli that activate the SNS (Anderson et al. 1987, 1991; Vallbo et al. 1979; Victor et al. 1987a, 1987b; Wallin 1984). This approach has the theoretical advantage of avoiding the potential difficulties posed by the relative "downstream" characteristics of plasma catecholamine, norepinephrine kinetic, or urinary excretion estimates of overall SNS activity. One limitation of the microneurographic method, however, is the fact that it provides a selective index of skeletal muscle SNS outflow, usually in one limb. Because SNS outflow is not uniform to all organ systems (see below), muscle SNS activity may or may not provide an accurate index of systemic SNS activity. In addition, this method is somewhat invasive and technically difficult. To our knowledge this approach has not been employed to assess SNS function in individuals with anxiety or affective disorders.

REGIONAL PATTERNS OF SYMPATHETIC NERVOUS SYSTEM RESPONSE

The total urinary excretion of norepinephrine and its metabolites and the measurement of plasma norepinephrine kinetics in arterial or arterialized blood are likely to reflect primarily SNS activity of the skeletal musculature and kidney, because these two organ systems disproportionately contribute to plasma norepinephrine appearance (Esler et al. 1988, 1989). Skeletal muscle SNS activity is also likely to be overrepresented in measurements of SNS activity assessed by microneurographic methods. Thus, currently available clinical methods do not necessarily provide an index of systemic SNS activity. In fact, the concept of "total body" SNS activity may represent a physiological oxymoron.

Although SNS activation has traditionally been viewed as an "all or none" system (Cannon 1929, 1939)—and this is generally true for severe stressors such as hypovolemic shock, profound hypoglycemia, or maximal exercise (Cryer 1980)—it is apparent that the SNS is capable of differential activation (Folkow 1982; Vallbo et al. 1979) and that the capacity for selective SNS responsiveness is orchestrated within the CNS (Brown and Fisher 1984, 1985; Vallbo et al. 1979). The remarkable specificity of SNS responses is evident in recent studies in dogs from our laboratories that demonstrated that SNS nerves to the pancreas are stimulated by CNS neuroglucopenia (induced by 2-deoxyglucose) but not by profound hypotension or hypoxemia. This differential response occurred despite the fact that all three stressors produce similar elevations of systemic norepinephrine, presumably reflecting equivalent activation of the cardiovascular component of the SNS (Havel et al. 1988). As described by Folkow (1982) and Hilton (1982), the adaptive nature of differential SNS activation is particularly evident during the "defense reaction," when cardiac, splanchnic, renal, and cutaneous SNS activity is increased but sympathetic vasoconstrictor fibers to skeletal muscle are inhibited. This pattern of SNS response increases cardiac output and blood pressure and increases neurogenic constriction of capacitance and most resistance vessels, except to the heart, skeletal muscle, and brain, where blood flow increases. Such hemodynamic adjustments optimally prepare the organism for "fight or flight." It is important to point out, however, that qualitatively similar responses have been demonstrated in humans in less threatening circumstances that simply require attention, vigilance, and concentration, such as mental arithmetic or other cognitive challenges (Esler et al. 1989; Folkow 1982; Goldstein et al. 1987; Hjemdahl et al. 1984).

Microneurographic measurements provide evidence of differential SNS activation in humans. Direct measurements of peripheral SNS nerve activity reveal that resting SNS activity in sympathetic nerves to skeletal muscle is regulated by baroreceptor activity (Vallbo et al. 1979; Wallin 1984), whereas SNS activity in cutaneous sympathetic nerves is not entrained to the cardiac cycle (Vallbo et al. 1979). Moreover, muscle SNS activity increases during the Valsalva maneuver, but cutaneous SNS activity is unaffected (Vallbo et al. 1979). Alternatively, cooling of the skin increases SNS discharge in cutaneous SNS nerves but does not influence muscle SNS nerve activity (Vallbo et al. 1979). Anderson and associates (1987) have shown that mental stress in humans causes a dissociation of arm and leg muscle SNS nerve activity with increased outflow to the leg but not to the arm. Victor and associates (1987b) have shown that the cold pressor test evokes an immediate elevation in heart rate, thought to be sympathetically mediated because it is abolished by beta-adrenergic blockade, but that activity in muscle SNS nerves does not increase until approximately 30 seconds later.

The dissociation of cardiac SNS activity from outflow to other organ systems is particularly interesting. Using isotope dilution techniques, Meredith and co-workers (1991) examined systemic and regional cardiac SNS activity in patients with cardiac disease who had survived spontaneous ventricular fibrillation. They observed no difference in overall plasma norepinephrine appearance rate in this group compared with a cardiac control group, but found a selective, fourfold increase in *cardiac* SNS activity in the ventricular fibrillation group. Conversely, Esler et al. (1991a) recently employed both plasma norepinephrine kinetic and microneurographic techniques to demonstrate that *suppression* of systemic plasma norepinephrine appearance and regional SNS input to the kidney and forearm skeletal muscle following desipramine administration was associated with an *increase* in cardiac norepinephrine appearance, possibly reflecting an increase in SNS input to the heart. These studies illustrate the capacity of the SNS for regional selectivity and, because the relative contribution of the heart to systemic plasma norepinephrine appearance is small (Esler et al. 1988), demonstrate that significant changes in cardiac SNS activity may not be detected by plasma norepinephrine, norepinephrine kinetic, or microneurographic methods.

CLINICAL STUDIES OF SYMPATHETIC NERVOUS SYSTEM ACTIVITY IN PTSD

Heart Rate and Blood Pressure

As previously noted, clinical symptoms of PTSD are suggestive of increased autonomic arousal and responsiveness. The review of the psychophysiological literature by McFall and Murburg (Chapter 7, this volume) indicates that individuals with PTSD may exhibit increased resting heart rate and systolic blood pressure compared with healthy control subjects. If these findings are in fact related to the presence of PTSD itself and not due to medication or medication withdrawal effects, they are compatible with either a generalized increase in SNS tone, a selective increase in cardiac SNS activity, or, as pointed out previously, a delayed return of the SNS to a basal state following excitation, resulting in an apparent elevation of basal heart rate. A reduction in parasympathetic tone, mediated either directly or as a reciprocal response to increased SNS tone, could also contribute to the heart rate findings. The presence of increased SNS and/or adrenomedullary activity documented in some patients with anxiety disorders and major depression (see Veith 1991 for review) could account for the failure to find differences between PTSD patients and some psychiatric control populations. PTSD patients also display accentuated cardiovascular responses to trauma-related cues compared with both normal subjects and psychiatric control subjects, indicating enhanced SNS activation under these circumstances.

Urinary Catecholamine Excretion

Davidson and Baum (1986), Kosten et al. (1987), and Yehuda, Giller, and colleagues (Chapter 10, this volume) have reported elevated 24-hour urinary catecholamine excretion in traumatized populations or PTSD patients, although this has not been a consistent finding (Pitman and Orr 1990). It is noteworthy that so few studies have examined urinary catecholamine excretion in PTSD patients. The interpretation of the findings of Kosten et al.

(1987) is complicated by the fact that some of their PTSD patients were not drug free and others had been off antidepressants and anxiolytics for only a short time, and there was no normal control population. In addition, none of the studies reporting increased urinary catecholamine excretion in PTSD exclude the possibility that differences among populations in activity (and, in the case of Yehuda et al.'s dopamine findings, diet) contributed to the apparent increases in catecholamine excretion among the subject groups. Nevertheless, these findings are compatible with an increase in the integrated activity of the SNS (encompassing both periods in the "basal" state and phasic responses to provocative internal and external stimuli) over a 24-hour period.

Plasma Catecholamines

It is particularly remarkable that only three studies have examined plasma catecholamines in PTSD (McFall et al. 1990; Murburg et al., Chapter 9; Hamner et al., Chapter 11, this volume). These preliminary studies suggest the presence of normal resting SNS function in PTSD. In addition, these findings suggest intact SNS responsiveness to exercise and noncombat experimental cues in combat veterans with PTSD. Our group (McFall et al. 1990; see also Murburg et al., Chapter 9, this volume) observed an approximately 30% greater plasma epinephrine response to viewing a combat film in combat veterans with PTSD compared with a veteran control group. The time needed for recovery of plasma epinephrine to baseline was prolonged, suggesting a sustained release (assuming no defect in plasma epinephrine clearance exists in PTSD patients). Because this study employed arterialized venous sampling, which closely approximates arterial blood (Veith et al. 1984), the apparent lack of a corresponding systemic plasma norepinephrine response is not likely an artifact of the sampling site. This finding, which requires confirmation, suggests that combat veterans with PTSD exhibit a modestly heightened SNS responsiveness to combat-related cues that might be selective for the adrenomedullary component of the SNS. Several factors must be considered, however, before this interpretation can be accepted.

The apparent absence of increased resting SNS tone and a

possible increase in adrenomedullary responsiveness to experimental stress observed in the limited number of PTSD subjects studied thus far appear to contradict the cumulative urinary excretion data. As noted in the preceding discussion, however, it is conceivable that a selective increase in SNS outflow to the heart could occur in PTSD, possibly accounting for an elevation of integrated norepinephrine excretion over prolonged periods, without a notable increase in plasma norepinephrine or norepinephrine appearance. Additional support for this speculation derives from the fact that a selective increase in cardiac SNS activity, rather than a hormonal effect of epinephrine, is a more likely explanation for the experimentally induced increase in heart rate and blood pressure observed in our study (McFall et al. 1990; Murburg et al., Chapter 9, this volume). The modest increase in plasma epinephrine (approximately 15 to 35 pg/ml) observed following exposure to the combat film would be expected to have only minimal hormonal effects on cardiovascular function (Cryer et al. 1980; Clutter et al. 1980). One must also consider the possibility that PTSD might be characterized by phasic, not continuous, elevations in systemic or cardiac SNS activity, which could account for a cumulative increase in urinary catecholamine excretion in the face of an apparently normal level of SNS activity measured by plasma catecholamines or systemic catecholamine kinetics. Finally, it is possible that experimentally induced stress reponses may not achieve the intensity of "naturally occurring" stress responses in vivo, making it difficult to accurately assess SNS responsiveness in the laboratory.

The notion that SNS activation is an important physiological component of PTSD deserves further study. The current, admittedly preliminary, findings in this area argue *against* the presence of a substantial, generalized disturbance of SNS tone or function in PTSD. The findings suggest, instead, that if a disturbance of SNS function is present in PTSD, it is more likely to manifest itself as an episodic, phasic increase in SNS output to the heart and adrenal. Although technically difficult, assessment of regional cardiac SNS activity during cardiac catheterization by isotope dilution techniques might be required to confirm this hypothesis (Esler et al. 1989, 1991a), or, possibly, the use of positron-emission tomography techniques (Goldstein et al. 1990). In addition, if it is concluded that laboratory stressors fail to achieve the full intensity of stress responses in vivo, measurement of plasma catecholamines by continuous blood sampling techniques (Dimsdale and Moss 1980) might more likely "capture" episodes of SNS activation, if SNS outflow is not restricted to the heart.

REFERENCES

Abumrad NN, Rabin D, Diamond MP, et al: Use of a heated superficial hand vein as an alternative site for the measurement of amino acid concentrations and for the study of glucose and alanine kinetics in man. Metabolism 30:936–940, 1981

Anderson EA, Wallin BG, Mark AL: Dissociation of sympathetic nerve activity in arm and leg muscle during mental stress. Hypertension 9 (suppl III):114–119, 1987

Anderson EA, Sinkey CA, Mark AL: Mental stress increases sympathetic nerve activity during sustained baroreceptor stimulation in humans. Hypertension 17 (suppl III):43–49, 1991

Barnes RF, Raskind MA, Gumbrecht G, et al: The effects of age on the plasma catecholamine response to mental stress in man. J Clin Endocrinol Metab 54:64–69, 1982

Best JD, Halter JB: Release and clearance rates of epinephrine in man: importance of arterial measurements. J Clin Endocrinol Metab 55:263–268, 1982

Brown MR, Fisher LA: Brain peptide regulation of adrenal epinephrine secretion. Am J Physiol 247:E41–E46, 1984

Brown MR, Fisher LA: Corticotropin-releasing factor: effects on the autonomic nervous system and visceral systems. Federation Proceedings 44:243–248, 1985

Cannon WB: Bodily Changes in Pain, Hunger, Fear and Rage. New York, D Appleton, 1929

Cannon WB: The Wisdom of the Body. New York, WW Norton. 1939

Carson ER, Cobelli C, Finkelstein L: Mathematical Modeling of Metabolic and Endocrine Systems. New York, Wiley, 1983

Charney DS, Menkes DB, Heninger GR: Receptor sensitivity and the mechanism of action of antidepressant treatment. Arch Gen Psychiatry 38:1160–1180, 1981

Christensen NJ, Brandsburg O: The relationship between plasma catecholamine concentration and pulse rate during exercise and standing. Eur J Clin Invest 3:399–406, 1973

Clutter WE, Bier DM, Shah SD, et al: Epinephrine plasma metabolic clearance rates and physiologic thresholds for metabolic and hemodynamic actions in man. J Clin Invest 66:94–101, 1980

Cryer PE: Physiology and pathophysiology of the human sympathoadrenal system. N Engl J Med 303:436–444, 1980

Davidson LM, Baum A: Chronic stress and posttraumatic stress disorders. J Consult Clin Psychol 54:303–308, 1986

DeVito JL, Smith OA: Afferent projections to the hypothalamic area controlling emotional responses (HACER). Brain Res 252:213–226, 1982

Dimsdale JE, Moss J: Short-term catecholamine response to psychological stress. Psychosom Med 62:347–504, 1980

Eisenhofer G, Esler MD, Cox HS, et al: Differences in the neuronal removal of circulating epinephrine and norepinephrine. J Clin Endocrinol Metab 70:1710–1720, 1990

Eisenhofer G, Smolich JJ, Cox HS, et al: Neuronal reuptake of norepinephrine and production of dihydroxyphenylglycol by cardiac sympathetic nerves in the anesthetized dog. Circulation 84:1354–1363, 1991

Elam M, Yao T, Thorén P, et al: Hypercapnia and hypoxia: chemoreceptor-mediated control of locus coeruleus neurons and splanchnic sympathetic nerves. Brain Res 222:373–381, 1981

Elam M, Yao T, Svennson TH, et al: Regulation of locus coeruleus neurons and splanchnic sympathetic nerves by cardiovascular efferents. Brain Res 290:281–287, 1984

Esler M: Renal catecholamine metabolism. Miner Electrolyte Metab 15:16–23, 1989

Esler M, Jackman G, Bobik A, et al: Determination of norepinephrine apparent release rate and clearance in humans. Life Sci 25:1461–1470, 1979

Esler M, Jennings G, Korner P, et al: Assessment of human sympathetic nervous system activity from measurements of norepinephrine turnover. Hypertension 11:3–20, 1988

Esler M, Jennings G, Lambert G: Measurement of overall and cardiac norepinephrine release into plasma during cognitive challenge. Psychoneuroendocrinology 14:477–481, 1989

Esler M, Wallin G, Dorward PK, et al: Effects of desipramine on sympathetic nerve firing and norepinephrine spillover to plasma in humans. Am J Physiol 260:R817-R823, 1991a

Esler M, Ferrier C, Lambert G, et al: Biochemical evidence of sympathetic hyperactivity in human hypertension. Hypertension 17 (suppl III):29–35, 1991b

Folkow B: Physiological aspects of primary hypertension. Physiol Rev 62:347–504, 1982

Goldstein DS, McCarty R, Polinsky RJ, et al: Relationship between plasma norepinephrine and sympathetic neural activity. Hypertension 5:552–559, 1983

Goldstein DS, Eisenhofer G, Sax FL, et al: Plasma norepinephrine pharmacokinetics during mental challenge. Psychosom Med 49:591–605, 1987

Goldstein DS, Eisenhofer G, Stull R, et al: Plasma dihydroxyphenylglycol and the intraneuronal disposition of norepinephrine in humans. J Clin Invest 81:213–220, 1988

Goldstein DS, Chang PC, Eisenhofer G, et al: Positron emission tomographic imaging of cardiac sympathetic innervation and function. Circulation 81:1606–1621, 1990

Hagbarth KE, Vallbo AB: Pulse and respiratory grouping of sympathetic impulses in human muscle nerves. Acta Physiol Scand 74:96–108, 1968

Halter JB, Pflug A, Porte D Jr: Mechanism of plasma catecholamine increases during surgical stress in man. J Clin Endocrinol Metab 45:930–944, 1977

Havel PJ, Veith R, Dunning BE, et al: Pancreatic noradrenergic nerves are activated by neuroglucopenia but not by hypotension or hypoxia in the dog. J Clin Invest 82:1538–1545, 1988

Hilton SM: The defence-arousal system and its relevance for circulatory and respiratory control. J Exp Biol 100:159–174, 1982

Hjemdahl P, Freyschuss U, Juhlin-Dannfelt A, et al: Differential sympathetic activation during neutral stress evoked by the Stroop Test. Acta Physiol Scand 527(suppl):25–29, 1984

Hoeldtke RD, Cilmi KM, Reichard GA Jr, et al: Assessment of norepinephrine secretion and production. J Lab Clin Med 101:772, 1983

Iversen L, Salt P: Inhibition of catecholamine uptake 2 by steroids in the isolated rat heart. Br J Pharmacol 40:528–530, 1970

Kopin IJ: Catecholamine metabolism: basic aspects and clinical significance. Pharmacol Rev 37(4):333–364, 1985

Kopin IJ, Eisenhofer G, Goldstein D: Sympathoadrenal medullary system and stress. Adv Exp Med Biol 245:11–23, 1988

Kosten TR, Mason JW, Giller EL, et al: Sustained urinary norepinephrine and epinephrine in post-traumatic stress disorder. Psychoneuroendocrinology 12:13–20, 1987

Linares OA, Jacquez JA, Zech LA, et al: Norepinephrine metabolism in humans: kinetic analysis and model. J Clin Invest 80:1332–1341, 1987

Linares OA, Zech LA, Jacquez JA, et al: Effect of sodium-restricted diet and posture on norepinephrine kinetics in humans. Am J Physiol 254:E222-E230, 1988

McFall ME, Murburg MM, Roszell DK, et al: Psychophysiologic and neuroendocrine findings in post-traumatic stress disorder: a review of theory and research. Journal of Anxiety Disorders 3:243–257, 1989

McFall M, Murburg MM, Ko GN, et al: Autonomic responses to stress in Vietnam combat veterans with post traumatic stress disorder. Biol Psychiatry 27:1165–1175, 1990

Meredith IT, Broughton A, Jennings GL, et al: Evidence of a selective increase in cardiac sympathetic activity in patients with sustained ventricular arrhythmias. N Engl J Med 325:618–624, 1991

Morrow LA, Linares OA, Hill TJ, et al: Age differences in the plasma clearance mechanisms for epinephrine and norepinephrine in humans. J Clin Endocrinol Metab 65:508–511, 1987

Pacholczyk T, Blakely RD, Amara SG: Expression cloning of a cocaine- and antidepressant-sensitive human noradrenaline transporter. Nature 350:350–354, 1991

Paton D: The Mechanisms of Neuronal and Extraneuronal Transport of Catecholamines. New York, Raven, 1976, pp 95–153, 325, 354

Peskind ER, Raskind MA, Wilkinson CW, et al: Peripheral sympathectomy and adrenal medullectomy do not alter cerebrospinal fluid norepinephrine. Brain Res 367:258–264, 1986

Pflug AE, Halter JB: Effect of spinal anesthesia on adrenergic tone and the neuroendocrine responses to surgical stress in man. Anesthesiology 55:120–126, 1981

Pitman RK, Orr SP: Twenty-four hour urinary cortisol and catecholamine excretion in combat-related post-traumatic stress disorder. Biol Psychiatry 27:245–247, 1990

Reis DJ, Granata AR, Joh H, et al: Brain stem catecholamine mechanisms in tonic and reflex control of blood pressure. Hypertension 6 (suppl II):7–15, 1984

Reis DJ, Morrison S, Ruggiero DA: The C1 area of the brainstem in tonic and reflex control of blood pressure: state of the art lecture. Hypertension 11 (suppl I):8–13, 1988

Rosen SG, Linares OA, Sanfield JA, et al: Epinephrine kinetics in humans: radiotracer methodology. J Clin Endocrinol Metab 69:753, 1989

Sawchenko PE, Swanson LW: Immunohistochemical identification of neurons in the paraventricular nucleus of the hypothalamus that project to the medulla or to the spinal cord in the rat. J Comp Neurol 205:260–272, 1982

Schwartz RS, Jaeger LF, Veith RC: The importance of body composition to the increase in plasma norepinephrine appearance rate in elderly men. J Gerontol 42:546–551, 1987

Selye H: The Physiology and Pathology of Exposure to Stress. Montreal, Acta, 1950

Silverberg AB, Shah SD, Hammond MW, et al: Norepinephrine: hormone and neurotransmitter in man. Am J Physiol 234:E252–E255, 1978

Smith OA, DeVito JL: Central neural integration for the control of autonomic responses associated with emotion. Annu Rev Neurosci 7:43–65, 1984

Smith OA, DeVito JL, Astley CA: Neurons controlling cardiovascular responses to emotion are located in lateral hypothalamus-perifornical region. Am J Physiol 259:R943–R954, 1990

Stoddard SL: Hypothalamic control and peripheral concomitants of the autonomic defense response, in The Neuroendocrinology and Neurobiology of Stress. Edited by Brown MR, Rivier C, Koob G. New York, Marcel Dekker, 1991, pp 231–253

Supiano MA, Linares OA, Smith MJ, et al: Age-related differences in norepinephrine kinetics: effect of posture and sodium-restricted diet. Am J Physiol 259:E422–E431, 1990

Swanson LW, Sawchenko PE: Paraventricular nucleus: a site for the integration of neuroendocrine and autonomic mechanisms. Neuroendocrinology 31:410–417, 1980

Trendelenburg U: A kinetic analysis of the extraneuronal uptake and metabolism of catecholamines. Rev Physiol Biochem Pharmacol 87:33–115, 1980

Vallbo AB, Hagbarth KE, Torebjork HE, et al: Somatosensory, proprioceptive, and sympathetic activity in human peripheral nerves. Physiol Rev 59:919–957, 1979

van der Kolk BA, Boyd H, Krystal J, et al: Post-traumatic stress disorder as a biologically based disorder: implications of the animal model of inescapable shock, in Post-Traumatic Stress Disorder: Psychological and Biological Sequelae. Edited by van der Kolk BA. Washington DC, American Psychiatric Press, 1984, pp 124–134

Van Loon GR: Plasma dopamine: regulation and significance. Federation Proceedings 42:3012–3018, 1983

Veith RC: Sympathetic nervous system disturbances in psychiatric illness, in The Neuroendocrinology and Neurobiology of Stress. Edited by Brown MR, Rivier C, Koob G. New York, Marcel Dekker, 1991, pp 395–435

Veith RC, Best JD, Halter JB: Dose-dependent suppression of norepinephrine appearance rate in plasma by clonidine in man. J Clin Endocrinol Metab 59:151–155, 1984

Veith RC, Featherstone JA, Linares OA, et al: Age differences in plasma norepinephrine kinetics in humans. J Gerontol 41:319–324, 1986

Victor RG, Leimbach WN Jr, Seals DR, et al: Effects of the cold pressor test on muscle sympathetic nerve activity in humans. Hypertension 9:429–436, 1987a

Victor RG, Seals DR, Mark AL: Differential control of heart rate and sympathetic nerve activity during dynamic exercise. J Clin Invest 79:508–516, 1987b

von Euler US: Identification of the sympathomimetic ergone in adrenergic nerves of cattle (sympathin H) with laevo-noradrenalin. Acta Physiol Scand 16:63–74, 1948

Wallin BG: Muscle sympathetic activity and plasma concentrations of noradrenaline. Acta Physiol Scand 527:25–29, 1984

Williams M, Young JB, Rosa RM, et al: Effect of protein ingestion on urinary dopamine excretion. J Clin Invest 78:1687–1693, 1986

Ziegler MD, Lake CR, Wood JH, et al: Norepinephrine in cerebrospinal fluid: basic studies, effects of drugs, and disease, in Neurobiology of Cerebrospinal Fluid. Edited by Wood JH. New York, Plenum, 1980, pp 141–152

Comment

Determining the Applicability of Animal Models of Stress to the Study of PTSD

Rachel Yehuda, Ph.D.
Seymour M. Antelman, Ph.D.

The chapters in this volume have carefully summarized the existing knowledge of catecholamine alterations in PTSD and have examined general features of the catecholaminergic system under basal conditions and in response to "stress." Some authors have described specific animal models of stress in order to make connections between the biological and behavioral consequences of stress in animals and those seen in PTSD. These models include chronic stress, fear conditioning, sensitization, uncontrollable stress, and learned helplessness (see Aston-Jones et al., Chapter 2; Simson and Weiss, Chapter 3; Antelman and Yehuda, Chapter 4; Zacharko, Chapter 5; Charney et al., Chapter 6; McFall and Murburg, Chapter 7; Murburg et al., Chapter 9). The attempt to "model" symptoms and biological alterations in PTSD follows a well-established tradition within the field of neuroscience and psychiatry. Animal modeling offers the opportunity to study the biology of a disorder in a systematic way and, ultimately, allows testing of pharmacological and other prospective "treatments," which might be difficult in humans.

Support of this work was provided by National Institute of Mental Health Grants MH49536-01 (RY), MH49555-01 (RY), and MH24114 (SMA), and National Institute on Alcohol Abuse and Alcoholism Grant P50AA08746 (SMA).

335

In most psychiatric disorders, animal models have been limited because they have not been based on a knowledge of the primary etiological agent(s) producing the disorder of interest. As such, the majority of animal models of psychiatric illness have usually been much more simplistic than the disease state they have purported to reflect. In examining PTSD, there is a greater potential to model the disorder accurately because the major precipitating factors are known (i.e., PTSD occurs in response to severe and unusual stressful or traumatic situations). However, in choosing the appropriate models to study, several points are worthy of consideration.

First, PTSD—a fairly circumscribed biobehavioral syndrome—can be induced by a wide range of stressors, whereas animal studies of stress have shown marked biobehavioral differences depending on the type of stressor studied (e.g., controllable, escapable, acute, chronic, predictable, physiological, psychological). Second, differential responsiveness to stress can be influenced by factors other than the actual stressor, such as state of the organism during stress, past stress history of the organism, and the species and strain of animal studied. Therefore, in studying the relationship between PTSD and stress, factors other than the actual stressor need to be addressed. These considerations make the task of animal modeling more complex than simply establishing prima facie comparisons between PTSD and the sequelae of "stress."

Indeed, the task of animal modeling in PTSD is not to select the perfect animal replica of the human disorder from among the many different stress paradigms—most investigators would agree that it would be unlikely that such a paradigm could be found. Rather, animal modeling of PTSD requires the ability to identify the aspect of the clinical syndrome being modeled and then determining the relative importance of the particular feature being modeled in the context of the overall clinical syndrome. It is a given that different animal models of stress may simulate different aspects of PTSD. However, some animal models may simulate more important aspects of PTSD than might others. To describe the relative utility of a particular animal model of stress in modeling PTSD, there must be some rank-ordering of the factors that are relevant to the clinical disorder.

In considering relevant animal models of PTSD, we believe that a first, critical step is to differentiate between, on the one hand, factors that are essential for the *induction* of PTSD, and, on the other, those that can influence the *manifestations* or course of the disorder. Although many factors appear to contribute to the form and/or intensity with which the stress response eventually manifests itself in humans and animals, only a few of these factors are relevant to its *induction*. Failure to make a distinction between factors influencing the induction versus manifestation of PTSD may result in the uncritical acceptance of animal models that rely principally on a superficial face validity and that ultimately prevent an understanding of the biological and behavioral correlates of PTSD.

FACTORS RELEVANT TO THE INDUCTION OF PTSD

The following guidelines may help to identify the factors that most likely influence the induction of PTSD:

1. *The stressor should be capable of producing PTSD regardless of its duration.* The clinical syndrome of PTSD can develop in response to many different types of stressors, even some that are of very brief duration. Thus, the etiological characteristic of the stressor does not appear to be its actual duration, but some other factor, possibly the extent to which it is "outside of the range of usual human experience" or the degree of distress produced. Animal models of stress that are relevant to the induction of PTSD, then, are those in which long-term behavioral or neurochemical consequences are induced by even a very brief stressor.
2. *The stressor should produce long-term changes.* Even though PTSD symptoms can appear immediately following the trauma, the diagnosis of PTSD is made only if symptoms endure for at least 1 month. Thus, acute biological changes occurring only in the period immediately following the trauma that do not persist or recur in response to later provocation are not directly relevant to the biological and behavioral correlates of

PTSD. Although several biological systems show changes immediately following stress, many of these systems quickly return to their prestress state, suggesting that mechanisms involved in maintaining short-term homeostasis are probably not directly responsible for the induction of the more chronic sequelae that lead to the development of PTSD. However, acute biological responses to trauma may sensitize stress-adaptive systems toward future dysregulation, or may only occur in individuals who will subsequently develop a more long-term syndrome. As such, the acute and short-term biological and behavioral responses to stress are important topics of investigation that need to be followed up by studies of long-term responses to stress.

3. *The stressor should induce bipolar biobehavioral alterations.* The syndrome of PTSD includes both enhanced (intrusive/reexperiencing) and reduced (avoidance and/or numbing) responsiveness to trauma-related stimuli. Although the avoidance symptoms may predominate immediately after the trauma and recur later as a coping response to the intrusive symptoms that subsequently appear, in current formulations of PTSD both symptom clusters must be present simultaneously to fulfill the diagnostic criteria for the disorder. Animal models relevant to the induction of PTSD should therefore exhibit the capacity for such bipolar manifestations, ideally manifesting a cycling between excitatory and inhibitory biobehavioral changes.

FACTORS RELEVANT TO THE MANIFESTATIONS OR COURSE OF PTSD

The following factors appear to be relevant to influencing the course of PTSD:

1. *Characteristics of a particular stressor (i.e., controllability vs. uncontrollability).* Because PTSD can occur in response to a wide range of stressors, choosing an animal model of stress based solely on the characteristics of a particular stressor and/or the "unique" behavioral and neurochemical aftermath conferred

by it is of limited value in understanding what causes PTSD. However, biological and behavioral differences conferred by different types of stressors may add to an understanding of how PTSD is manifested. One of the more popular distinctions that have been made in the animal stress literature (as well as the PTSD literature) is the distinction between uncontrollable and controllable stress. Animals subjected to uncontrollable stress (such as inescapable shock) show behavioral symptoms and biological changes that are distinct from those seen in animals subjected to controllable stress. The appeal of the uncontrollable stress paradigm to those investigators attempting to derive animal models of PTSD is that it appears to have "face validity," because traumas known to give rise to PTSD—such as rape, natural disasters, or combat—occur without control of the individual. Indeed, this paradigm has repeatedly been proposed as perhaps the best single animal model of PTSD. Upon closer examination, however, it becomes clear that not all traumatic experiences involve uncontrollability. Therefore, although factors having to do with controllability may certainly explain salient features of the stress responsiveness and coping strategies in traumatized individuals, these factors are not necessarily relevant to the induction of the PTSD syndrome.

2. *Chronicity of the stressor.* We have already noted above that duration of the stressor does not seem to be directly relevant to predicting the induction of PTSD. However, this factor may play a role in determining how PTSD is manifested. There has been much attention on animal models of PTSD that focus on long-lasting, chronic stressors, and, as a result, the role of "conditioning" has become an important consideration to animal modelers of PTSD. The paradigm of inescapable shock ("learned helplessness"), for example, involves a continuous series of shocks from which escape is *not* possible, followed by exposure to a severe stressor from which escape *is* possible. The first half of the paradigm relies on repeated conditioning to teach animals that attempts to escape severe physical stress will fail. Only animals that have been previously exposed to the chronic regimen of inescapable shock have trouble learning to escape even when this option is presented, and often

exhibit marked passivity and apparent numbing and resultant biological manifestations (i.e., catecholamine depletion).

Although it is clear that this paradigm may not have widespread applicability in understanding the factors that give rise to the syndrome of PTSD (because not all traumas are inescapable and chronic), this model may be useful in simulating certain types of trauma. Specifically, the model is reminiscent of the trauma of combat exposure (i.e., basic training followed by subsequent chronic high intensity stressors from which there may often not be escape, and/or followed by experiences from which escape is possible). Examining the role of factors such as "controllability" in animals, therefore, could theoretically contribute to an understanding of the significant differences that have been observed across clinical groups (i.e., combat veterans vs. rape victims) in manifestations of PTSD such as form, intensity, chronicity of illness, level of impairment, or comorbidity (which appear to be particularly common among war veterans but not necessarily other traumatized groups).

3. *Interindividual variability in response to a stressor.* Although exposure to trauma remains the most salient predictor of who will develop PTSD, one of the most perplexing aspects in clinical studies of this disorder is the fact that not all individuals who are exposed to extreme trauma develop symptoms. This observation has prompted a wealth of studies examining the effect of prior stress history, premorbid psychiatric functioning and character structure, family studies, and coping skills on PTSD phenomenology. It is now clear that many of the above factors may influence both the induction and the manifestations of this disorder. The major implication of interindividual variability in response to stress for animal modeling in PTSD is in establishing the fact that other variables clearly do play a role in predicting vulnerability and modulating the response to trauma. A major application of animal modeling in further exploring the biological underpinnings of PTSD is to identify paradigms in which interindividual variability to a stressor can be initially demonstrated, and then systematically evaluate their impact on the syndrome of PTSD.

CONCLUSIONS

Although the enormous interspecies differences in genetic, anatomic, and physiological features necessarily limit the ability of any animal model to explain a human disorder, the animal stress literature provides a rich source of information with potential relevance to PTSD. Given the number of stress paradigms and their unique behavioral and biochemical consequences, it is, however, important to choose judiciously among the various options. By distinguishing between the factors that induce PTSD and those that influence the way the disorder is manifested, it will be possible for investigators to more successfully pair animal models of stress with the specific clinical syndrome of PTSD and evaluate the overall relevance of these models to PTSD.

Afterword

Matthew J. Friedman, M.D., Ph.D.

The publication of this book is a strong indication that neurobiological research on PTSD has progressed beyond its descriptive show-and-tell infancy to an adolescence marked by elegant brain research, debates over the appropriateness of different animal models, and hypothesis-driven clinical studies. During the past 10 years it has been established, beyond doubt, that PTSD is associated with psychophysiological and neurobiological abnormalities. Such findings, along with rediscovery of Abram Kardiner's prescient and seminal work (Kardiner 1941; Kardiner and Spiegel 1947), have generated provocative empirical results and theoretical models. The accumulating evidence suggests that PTSD is an extremely complex disorder marked by dysregulation in a number of fundamental neurobiological systems necessary for survival during conditions of extreme stress. Such neurobiological systems are involved in learning, memory, coping, and adaptation. It remains to be shown whether central nervous system (CNS) functions that respond to the normal vicissitudes of life are homologous to or distinctly different from those neurobiological operations set in motion by traumatic stress.

Dr. Michele Murburg has attempted to restrict our focus to one of the major systems through which the pathophysiology of PTSD is expressed. She has shown us the many layers of inquiry needed to explicate catecholaminergic brain mechanisms affected by traumatic stress. In that regard, the book is a comprehensive compilation that achieves a good balance between animal and clinical research as well as between methodological and theoretical issues. Given the depth, breadth, and complexity of information presented in this book, I will attempt to synthesize this material by reviewing it in the context of 12 questions addressed by the authors from their various perspectives.

343

What Have We Learned About How Adrenergic Mechanisms Are Altered by Exposure to Trauma?

The locus coeruleus (LC) not only exhibits a basal level of tonic activity but is influenced prominently by a variety of phasic inputs (Aston-Jones et al., Chapter 2; Simson and Weiss, Chapter 3). One of the major inputs to the LC is the nucleus paragigantocellularis (PGi), which is the hub of a network that can simultaneously process information to the LC and peripheral sympathetic nervous system (SNS). It is of great interest that a major source of input to the PGi is the central nucleus of the amygdala, which is involved in conditioned emotional responses and in fear-potentiated startle. Simson and Weiss (Chapter 2) emphasize also that the LC responds to phasic rather than tonic input. Under conditions of inescapable stress the authors demonstrate increased LC activation, which they attribute to a "functional blockade" of alpha$_2$ autoreceptors resulting from depletion (or decreased availability) of norepinephrine. Although such a "blockade" might account for the initial disinhibition of the LC, such a mechanism probably could not be sustained over time under conditions of chronic stress. Instead, one would predict that alpha blockade–induced LC disinhibition should result in downregulation of alpha$_2$ receptors (as discussed by Perry and Lerer et al. in Chapters 12 and 13, respectively).

Charney et al. (Chapter 6) make the link from animal to clinical research, reviewing psychophysiological findings on SNS activation, elevated urinary catecholamine levels, and, most intriguingly, yohimbine-enhanced responses in PTSD patients. Lerer et al. (Chapter 13) and Perry (Chapter 12) report on downregulation of (lymphocyte) beta- and (platelet) alpha$_2$-adrenergic receptors in traumatized war veterans and children. Yehuda and co-workers (Chapter 10) demonstrate elevated urinary catecholamines in war veterans and Holocaust survivors with PTSD. Rausch et al. (Chapter 14) show excessive startle response among war veterans with PTSD. Murburg, McFall, and associates (Chapters 8 and 9) report on an increased phasic sympathoadrenal response among war veterans with PTSD to trauma-related stimuli but no alterations in basal SNS tone. Hamner et al. also found no alterations in basal or postexercise stress plasma norepinephrine levels between PTSD patients and control subjects. Their finding that 3-methoxy-4-hydroxyphenylglycol (MHPG) levels are markedly elevated among PTSD patients, compared with control subjects, following exercise suggests increased sensitivity to norepinephrine activation among PTSD patients.

What Other Systems Are Probably Affected and Need to Be Studied (and Have Books Devoted to Them)?

Several chapters address dopaminergic mechanisms. Zacharko's finding (see Chapter 5) that chronic stress exposure reduces the rewarding value of mesocorticolimbic electrical self-stimulation may have clinical relevance to the high prevalence of depressive symptoms among patients with PTSD. Zacharko's work is also of great interest because it demonstrates the importance of 1) the monitoring of such changes longitudinally, 2) an animal's preexposure stress history, and 3) genetic factors (strain differences) that may produce different responses to inescapable shock. Charney et al. (Chapter 6) review animal research on dopaminergic mechanisms and link such findings to PTSD hypervigilance symptoms. Yehuda et al. (Chapter 10) show that urinary dopamine levels are elevated, along with norepinephrine levels, among war veterans and Holocaust survivors with PTSD compared with control subjects.

The review by Charney et al. indicates that inescapable stress also induces alteration in opioid, benzodiazepine, and hypothalamic-pituitary-adrenocortical (HPA) mechanisms. Corticotropin-releasing factor (CRF), benzodiazepines, and opioids influence the PGi-LC system (Aston-Jones et al., Chapter 2), and opioids also significantly affect the dopaminergic mesocorticolimbic reward system (Zacharko, Chapter 5). Two potentially important systems mentioned in passing but never addressed in this book are the serotonergic system, which is targeted by some very promising drugs such as fluoxetine, and the NMDA system, which is implicated in learning, extinction, and memory and may also mediate sensitization following traumatic exposure. Dr. Murburg's book certainly whets our appetite for other books that will focus on any of these important nonadrenergic systems.

Are the Abnormalities in PTSD Tonic or Phasic Alterations in Catecholamine Function?

Evidence presented by several authors indicates that adrenergic abnormalities are phasic rather than tonic. The LC itself is much more responsive to phasic input (Aston-Jones et al., Chapter 2; Simson and Weiss, Chapter 3). Careful clinical studies on the cardiovascular system indicate that phasic, but not basal, pulse rate, blood pressure, and plasma catecholamine levels differentiate PTSD patients from control subjects (Murburg et al., Chapter 9; Hamner et al., Chapter 11; Perry, Chapter 12). This is an important finding that might appear contrary to reports of elevated 24-hour urinary catecholamine levels described in this book (Yehuda et al., Chapter 10) and elsewhere (Kosten et al. 1987). It also might appear contrary to the elevated basal levels of cardiovascular tone reported by many authors, as reviewed by Blanchard (1990) and as reported by Perry in Chapter 12 regarding basal heart rate of children with PTSD. As noted by Murburg et al., however, 24-hour urinary results simply reflect net SNS activity over time and cannot distinguish tonic from phasic changes. These authors argue further that plasma and urinary measurements of catecholamines represent different physiological processes. Veith and Murburg suggest that conflicting results regarding cardiovascular indices may result primarily from methodological differences between investigations.

I believe that given the nature of PTSD we must question the definitions of tonic versus phasic in that context. If, in the course of a day, a PTSD patient is frequently experiencing phasic responses (in the form of waking recollections, nocturnal traumatic nightmares, exposure to trauma-mimetic stimuli, and stimulus generalization/sensitization to more ordinary stressful events), such an accumulation of diurnal phasic catecholamine activity will appear to represent a tonic abnormality under certain experimental conditions and a phasic one under others.

What Is the Nature of the Physiological and Neurobiological Equilibrium That Is Present in PTSD?

Bruce McEwen (personal communication, 1992) has observed that when a playground seesaw is perfectly balanced by two

40-pound children, it is in equilibrium. When the seesaw is perfectly balanced by two 4,000-pound elephants, it is also in equilibrium. The first example represents a *homeostatic* equilibrium, because it is well within the normal response capacity of the system. The second example, according to McEwen, is an *allostatic* equilibrium that exerts tremendous pressure on the system, which may require abnormal compensatory mechanisms that the system may not be able to sustain indefinitely. There is evidence that basal catecholamine function in chronic PTSD is an allostatic rather than a homeostatic equilibrium. The excessive phasic responsiveness reported in several chapters is reminiscent of the latent rebound hyperexcitability present in drug-addicted individuals that is unmasked during acute withdrawal of drugs. Furthermore, evidence from several authors suggests that PTSD patients pay a neurobiological price to achieve a baseline equilibrium that would meet McEwen's definition of allostasis. Simson and Weiss (Chapter 3) report that inescapable stress produces excessive LC excitability, which they attribute to functional blockade of $alpha_2$ receptors. Zacharko (Chapter 5) reports that the mesocorticolimbic reward system is less efficacious following inescapable stress. Clinical studies show lower resting MHPG levels (Hamner et al., Chapter 11), higher urinary norepinephrine and dopamine levels (Yehuda et al., Chapter 10), and down-regulation of platelet $alpha_2$- and lymphocyte beta-adrenergic receptors (Perry, Chapter 12; Lerer et al., Chapter 13). Whether or not tonic physiological or neurobiological alterations actually occur in PTSD patients, it is the allostatic baseline state that serves as substrate for the phasic abnormalities discussed previously. One might even carry these speculations one step further and hypothesize that recovery in PTSD represents a more favorable allostatic equilibrium rather than a return to normal homeostasis. This speculation is based on Yehuda et al.'s data (Chapter 10) showing that Holocaust survivors without PTSD show a (nonsignificant) trend toward lower urinary norepinephrine and dopamine levels than do age- and sex-matched controls. This finding is also consistent zwith Lavie and Kaminer's (1989) report that well-functioning Holocaust survivors without PTSD show less dream recall than do normal control subjects (who, in turn, show less recall than do Holocaust survivors with PTSD).

What Are Current Candidate Animal Models and How Well Do They Fit Research Findings and Clinical Phenomenology?

Since publication of van der Kolk et al.'s (1985) inescapable stress (IES) hypothesis of PTSD, it has been the most frequently cited animal model of this disorder. Indeed, the data reported by Simson and Weiss (Chapter 3) and by Zacharko (Chapter 5) were generated from animals subjected to an IES experimental paradigm. Charney et al. (Chapter 6) show us that there are other candidate animal models that may be as appropriate as, or more appropriate than, IES, including fear conditioning, failure of extinction, and behavioral sensitization/stress sensitivity. Antelman and Yehuda (Chapter 4) offer a delayed sensitization (i.e., time-dependent change [TDC]) model that has a distinct advantage over IES with regard to its capacity to explain the persistence of PTSD symptoms, delayed-onset PTSD, the worsening of untreated PTSD over time, and the development of PTSD after exposure to a single brief traumatic event. Yehuda and Antelman (Chapter 16) courageously take the next step and begin to set down guidelines for animal models of PTSD by identifying those factors that are essential for the induction of PTSD and those that can influence the manifestation or course of the disorder.

In my opinion, because many different traumatic events can lead to PTSD (as many different etiological factors can lead to fever or edema), there may not be a single best model for PTSD. Whereas a sensitization model may be best for PTSD following a single brief exposure such as an automobile accident or certain natural disasters, IES may be better suited for protracted stress such as that produced by war, incest, or torture. TDC and IES are not mutually exclusive and may both be operative under certain circumstances. I believe that any adequate animal model will incorporate the following points: 1) that traumatic exposure is a necessary, not a sufficient, condition for development of PTSD, because all exposed organisms do not develop the disorder; 2) that recovery (or at least attenuation of symptoms) does occur frequently following clinical expression of the full PTSD syndrome (e.g., lifetime prevalence rates are at least twice as great as current prevalence rates); and 3) that the acute response to trauma may differ among organisms who recover in contrast to those who develop chronic PTSD following traumatic exposure.

Are There Important Methodological Issues That May Explain Conflicting Results?

I have covered much of this ground already with regard to the question of tonic versus phasic changes. Veith and Murburg (Chapter 16) provide an excellent methodological discussion of the many measurement problems that must be solved when monitoring cardiovascular physiology or plasma catecholamines. Similarly, some of the current controversies regarding urinary cortisol levels among PTSD patients (Mason et al. 1986; Pitman et al. 1991) may have more to do with methods of collection and choice of preservative reagents and biochemical analytic techniques than with observable differences.

What About Control Groups?

Lerer and associates (Chapter 13) provide a very instructive chapter. It seems to make a difference whether PTSD patients are compared with nontraumatized control subjects or with similarly traumatized groups without PTSD. Lerer et al. also mention their unpublished observations that "combat experience per se may influence alpha$_2$-adrenergic receptor function in platelets to an extent that differentiates Vietnam veterans with a combat history (with or without PTSD) from noncombatant individuals." Similarly, Yehuda et al. (Chapter 10) show that Holocaust survivors without PTSD have lower urinary catecholamine levels than control subjects, whereas Holocaust survivors with PTSD have higher levels than control subjects. Finally, McFall and Murburg report that combat-exposed veterans without PTSD had lower resting heart rate and blood pressure than did nonexposed control subjects. Besides the intrinsic interest of these deviations from "normal" found in traumatically exposed non-PTSD cohorts (with regard to questions about adaptation, recovery, and allostasis), such differences may have an important effect on data analysis and its implications.

Because of this problem, clinical studies with PTSD patients will be more interpretable if they include both nonexposed and non-PTSD traumatically exposed comparison groups.

Is the PTSD Diagnosis Meaningful With Regard to Alterations in Catecholamine Function?

It is now well established that psychometric and psychophysiological assessment of PTSD is both reliable and valid (Keane et al. 1987; Kulka et al. 1990). In this book strong evidence is presented that people who meet PTSD diagnostic criteria will exhibit abnormalities in catecholamine function as indicated by urinary catecholamine levels, SNS reactivity, and SNS baseline indices (Yehuda et al., Chapter 10; Murburg et al., Chapter 9; Hamner et al., Chapter 11; Perry, Chapter 12). Furthermore, it appears that psychometrically measured symptom severity is linearly correlated with the severity of catecholaminergic abnormalities. This is shown most explicitly by Yehuda et al., who found significant correlation between PTSD symptom severity and urinary norepinephrine and dopamine levels. I find the comparison between PTSD inpatients and PTSD outpatients most interesting in this regard, because the inpatients had significantly higher urinary catecholamine levels as well as higher PTSD symptom severity than the outpatients. This is consistent with preliminary (unpublished) results obtained at the National Center for PTSD indicating that among hospitalized Vietnam veterans with PTSD, the magnitude of urinary neurohormone abnormalities correlates with PTSD symptom severity (as measured by a number of psychometric instruments). Such data suggest that altered catecholamine function in PTSD may be useful as a dimensional as well as a categorical index of symptomatology. Finally, based on observations with Holocaust survivors and war veterans, it appears that these catecholaminergic abnormalities persist as long as PTSD symptoms persist.

Does the Nature of the Trauma Seem to Make a Difference?

Data reported in this book were obtained mostly on male war veterans but also on a small number of traumatized children and Holocaust survivors who were both male and female. Some comparisons across groups are possible. Both traumatized children and war veterans exhibit downregulation of alpha$_2$ receptors (Lerer et al., Chapter 13; Perry, Chapter 12) as well as augmentation of the acoustic startle reflex (Rausch et al., Chapter 14). Both Holocaust survivors and war veterans exhibit elevated urinary catecholamine levels (Yehuda et al., Chapter 10).

Obviously much more neurobiological research is needed with rape/incest, political torture, natural disaster, and industrial accident survivors with PTSD to determine the generalizability of these findings. Very few neurobiological data have been published to date on women with PTSD. Nor is there much information on racial/genetic factors that might influence the neurobiological expression of PTSD. Because all neurobiological research has been conducted on patients from Western industrialized nations, there is no information on PTSD patients from traditional nonindustrialized societies. This is particularly pertinent to cross-cultural questions concerning the applicability of the PTSD model to traumatized individuals from non-Western ethnocultural backgrounds (Friedman and Jaranson, in press; Marsella et al. 1993). If ethnocultural factors affect the phenomenological expression of posttraumatic symptoms (especially with regard to avoidant/numbing symptoms) in such a way that severely traumatized individuals from certain societies do not meet the DSM-III-R diagnostic criteria (American Psychiatric Association 1987), it may only be through neurobiological assessment that we can rule in or rule out the universality of a posttraumatic stress syndrome.

How Are We to Understand the Relationship Between PTSD and Major Depressive Disorder?

According to Lerer et al. (Chapter 13), 95% of the Israeli combat veterans with PTSD who were studied also met diagnostic criteria for major depressive disorder (MDD). Other studies have also shown high rates of comorbidity between PTSD and MDD in both community and treatment-seeking cohorts (Green et al. 1989; Kulka et al. 1990). Findings regarding HPA function show that PTSD patients have significantly lower 24-hour urinary cortisol levels (Mason et al. 1986) and significantly more lymphocyte glucocorticoid receptors (Yehuda et al. 1991b) than do MDD patients. Furthermore, whereas MDD patients often show non-suppression of the HPA system following dexamethasone, PTSD patients show supersensitive HPA suppression following doses of dexamethasone that do not affect normal subjects (Yehuda et al. 1991a). These HPA axis abnormalities suggest that when comorbid with PTSD, MDD is a different disorder than MDD presenting like classic melancholia (i.e., MDD without PTSD). Results reported in this book on catecholamine function in PTSD add more weight to this argument. PTSD patients show significantly fewer platelet alpha₂ receptors, whereas depressed patients show an equal or greater number of these receptors than do normal control subjects (Perry, Chapter 12; Lerer et al., Chapter 13). Murburg et al. (Chapter 8) monitored SNS function in PTSD patients with and without MDD because the authors expected that increased SNS activity previously reported among MDD patients would distinguish the two groups. However, they found no significant differences between the PTSD alone and the comorbid PTSD/MDD groups, suggesting that increased SNS activity does not occur when MDD is comorbid with PTSD. All of these findings on both HPA and catecholamine function suggest that the DSM-III-R (which relies exclusively on phenomenology) cannot be used to distinguish between true melancholia and a depressive manifestation of PTSD that has a distinctly different pathophysiology. Perhaps a clue to the underlying neurobiological abnormality can be found in Zacharko's results (see Chapter 5) suggesting that IES reduces the rewarding value of intracranial self-stimulation mediated by the mesocorticolimbic system.

What Are the Sequelae of Traumatic Exposure Among Young Children?

Perry (Chapter 12) provides an excellent review of current literature on traumatic exposure and raises two fundamental concerns. First, traumatic exposure before age 3 can produce altered development of the CNS and developmental delay, and can result in stable autonomic hyperarousal. These are important clinical observations that should be systematically investigated, using the animal model paradigms mentioned earlier, with animals at various stages of development. Second, Perry invokes a diathesis-stress model in which age of traumatization and family psychiatric history are the major predictive factors. (In Chapter 5, Zacharko has demonstrated how strain differences significantly influence an animal's response to an inescapable stress condition.) Perry reports that traumatized children from schizophrenic families are more likely to develop prepsychotic or psychotic symptoms, whereas children with an affective/anxiety family history are more likely to develop mood and anxiety symptoms. Besides the obvious implication of genetic factors, these findings also indicate that traumatic exposure may strongly influence the expression of other major psychiatric disorders besides PTSD.

What Do Those Findings Suggest About Treatment?

Because there have been so few randomized double-blind controlled trials of tricyclic antidepressants (TCAs) and monoamine oxidase inhibitors (MAOIs), Southwick et al.'s quantitative review of open as well as controlled trials (see Chapter 15) is very helpful. Their conclusion that TCAs and MAOIs seem to have specific efficacy on global and intrusive PTSD symptoms but appear ineffective against avoidant/numbing symptoms is consistent with less quantitative literature reviews (Friedman 1991, in press). Since hyperarousal symptoms were monitored infrequently (because most investigations relied on the Impact of Event Scale), it is too early to reach any conclusions in that regard. Southwick et al.'s analysis suggests that adequate pharmacotherapy for PTSD may necessitate the prescribing of several different classes of drugs to attenuate dysregulation in a number of neurobiological systems affected in PTSD. Indeed, basic research in this book supports this speculation, as opioids, benzodiazepines, and CRF profoundly affect (while serotonin and NMDA agonists may also influence) CNS mechanisms that mediate the organism's response to chronic stress (Aston-Jones et al., Chapter 2; Simson and Weiss, Chapter 3; Zarcharko, Chapter 5; Charney et al., Chapter 6). Finally, Perry demonstrates the efficacy of the alpha$_2$ agonist clonidine on PTSD and other symptoms among children who had been exposed to traumatic stress. Clearly, we have just begun to carefully evaluate different pharmacotherapeutic approaches to PTSD.

This book, *Catecholamine Function in PTSD: Emerging Concepts,* is a giant step forward. It helps us ask better questions, conceptualize clinical data from a basic neurobiological perspective, and develop animal models that may be more pertinent to PTSD. Dr. Murburg has made a significant contribution by compiling and synthesizing all of this material. She deserves thanks from all of us.

REFERENCES

American Psychiatric Association: Diagnostic and Statistical Manual of Mental Disorders, 3rd Edition, Revised. Washington, DC, American Psychiatric Association, 1987

Blanchard EB: Elevated basal levels of cardiovascular response in Vietnam veterans with PTSD: a health problem in the making? Journal of Anxiety Disorders 4:233–237, 1990

Friedman MJ: Biological approaches to the diagnosis and treatment of post-traumatic stress disorder. Journal of Traumatic Stress 4:67–91, 1991

Friedman MJ: Biological and pharmacological aspects of the treatment of PTSD, in Handbook of Post-Traumatic Therapy. Edited by Williams MB, Sommer JF. Westport, CT, Greenwood Press (in press)

Friedman MJ, Jaranson JM: The applicability of the PTSD concept to refugees, in In Peril and Pain: The Mental Health and Well-Being of the World's Refugees. Edited by Marsella AJ, Borneman TH, Orley J. Washington, DC, American Psychological Press (in press)

Green BL, Lindy JD, Grace MC, et al: Multiple diagnosis in posttraumatic stress disorder: the role of war stressors. J Nerv Ment Dis 177:329–335, 1989

Kardiner A: The Traumatic Neuroses of War (Psychosomatic Medicine, Monograph I-II). Washington, DC, National Research Council, 1941

Kardiner A, Spiegel H: The Traumatic Neuroses of War. New York, Paul Hoeber, 1947

Keane TM, Wolfe J, Taylor KL: Post-traumatic stress disorder: evidence for diagnostic validity and methods of psychological assessment. J Clin Psychol 43:32–43, 1987

Kosten TR, Mason JW, Giller EL, et al: Sustained urinary norepinephrine and epinephrine elevation in post-traumatic stress disorder. Psychoneuroendocrinology 12:13–20, 1987

Kulka RA, Schlenger WE, Fairbank JA, et al: Trauma and the Vietnam War Generation. New York, Brunner/Mazel, 1990

Lavie P, Kaminer H: Holocaust survivors' coping with bereavement as reflected in sleep and dreaming forty years later, in Biological Aspects of Non-psychotic Disorders. Abstract from the scientific proceedings of the World Federation of Biological Psychiatry, Jerusalem, 1989, No 147

Marsella AJ, Friedman MJ, Spain EH: Ethnocultural aspects of PTSD, in American Psychiatric Press Annual Review of Psychiatry, Vol 12. Edited by Oldham JM, Riba MB, Tasman A. Washington, DC, American Psychiatric Press, 1993, pp 157–181

Mason JW, Giller EL Jr, Kosten TR, et al: Urinary free-cortisol in posttraumatic stress disorder. J Nerv Ment Dis 174:145–149, 1986

Pitman RK, Orr SP, Meyerhoff JL, et al: Urinary cortisol excretion in PTSD. Paper presented at the 144th annual meeting of the American Psychiatric Association, New Orleans, LA, May 1991

van der Kolk BA, Greenberg M, Boyd H, et al: Inescapable shock, neurotransmitters, and addiction to trauma: toward a psychobiology of post-traumatic stress. Biol Psychiatry 20:314–325, 1985

Yehuda R, Giller EL Jr, Boisoneau D, et al: The low-dose DST in PTSD, in 1991 New Research Program and Abstracts, 144th annual meeting of the American Psychiatric Association, New Orleans, LA, May 1991a, NR324, pp 125–126

Yehuda R, Lowy MT, Southwick SM, et al: Lymphocyte glucocorticoid receptor number in posttraumatic stress disorder. Am J Psychiatry 148:499–504, 1991b

Index